Contemporary Diagnosis and Management of

Type 2 Diabetes®

Willa A. Hsueh, MD

Professor of Medicine
Chief, Division of Endocrinology, Diabetes, and Hypertension
David Geffen School of Medicine at UCLA
Los Angeles, California

Lisa Moore, MD

Gonda Research Fellow, Division of Endocrinology,
Diabetes, and Hypertension
David Geffen School of Medicine at UCLA

Michael Bryer-Ash, MD, FRCP

Associate Professor of Medicine
Medical Director, Gonda (Goldschmied) Diabetes Center
Clinical Director, Division of Endocrinology,
Diabetes, and Hypertension
David Geffen School of Medicine at UCLA
Staff Physician, West Los Angeles Veterans Administration
Medical Center

Second Edition

Published by
Handbooks in Health Care Co.,
Newtown, Pennsylvania, USA

This book has been prepared and is presented as a service to the medical community. The information provided reflects the knowledge, experience, and personal opinions of Willa A. Hsueh, MD, Professor of Medicine, Chief, Division of Endocrinology, Diabetes, and Hypertension, David Geffen School of Medicine at UCLA, Los Angeles; Lisa Moore, MD, Gonda Research Fellow, Division of Endocrinology, Diabetes, and Hypertension, David Geffen School of Medicine at UCLA; and Michael Bryer-Ash, MD, FRCP, Associate Professor of Medicine, Medical Director, Gonda (Goldschmied) Diabetes Center, Clinical Director, Division of Endocrinology, Diabetes, and Hypertension, David Geffen School of Medicine at UCLA.

This book is not intended to replace or to be used as a substitute for the complete prescribing information prepared by each manufacturer for each drug. Because of possible variations in drug indications, in dosage information, in newly described toxicities, in drug/drug interactions, and in other items of importance, reference to such complete prescribing information is definitely recommended before any of the drugs discussed are used or prescribed.

Acknowledgment
Ellen Kurek, a medical writer, contributed to the research and writing of this book. The authors also acknowledge the staff of the Gonda Diabetes Center for advice and assistance.

International Standard Book Number: 1-931981-27-2

Library of Congress Catalog Card Number: 2003116181

Table of Contents

Dedication

This book is dedicated with sincere appreciation to Leslie and Susan Gonda, and to the members of the Gonda (Goldschmied) family, to honor their commitment to research in diabetes mellitus and to providing outstanding care to patients with diabetes.

Chapter 1

Pathophysiology of Type 2 Diabetes: A Quartet of Abnormalities

ype 2 diabetes and the hyperglycemia and hyperinsulinemia that characterize it are established risk factors for cardiovascular disease.[1] Obesity, dyslipidemia, and hypertension are also risk factors for cardiovascular disease and are associated with type 2 diabetes.[2] Kaplan considered obesity, particularly the upper-body, central, or android type, to be the key risk factor for cardiovascular disease and argued that it could account for the other cofactors by promoting dyslipidemia and peripheral insulin resistance. Because of its contribution to mortality related to atherosclerotic heart disease, Kaplan termed the risk-factor cluster of diabetes, obesity, hypertriglyceridemia, and hypertension 'the deadly quartet.'[3] The appropriateness of this term was documented by a follow-up study of patients who received an isolated coronary artery bypass graft, in whom the presence of the deadly quartet was associated with a mortality hazard ratio of 2.5 for men and 13.4 for women.[4]

This quartet of risk factors has been referred to by a variety of names, including syndrome X,[2] the cardiovascular metabolic syndrome, the dysmetabolic syndrome,[5] and the metabolic syndrome. Analysis of the syndrome's components indicates that obesity is the central feature over time, which supports the hypothesis that the syndrome's components are linked through obesity.[6] The common association of obesity with insulin resistance[7] has resulted in another proposed name: the insulin resistance syndrome.

Metabolic Abnormalities

Just as obesity plays a key role in the genesis of the other components of this syndrome, excess fat in obesity plays a key role in the genesis of the metabolic abnormalities that underlie the deadly quartet: disrupted fat metabolism, insulin resistance in skeletal muscle, increased hepatic glucose production, and decreased insulin secretion by pancreatic islet cells. The finding that insulin resistance increases with weight gain and decreases with weight loss indicates that fat accumulation is not just associated with insulin resistance but contributes to it.[7] Intra-abdominal fat, in particular, is associated with insulin resistance, and obese patients with diabetes are likely to have such fat. This fat is not only insulin resistant[8] and thus less sensitive to the suppression of lipolysis by insulin,[9] but also more responsive to the adrenergic agonists that stimulate lipolysis. As a result, more free fatty acids (FFAs) may be released into the portal circulation of these patients.[3,9] In the liver, these nonesterified FFAs promote secretion of very low density lipoprotein (VLDL), which is normally inhibited by insulin, an effect that is lost in the insulin-resistant state. Hepatic nonesterified FFAs also cause small, dense, atherogenic low-density lipoprotein to form; reduce apolipoprotein B degradation; and impair triglyceride removal by adipose lipoprotein lipase, resulting in diabetic dyslipidemia. High levels of FFAs also inhibit hepatic insulin extraction, possibly via a signal generated through the action of glucagon-like peptide-1.[10] Decreased hepatic insulin extraction increases hepatic gluconeogenesis,[8] contributing to hyperglycemia, and allows more insulin to be shunted into peripheral tissue, promoting peripheral hyperinsulinemia. Decreased hepatic insulin extraction worsens at the increased levels of plasma free testosterone that characterize android obesity.[3]

Increased FFA levels increase triglyceride levels within skeletal muscle cells, which may cause the cells to resist insulin action by generating an insulin-resistance signal or by interfering with the normal action of insulin. FFAs may also cause muscle insulin resistance by increasing cytosolic levels of long-chain acyl-coenzyme A (acyl-CoA) and diacyl glycerol, which activate protein kinase C, some isoforms of which inhibit insulin action via serine phosphorylation of the insulin receptor and its substrates.[7] Acyl-CoA may impair insulin action by promoting the accumulation of ceramide in muscle cells.[11] FFAs may also induce skeletal muscle insulin resistance by activating the hexosamine pathway or by changing the fatty acid composition of membrane phospholipids, thereby impairing membrane fluidity.[7]

β-Cell Dysfunction

However, if enough insulin can be secreted to counteract the effect of peripheral insulin resistance and increased hepatic glucose output, these pathophysiologic abnormalities are insufficient to cause type 2 diabetes. For type 2 diabetes to develop, β-cell failure must progress to the point at which elevated insulin secretion can no longer counteract these abnormalities and hyperglycemia ensues. Disrupted fat metabolism also plays a key role in β-cell failure. Chronically elevated FFA and glucose levels create a toxic environment that impairs β-cell function and further exacerbates insulin resistance. Normally, FFAs are the substrates for up to half of all basal insulin production and are promoters of glucose-stimulated insulin secretion, but chronically elevated FFA levels blunt the responsiveness of β cells to glucose. This blunting may originate in downregulated expression of acetyl-CoA carboxylase, which catalyses malonyl CoA formation, a key regulator of FFA oxidation. Decreased levels of malonyl CoA double or triple FFA oxidation and suppress glucose-stimulated insulin secretion.

Elevated FFA levels seem to decrease insulin gene expression in islet cells only at high glucose levels, so hyperglycemia may be required for lipid-induced β-cell injury. Hyperlipidemia injures β cells by inducing over-expression of the hexosamine pathway's rate-limiting enzyme, glucose fructosamine amidotransferase (GFAT), which not only impairs β-cell function by inducing oxidative stress, but also increases insulin resistance in skeletal muscle and promotes hepatic fatty acid synthesis. β-cell exhaustion may also result from long-term hypersecretion of insulin.[12] Islet cells produce amyloid in tandem with insulin; therefore, increased insulin production increases amyloid production and also promotes β-cell dysfunction.[13] Moreover, a genetic tendency toward increased β-cell apoptosis may intensify loss of insulin secretory capacity in some patients. Even in patients with intact β cells, hyperinsulinemia may not be able to compensate for insulin resistance until FFA levels are decreased by weight loss.[12]

Diet and Exercise

Weight loss has been stressed as a means of counteracting insulin resistance in obese patients. Because of the role of fat and FFAs in the pathophysiology of type 2 diabetes, caloric restriction through reduced fat consumption has been recommended as a weight loss strategy. Consumption of saturated fat has been a key target for reduction because saturated fat has the most detrimental effect on insulin action. Reduced intake of *trans*-fatty acids may also be important because incorporation of these acids into cell membranes may impair insulin-stimulated glucose transport.[14] In the Nurses Health

Study,[15] consumption of *trans*-fatty acids was associated with increased incidence of type 2 diabetes. However, because low-fat/high-carbohydrate diets can worsen hyperglycemia and hyperinsulinemia in hypertensive patients, reduction in saturated fat and *trans*-fatty acid intake to promote weight loss and enhance insulin sensitivity should be accompanied by increased consumption of unsaturated fats, particularly ω-3 fatty acids. ω-3 fatty acids have been shown to prevent insulin resistance in animal studies.[3] ω-3 fatty acids suppress VLDL secretion and prevent continuously elevated insulin levels from stimulating hepatic secretion of VLDL-triacylglycerol, which impairs glucose-stimulated insulin secretion by β cells and promotes insulin resistance in muscle cells.[16] The long-chain polyunsaturated fatty acids (LCPUFAs) formed from ω-3 fatty acids promote the survival of pancreatic β cells by inhibiting eukaryotic translation initiation factor-2, thereby enhancing glucose homeostasis and preventing the development or worsening of type 2 diabetes.[17]

Similar to diet, exercise can help decrease insulin resistance by promoting weight loss. Even in the absence of weight loss, exercise can decrease insulin resistance[3] by enhancing insulin-stimulated glucose uptake and glycogen synthase activity in skeletal muscle.[7] However, patients with type 2 diabetes have decreased maximal oxygen consumption and oxygen uptake kinetics, which decrease exercise performance and thereby make regular exercise difficult.[18] Low aerobic capacity is also associated with decreased ability to oxidize excess dietary fat, which predicts weight gain and deterioration of insulin sensitivity.[19] The thiazolidinedione (TZD) class of insulin-sensitizing agents may counteract these effects by improving exercise capacity in these patients. TZDs can also counteract central obesity and its diabetogenic effects by redistributing fat from the liver and viscera to the subcutaneous periphery.[18]

Inflammatory Factors

In addition to their other benefits, exercise, TZDs, and ω-3 fats can counteract inflammation, which is gaining recognition as an important aspect of the pathophysiology of type 2 diabetes and cardiovascular disease. These anti-inflammatory effects may also help to counteract insulin resistance. For example, exercise enhances production of antiatherogenic cytokines and decreases serum levels of such markers of inflammation as fibrinogen and C-reactive protein (CRP). Consumption of ω-3 fats and other precursors of LCPUFAs suppresses formation of inflammatory cytokines such as tumor necrosis factor-α (TNF-α).[17] TNF-α also promotes increased FFA secretion and gluconeogenesis.[20] Several inflammatory cytokines such as TNF-α are secreted in increased amounts by excess adipose tissue[21] and are thus termed adipocytokines. Inflammatory cytokines seem to be involved in the development of each component of the metabolic syndrome as well as atherosclerotic cardiovascular disease. TZDs can help suppress inflammatory cytokine production by macrophages and adhesion molecule expression in vascular endothelial cells by activating peroxisome proliferator-activated receptor-γ (PPAR-γ) and thereby increasing levels of plasma adiponectin, an antiatherogenic cytokine.[17] Adiponectin appears to increase insulin sensitivity, possibly by interrupting the interaction between receptors in muscle and liver tissues and substances that interfere with insulin action, such as TNF-α, as well as by enhancing fatty acid oxidation in these tissues and thereby decreasing their triglyceride content.[9] In obese patients and patients with type 2 diabetes, adiponectin levels are decreased. Similar to TZDs, LCPUFAs, which are endogenous PPAR-γ ligands, may increase adiponectin levels and reduce production of inflammatory cytokines, inflammation, and insulin resistance in these patients.

Adipocytes release a variety of factors, including adiponectin, that modulate energy balance and affect in-

10

sulin resistance. These factors include resistin, which has been shown in animal studies to decrease insulin sensitivity in peripheral tissue. Studies in mice have found that while resistin levels increase during adipocyte differentiation, resistin appears to inhibit adipogenesis and thus may regulate fat mass through negative feedback. A human homologue of resistin has been found.[22]

Another adipocyte hormone, leptin, decreases adipose tissue mass by promoting fatty acid oxidation and helps to confine triglyceride storage to adipocytes and thereby protect other cell types from lipotoxicity. Leptin also regulates the rate of gluconeogenesis by modulating gluconeogenic enzyme expression, which may limit hepatic triglyceride formation. Sensitivity to leptin appears to be decreased in obesity and type 2 diabetes, thereby promoting hypertriglyceridemia and insulin resistance.[23] In addition, leptin crosses the blood-brain barrier and acts in the hypothalamus to modulate neuroendocrine and autonomic activity and thereby decrease food intake and increase energy expenditure.[22] LCPUFAs affect leptin gene expression and cerebral anandamide levels and thereby regulate food intake. They also regulate cholesterol metabolism by inhibiting enzyme activity.

Inflammatory agents such as TNF-α, interleukin-1 (IL-1), and interleukin-6 (IL-6) are markers of the acute-phase immune response, as are CRP, plasminogen activator inhibitor-1 (PAI-1), fibrinogen, and lipoprotein (a). Their presence in type 2 diabetes and cardiovascular disease indicates that long-term activation of the innate immune response to harmful molecules may contribute to the pathophysiology of these conditions. Because periodontal disease is one of the foremost chronic infections linked with cardiovascular disease and is common in type 2 diabetes, periodontal bacteria and other microorganisms may be triggers of this innate immune response.[24] The inflammatory immune response to chronic infection may stimulate the production of cytokines that promote insulin resistance, such as TNF-α.[25] In addition, in type 2 diabetes, altered proteins such as advanced glycosylation end products, which are a by-product of hyperglycemia, may stimulate the production of inflammatory cytokines, as does glucose itself.[24]

One of the effects of the cytokines IL-1 and IL-6 is to stimulate pituitary release of cortisol. At high levels, cortisol contributes to insulin resistance, hypertension, and central obesity[24] by impairing adipocyte differentiation and proliferation, decreasing the number of adipocytes and the total amount of fat they store, and increasing adipocyte size. These changes promote insulin resistance by allowing dietary fat to accumulate in liver, muscle, and β cells[19] and by inducing production of cytokines such as TNF-α. TZDs counteract these effects by promoting adipocyte differentiation.[26] Patients with Cushing's syndrome, which results from elevated cortisol levels related to disturbances of the hypothalamo-pituitary-adrenal (HPA) axis, typically develop the metabolic syndrome. It may logically follow that other conditions that increase cortisol levels, such as stress, contribute to the metabolic syndrome. However, although acute stress activates the HPA axis and can adversely affect glucose metabolism, the causal link between chronic stress and sustained perturbation of the HPA axis remains unproved. The absence of evidence that cortisol production is consistently elevated in patients with the metabolic syndrome indicates that the link between chronic stress, cortisol levels, and the metabolic syndrome may be more complex. For example, the metabolic syndrome has been associated with disturbances in the normal diurnal variation in cortisol levels, which may be related to disturbed sex steroid and growth hormone secretion and hence to visceral obesity and insulin resistance.[27] Growth hormone deficiency is particularly associated with obesity, and adult cancer survivors with treatment-related childhood growth hormone deficiency have a high prevalence of the metabolic syndrome,[28] which suggests that low levels of growth hormone may promote the metabolic syndrome. Disturbances in growth hormone and sex steroid levels may lead to the metabolic syndrome by impairing glucose homeostasis and increasing adipocyte size.[19]

Endothelial Dysfunction

The definition of the metabolic syndrome formulated by the World Health Organization (WHO) includes microalbuminuria as well as obesity, hypertension, and dyslipidemia.[29] Thus defined, the metabolic syndrome has been found to confer a threefold increased risk of coronary heart disease and stroke compared with type 2 diabetes or impaired glucose tolerance alone.[30] Moreover, in a large family study of patients with type 2 diabetes in Scandinavia, microalbuminuria was found to confer the greatest risk of cardiovascular death of any component included in the WHO definition. Microalbuminuria is also an indicator of endothelial dysfunction.[29] Thus, the paramount role of microalbuminuria among the components of the metabolic syndrome in increasing the risk of cardiovascular mortality indicates that endothelial dysfunction is a critical aspect of the pathophysiology of the metabolic syndrome. Endothelial dysfunction may be the linchpin of this syndrome because insulin action depends on endothelial cells to transport insulin to muscle and fat via the interstitial fluids that bathe these target tissues. In addition to promoting insulin resistance, endothelial dysfunction may promote hypertension and atherosclerosis by shifting the balance between the production of promoters and inhibitors of vascular smooth muscle cell proliferation toward promoters.[31]

The primary factor in endothelial dysfunction appears to be insulin resistance, which impairs insulin-dependent production of nitric oxide (NO).[32] Agents that enhance insulin sensitivity, such as the TZDs, can improve the endothelium-dependent vascular response to insulin, which may slow or delay the progression of vascular disease. For example, 4 mg rosiglitazone (Avandia®) daily for 6 weeks was shown to more than double brachial artery vasoactivity (from 4% to 10%, P <0.05) in a study group that included obese patients without diabetes. Metformin (Glucophage®) does not have a direct effect on peripheral insulin sensitivity like that of the TZDs, but it has also been shown to improve endothelial function in patients with type 2 diabetes at a dosage of 500 mg twice daily for 12 weeks.[18] Because glucose has been shown to elevate blood pressure when endothelial dysfunction is present,[33] combining insulin sensitizers with a diet featuring foods with a high glycemic index to stabilize glucose levels may help to control hypertension.

Hypertension

Nitric oxide is considered the most important endothelium-derived relaxing factor,[34] and its impaired production may partly account for hypertension in the metabolic syndrome. Such hypertension may also stem from hyperinsulinemia, which promotes renal retention of sodium, induces smooth muscle hypertrophy, and increases activation of the sympathetic nervous system and intracellular calcium levels.[3] However, results of studies of the association between fasting or post-glucose-load insulin levels and blood pressure have been mixed.[33] Obesity may promote hypertension indirectly by promoting insulin resistance as well as directly by secretion of angiotensin II from adipose tissue.[19] Obesity-related increases in FFA levels also directly promote hypertension by increasing vascular reactivity and endothelial dysfunction.[9]

A stronger correlation exists between insulin resistance and cardiovascular disease than between hyperinsulinemia and such disease.[32] Insulin resistance may promote atherosclerotic cardiovascular disease by making insulin more mitogenic as well as by reducing levels of NO, which has antiatherogenic effects. Insulin resistance promotes a shift in the cellular response to insulin away from the metabolic activity associated with phosphatidylinositol 3-kinase pathway activation and toward mitogenic activity associated with mitogen-activated protein kinase pathway activation.[18,35,36] The underlying abnormality found in atherosclerotic vessel walls seems to be less available NO but more superoxide anions. In the vascular wall, oxidized low-density lipoprotein promotes formation of free radicals, which can oxidize NO to nitrite, nitrate, and peroxynitrite, a known tissue toxin that generates more free radicals and activates cytokines.[34]

Plasminogen Activator Inhibitor-1

Cytokines have many adverse effects on endothelium. They promote the synthesis of adhesion molecules and chemoattractants that cause leukocyte recruitment, leading to atherogenesis; induce thrombosis;[18] and promote rupture of atherosclerotic plaque, which can lead to occlusion and ischemia.[21] These prothrombotic effects may be enhanced by insulin. In vitro, in the presence of insulin, cytokines such as TNF-α induce cellular production of PAI-1,[8] which has been implicated in impaired fibrinolysis and enhanced thrombosis. An increased PAI-1 level is the most prominent of the emerging cardiovascular risk factors associated with the main components of the metabolic syndrome.[1] Similar to insulin, proinsulin has been shown to increase PAI-1 levels in vitro, and an association between elevated proinsulin levels and the metabolic syndrome has been found.[37] Furthermore, insulin itself potentiates angiotensin-II-stimulated PAI-1 production,[32] and in Framingham Offspring Study participants, serum levels of PAI-1 and the hemostatic factor tPA were found to increase with increasing insulin levels in glucose-tolerant and glucose-intolerant patients.[18]

Visceral fat appears to be an important producer of PAI-1 in insulin-resistant patients, and this mechanism appears to account for much of central obesity's contribution to the development of ischemic heart disease in the metabolic syndrome.[8] Insulin sensitizers such as the TZDs have been shown to reduce PAI-1 levels in patients with type 2 diabetes. TZDs may therefore decrease the risk of cardiovascular complications in patients with type 2 diabetes by increasing fibrinolysis and decreasing thrombotic risk. Moreover, because activation of the renin-angiotensin system seems to stimulate PAI-1 production in adipocytes, the use of agents that inhibit this system may also help to decrease thrombotic risk by enhancing fibrinolysis.[18] Aerobic fitness is also associated with enhanced fibrinolysis.[38] Thus, combining TZD and angiotensin-inhibitor therapy with regular aerobic exercise and a weight-reducing diet to reduce the number of PAI-1 producing adipocytes provides a multi-pronged approach to reducing the elevated risk of cardiovascular events in the metabolic syndrome.

References

1. Deedwania PC: Mechanism of the deadly quartet. *Can J Cardiol* 2000;16(suppl E):17E-20E.

2. Hauner H: Insulin resistance and the metabolic syndrome—a challenge of the new millennium. *Eur J Clin Nutr* 2002;56(suppl 1):S25-S29.

3. Kaplan N: The deadly quartet. Upper-body obesity, glucose intolerance, hypertriglyceridemia, and hypertension. *Arch Intern Med* 1989;149:1514-1520.

4. Sprecher DL, Pearce GL: How deadly is the "deadly quartet"? A post-CABG evaluation. *J Am Coll Cardiol* 2000;36:1159-1165.

5. Groop L, Orho-Melander M: The dysmetabolic syndrome. *J Intern Med* 2001;250:105-120.

6. Maison P, Byrne CD, Hales CN, et al: Do different dimensions of the metabolic syndrome change together over time? Evidence supporting obesity as the central feature. *Diabetes Care* 2001;24:1758-1763.

7. Boden G: Pathogenesis of type 2 diabetes: insulin resistance. *Endocrinol Metab Clin North Am* 2001;30:801-815.

8.   Anwar AJ, Barnett AH, Kumar S: The metabolic syndrome and vascular disease. In: Johnstone MT, Veves A, eds: *Diabetes and Cardiovascular Disease*. Totowa, NJ: Humana Press, 2001, pp 3-22.

9.   Goldstein BJ: Insulin resistance as the core defect in type 2 diabetes mellitus. *Am J Cardiol* 2002;90:3G-10G.

10.   Bergman RN, Van Citters GW, Mittelman SD, et al: Central role of the adipocyte in the metabolic syndrome. *J Investig Med* 2001;49:119-126.

11.   Kraegen EW, Cooney GJ, Ye JM, et al: The role of lipids in the pathogenesis of muscle insulin resistance and beta cell failure in type II diabetes and obesity. *Exp Clin Endocrinol Diabetes* 2001;109(suppl 2):S189-S201.

12.   LeRoith D: Beta-cell dysfunction and insulin resistance in type 2 diabetes: role of metabolic and genetic abnormalities. *Am J Med* 2002;113(suppl 6A):3S-11S.

13.   Hayden MR: Islet amyloid, metabolic syndrome, and the natural progressive history of type 2 diabetes mellitus. *JOP* 2002;3: 126-138.

14.   Kahn BB: Glucose transport: pivotal step in insulin action. *Diabetes* 1996;45:1644-1654.

15.   Marshall JA, Bessesen DH: Dietary fat and the development of type 2 diabetes. *Diabetes Care* 2002;25:620-622.

16.   Zammit VA, Waterman IJ, Topping D, et al: Insulin stimulation of hepatic triacylglycerol secretion and the etiology of insulin resistance. *J Nutr* 2001;131:2074-2077.

17.   Das UN: Obesity, metabolic syndrome X, and inflammation. *Nutrition* 2002;18:430-438.

18.   Reusch JE: Current concepts in insulin resistance, type 2 diabetes mellitus, and the metabolic syndrome. *Am J Cardiol* 2002; 90(suppl 5A):19G-26G.

19.   Ravussin E, Smith SR: Increased fat uptake, impaired fat oxidation, and failure of fat cell proliferation result in ectopic fat storage, insulin resistance, and type 2 diabetes. *Ann N Y Acad Sci* 2002;967:363-378.

20.   Grimble RF: Inflammatory status and insulin resistance. *Curr Opin Clin Nutr Metab Care* 2002;5:551-559.

21.   Grundy SM: Obesity, metabolic syndrome, and coronary atherosclerosis. *Circulation* 2002;105:2696-2698.

22. Shuldiner AR, Yang R, and Gong D-W: Resistin, obesity, and insulin resistance - the emerging role of the adipocyte as an endocrine organ. *N Engl J Med* 345:1345-1346.

23. Al-Daghri N, Bartlett WA, Jones AF, et al: Role of leptin in glucose metabolism in type 2 diabetes. *Diabetes Obes Metab* 2002;4:147-155.

24. Pickup JC, Crook MA: Is type II diabetes mellitus a disease of the innate immune system? *Diabetologia* 1998;41:1241-1248.

25. Lamster IB, Lalla E: Periodontal disease and diabetes mellitus: discussion, conclusions, and recommendations. *Ann Periodontol* 2001;6:146-149.

26. Kadowaki T, Hara K, Kubota N, et al: The role of PPARgamma in high-fat diet-induced obesity and insulin resistance. *J Diabetes Complications* 2002;16:41-45.

27. O'Rahilly SP: The metabolic syndrome: all in the mind? *Diabetic Med* 1999;16:355-357.

28. Talvensaari K, Knip M: Childhood cancer and later development of the metabolic syndrome. *Ann Med* 1997;29:353-355.

29. Isomaa B, Almgren P, Tuomi T, et al: Cardiovascular morbidity and mortality associated with the metabolic syndrome. *Diabetes Care* 2001;24:683-689.

30. Groop LC: Pathogenesis of insulin resistance in type 2 diabetes: a collision between thrifty genes and an affluent environment. *Drugs* 1999;58(suppl 1):11-12.

31. Hsueh WA, Anderson PW: Hypertension, the endothelial cell, and the vascular complications of diabetes mellitus. *Hypertension* 1992;20:253-263.

32. Fagan TC, Deedwania PC: The cardiovascular dysmetabolic syndrome. *Am J Med* 1998;105(suppl 1A):77S-82S.

33. Cubeddu LX, Hoffmann IS: Insulin resistance and upper-normal glucose levels in hypertension: a review. *J Hum Hypertens* 2002;16(suppl 1):S52-S55.

34. Quyyumi AA: Endothelial function in health and disease: new insights into the genesis of cardiovascular disease. *Am J Med* 1998;105(suppl 1A):32S-39S.

35. Hseuh WA, Law RE: Diabetes is a vascular disease. *J Investig Med* 1998;46:387-390.

36. Hsueh WA, Law RE: Insulin signaling in the arterial wall. *Am J Cardiol* 1999;84:21J-24J.

37.   Haffner SM, Hanley AJ: Do increased proinsulin concentrations explain the excess risk of coronary heart disease in diabetic and prediabetic subjects? *Circulation* 2002;105:2008-2009.

38.   American Diabetes Association: Position statement: diabetes mellitus and exercise. *Diabetes Care* 2001;24(suppl 1).

Chapter 2

The Spectrum of Insulin Resistance: Where Does Disease Begin?

Type 2 diabetes develops from the interplay between increasing insulin resistance in skeletal muscle and liver, increasing hepatic glucose output, and decreasing insulin secretion caused by progressive pancreatic β-cell dysfunction owing to lipotoxicity, glucose toxicity, and other factors. As a result, type 2 diabetes develops in stages that correspond to the relative predominance of each of these physiologic factors as they relate to defects in insulin-mediated glucose uptake in skeletal muscle (Figure 2-1).

In the earliest stage, insulin resistance is associated with hyperinsulinemia and, in general, excess visceral adiposity. The production of adipokines by adipose tissue is increasingly recognized as one important mediator of this relationship. Substances produced by fat, such as free fatty acids, tumor necrosis factor-α, and leptin, suppress insulin-mediated glucose uptake. The greater the visceral adiposity, the higher the circulating levels of adipose-derived products. Genetic and environmental factors interact to determine adiposity and insulin resistance, as well as β-cell insulin secretion. With increasing age, components of the

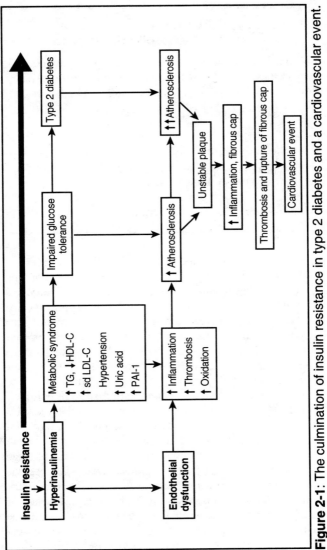

Figure 2-1: The culmination of insulin resistance in type 2 diabetes and a cardiovascular event.

Table 2-1: NCEP Criteria
for the Metabolic Syndrome

The metabolic syndrome can be diagnosed in patients who meet at least three of the following criteria:

- Fasting plasma glucose ≥110 mg/dL
- Serum triglyceride ≥150 mg/dL
- Serum high-density lipoprotein <40 mg/dL
- Blood pressure ≥130/85 mm Hg
- Waist circumference >102 cm (40 in) for women and >94 cm (37 in) for men

NCEP = National Cholesterol Education Program

metabolic syndrome appear, defined by the National Cholesterol Education Program (NCEP) as the presence of three of the five criteria shown in Table 2-1. Twenty percent to 30% of the US population has the metabolic syndrome.[1] In the next stage, pancreatic insulin production cannot keep up with insulin resistance in skeletal muscle and liver, resulting in the transition from normal glucose tolerance (NGT) to impaired glucose tolerance (IGT).[2] This stage is characterized by postprandial hyperglycemia (140 to 199 mg/dL), which is also associated with fasting hyperglycemia (100 to 125 mg/dL), although postprandial glucose is a more sensitive index of IGT. Because glucose uptake into muscle requires three to four times the amount of insulin needed to inhibit glucose production by the liver, in this stage, enough insulin is secreted to suppress hepatic glucose output and prevent the fasting plasma glucose (FPG) concentration from surpassing normal levels. However, as hepatic insulin resistance worsens, the liver begins to produce glucose in increasing amounts, which leads to the gradual increase in FPG that results in impaired fasting glucose (IFG).[3]

Table 2-2: Key Glycemic Levels

Normal fasting glucose	65 to 109 mg/dL (3.6 to 6.0 mmol/L)
Impaired fasting glucose	110 to 125 mg/dL (6.1 to 6.9 mmol/L)
Impaired glucose tolerance	140 to 199 mg/dL) (7.8 to 11.0 mmol/L) (2 hours post OGTT)
Diabetes	
Fasting plasma glucose	≥126 mg/dL (7.0 mmol/L)
or	
Postprandial glucose	≥200 mg/dL (11.1 mmol/L)
or	
Random glucose	≥200 mg/dL (11.1 mmol/L) with symptoms

OGTT = oral glucose tolerance test

Reprinted with permission from Reasner et al, *Am Fam Phys* 2001;63:1687-1694.

The transition to type 2 diabetes occurs as progressive β-cell dysfunction and liver insulin resistance develop.[2] Increasing pancreatic failure also leads to a steep increase in hepatic glucose output during sleep, which results in the level of fasting hyperglycemia that characterizes type 2 diabetes.[3] Table 2-2 provides the key glycemic ranges that define the stages in the development of type 2 diabetes, and Table 2-3 provides a more detailed description of these stages, as well as approaches to deal with glucose control and insulin resistance.

Table 2-3: Progression of Type 2 Diabetes

Factors	NGT	IGT/IFG
Hb A$_{1c}$ (%)	<5.5	5.5 to 6.1
FPG (mg/dL)	<110 (6.1 mmol/L)	110 to 125 (6.1 to 6.9 mmol/L)
Insulin resistance	Moderate	Moderate
Insulin levels	↑↑↑*	↑↑
Treatment	Diet + exercise	Diet + exercise + metformin

NGT = normal glucose tolerance; IGT = impaired glucose tolerance; IFG = impaired fasting glucose; Hb A$_{1c}$ = glycated hemoglobin; FPG = fasting plasma glucose; NL = normal

The diagnosis of diabetes can be made by fasting or postprandial glucose (Table 2-3). It is important to identify patients with IGT or IFG, which constitute prediabetes. Approximately 30% of patients in these categories go on to develop frank diabetes and increased risk for not only atherosclerosis, but also microvascular complications. The progression of prediabetes to diabetes can be attenuated, and, with intervention, the atherosclerosis risk can be decreased. A postprandial plasma glucose level identifies about 20% more patients with prediabetes or diabetes than a fasting level. Therefore, if the fasting level is normal, but carbohydrate intolerance is suspected, an oral glucose tolerance test (OGTT) should be performed.

Type 2 Diabetes (mild lack of control)	Type 2 Diabetes (moderate lack of control)	Type 2 Diabetes (insulin deficiency)
6.2 to 7.5	7.6 to 10.0	>10.0
126 to 160 (7.0 to 8.9 mmol/L)	161 to 240 (8.9 to 13.3 mmol/L)	>240 (13.3 mmol/L)
Moderate	Moderate-severe	Severe
↑ or NL	↓ or ↓↓	↓↓↓
Insulin sensitizers (thiazolidinediones or metformin)	Insulin sensitizers + insulin secretagogue	Insulin sensitizers + insulin

* The number of arrows indicates the magnitude of the change in insulin secretion (ie, ↑ = increased, ↓ = decreased).

Adapted from Reasner et al, *Am Fam Phys* 2001;63:1687-1694.

Scientific Basis for Glycemic Cut Points Separating Stages of Insulin Resistance

Whether based on OGTT or FPG results, the glycemic cut points that define diabetes are based on evidence that the degree of glycemia exceeding these levels is associated with a high risk of developing microvascular complications: retinopathy, nephropathy, and neuropathy.[4-6] In addition, plasma glucose levels after OGTT are bimodally distributed in many populations at high risk for type 2 diabetes, which indicates a clear separation between nondiabetic and diabetic levels of glucose tolerance. In contrast, no bimodal distribution exists in the continuum of plasma glucose values after OGTT to indicate the cut point between NGT and IGT.[7] Moreover, this cut point does not have as clear a pathophysiologic basis as the diabetes cut point.[5] Nevertheless, although the glycemic level that represents the upper limit of normal may be somewhat arbitrary, it suggests a level of glucose at which acute-phase insulin secretion in response to intravenous glucose administration is lost[4] and therefore defines an important pathophysiologic defect in diabetes.

Nondiabetic Insulin Resistance and Risk of Complications

Impaired glucose tolerance or IFG confers a greater risk of atherosclerotic complications.[8] In the Baltimore Longitudinal Study of Aging, the incidence of coronary artery disease and all-cause mortality increased substantially and almost linearly as FPG increased from 110 to 120 mg/dL, which is the lower portion of the glycemic range that defines IFG.[4] The risk of macrovascular complications has even been found to increase with increasing FPG within the normal range.[5] Several recent studies using current glycemic cut points have confirmed the increased risk of macrovascular complications in patients with IGT or IFG.[9] However, increased cardiovascular risk has not been found in insulin-resistant nondiabetic patients in all studies using updated definitions.[7] The metabolic syndrome itself, as defined by NCEP or by World Health Organization criteria, has been clearly associated with increased cardiovascular effects and mortality and even all-cause mortality when patients were followed for a period of 12 years.[10] Endothelial dysfunction has been detected in insulin-resistant subjects even before the onset of the metabolic syndrome, suggesting that the presence of insulin resistance and hyperinsulinemia contributes to vascular injury.[11] Chronic insulin infusion into normal humans (>6 hours) has resulted in endothelial dysfunction, so the long-term impact of hyperinsulinemia on the vasculature remains to be determined.[12] Taken together, these studies suggest that aggressive treatment of traditional atherosclerotic risk factors (eg, low-density lipoprotein cholesterol, blood pressure, triglyceride, high-density lipoprotein cholesterol, smoking) may be useful in diabetic and prediabetic patients and, potentially, in patients with the metabolic syndrome or only visceral adiposity. Lifestyle changes that improve insulin sensitivity are also important.

A continuous relation may also exist between the degree of nondiabetic insulin resistance and risk of microvascular complications.[5] Several clinical studies have found an elevated incidence of complications in patients with IGT, IFG, or both, compared with the incidence of complications in those with NGT. Other studies have found that incidence of complications even increases within the NGT range. For example, in several key population studies, including the Third National Health and Nutrition Examination Survey, no absolute threshold in the association between glycemia and risk of retinopathy was found because some retinopathy was found at all glycemic levels.[4] Furthermore, in insulin-resistant patients, IGT may confer greater risk of retinopathy regardless of FPG. For instance, in a Japanese study, the incidence of retinopathy was found to be greater in patients with IGT than in those without IGT even at similar FPGs, which illustrates the value of OGTT in predicting the development of diabetic complications, particularly in high-risk patients.[13] In addition, a 25% prevalence of IGT or IFG was found in patients with idiopathic polyneuropathy, which is significantly greater than that in the general population and illustrates the importance of OGTT in these patients.[14]

Nondiabetic Insulin Resistance Confers a Strong Risk of Type 2 Diabetes

The association between IGT and risk of developing type 2 diabetes has been documented in a wide range of racial and ethnic populations. In the San Antonio Heart Study, the relative risk of developing type 2 diabetes conferred by IGT ranged from 4.3 to 7.0 depending on race and sex.[7] By some estimates, as many as half of all individuals with IGT will develop type 2 diabetes after 10 years of follow-up,[15] and this rate is considerably higher in groups with a high prevalence of diabetes.[5] Patients with IFG also have increased rates of late development of diabetes.[16] Women with a history of gestational diabetes have the highest incidence of developing permanent diabetes later in life (75% over 10 years).[17] These patients need lifestyle recommendations as well as lifelong follow-up to prevent diabetes.

The possibility that a continuous relation exists between nondiabetic levels of glycemia and risk of developing type 2 diabetes and its complications highlights the importance of identifying and treating patients predisposed to increasing insulin resistance as early as possible. Addressing IGT in its earliest stages with diet and exercise and, if necessary, adding treatment with agents that decrease postprandial hyperglycemia can prevent complications in many patients, even if it cannot prevent type 2 diabetes from eventually developing. Even in patients with well-established IGT, using metformin (Glucophage®) to decrease hepatic glucose output and thus forestall the development of IFG and overt diabetes could be expected to prevent complications.

Such interventions may be particularly important in patients with other risk factors for progression to type 2 diabetes besides hyperglycemia and hyperinsulinemia related to glucose intolerance and insulin resistance. These risk factors include obesity, elevated plasma triglyceride levels, or age older than 45 years. In particular, android or central obesity, as indicated by a high ratio of waist circumference to hip circumference, confers an eightfold increase in risk of progression to type 2 diabetes in middle-aged patients.[15] Therefore, early

Table 2-4: Prevention of Diabetes in IGT

Study	Therapy	RR	Reference
Diabetes Prevention Program Research Group	Diet + exercise	58%	18
	Metformin	31%	
Finnish Diabetes Prevention Study Group	Diet + exercise	58%	19
DA Qing IGT and Diabetes Study	Diet	36%	20
	Exercise	38%	
	Diet + exercise	58%	
STOP-NIDDM trial	Acarbose	25%	21

IGT = impaired glucose tolerance

RR = risk reduction

STOP-NIDDM = Study to Prevent Non-Insulin-Dependent Diabetes

intervention is particularly crucial for individuals with IGT and central obesity at midlife. However, although body mass index was an independent predictor of progression to type 2 diabetes in many studies, it was not as consistently associated with progression after adjustment for other risk factors as was glycemia. This finding illustrates the need to aggressively treat abnormal glucose tolerance even when unaccompanied by other risk factors for progression to type 2 diabetes.[7] Impaired glucose tolerance and IFG should be addressed at their earliest stages with diet and exercise to prevent diabetes (Table 2-4). Metformin has been shown to be helpful in the Diabetes Prevention Program in adult subjects aged less than 60 years (mean age 51 years).[18]

References

1.   Ford ES, Giles WH, Dietz WH: Prevalence of the metabolic syndrome among US adults: findings from the third National Health and Nutrition Examination Survey. *JAMA* 2002;287:356-359.

2.   Nijpels G: Determinants for the progression from impaired glucose tolerance to non-insulin-dependent diabetes mellitus. *Eur J Clin Invest* 1998;29(suppl 2):8-13.

3.   Reasner CA, Defronzo RA: Treatment of type 2 diabetes mellitus: a rational approach based on its pathophysiology. *Am Fam Physician* 2001;63:1687-1688, 1691-1692, 1694.

4.   Report of the expert committee on the diagnosis and classification of diabetes mellitus. *Diabetes Care* 2003;26(suppl 1):S5-S20.

5.   Meigs JB, Nathan DM, Wilson PW, et al: Metabolic risk factors worsen continuously across the spectrum of nondiabetic glucose tolerance. The Framingham Offspring Study. *Ann Intern Med* 1998;128:524-533.

6.   Keen H: Impaired glucose tolerance—not a diagnosis. *Diabetes Metab Rev* 1998;14(suppl 1):S5-S12.

7.   Stern MP, Burke JP: Impaired glucose tolerance and impaired fasting glucose: risk factors or diagnostic categories. In: LeRoith D, Taylor SI, Olefsky JM, eds. *Diabetes Mellitus: A Fundamental and Clinical Text*, 2nd ed. Philadelphia, PA, Lippincott Williams & Wilkins, 2000.

8.   Hsueh WA, Law RE: Cardiovascular risk continuum: implications of insulin resistance and diabetes. *Am J Med* 1998;105(suppl 1A):4S-14S.

9.   Lim SC, Tai ES, Tan BY, et al: Cardiovascular risk profile in individuals with borderline glycemia: the effect of the 1997 American Diabetes Association diagnostic criteria and the 1998 World Health Organization Provisional Report. *Diabetes Care* 2000;23:278-282.

10. Lakka HM, Laaksonen DE, Lakka TA, et al: The metabolic syndrome and cardiovascular disease mortality in middle-aged men. *JAMA* 2002;288:2709-2716.

11. Inoue T, Matsunaga R, Sakai Y, et al: Insulin resistance affects endothelium-dependent acetylcholine-induced coronary artery response. *Eur Heart J* 2000;21:895-900.

12. Arcaro G, Cretti A, Balzano S, et al: Insulin causes endothelial dysfunction in humans: sites and mechanisms. *Circulation* 2002;105:576-582.

13. Kuzuya T: Early diagnosis, early treatment and the new diagnostic criteria of diabetes mellitus. *Brit J Nutr* 2000;84(suppl 2):S177-S181.

14. Simmons Z, Feldman EL: Update on diabetic neuropathy. *Curr Opin Neurol* 2002;15:595-603.

15. Alberti KG: Impaired glucose tolerance: what are the clinical implications? *Diabetes Res Clin Pract* 1998:40(suppl):S3-S8.

16. Charles MA, Fontbonne A, Thibult N, et al: Risk factors for NIDDM in white population. Paris prospective study. *Diabetes* 1991;40:796-799.

17. Buchanan TA, Xiang AH, Peters RK, et al: Preservation of pancreatic beta-cell function and prevention of type 2 diabetes by pharmacological treatment of insulin resistance in high-risk Hispanic women. *Diabetes* 2002;51:2796-2803.

18. Knowler WC, Barrett-Connor E, Fowler SE, et al: Reduction in the incidence of type 2 diabetes with lifestyle intervention or metformin. *N Engl J Med* 2002;346:393-403.

19. Tuomilehto J, Lindstrom J, Eriksson JG, et al: Prevention of type 2 diabetes mellitus by changes in lifestyle among subjects with impaired glucose tolerance. *N Engl J Med* 2001;344:1343-1350.

20. Li G, Hu Y, Yang W, et al: Effects of insulin resistance and insulin secretion on the efficacy of interventions to retard development of type 2 diabetes mellitus: the DA Qing IGT and Diabetes Study. *Diabetes Res Clin Pract* 2002;58:193-200.

21. Chiasson JL, Josse RG, Gomis R, et al: Acarbose for prevention of type 2 diabetes mellitus: the STOP-NIDDM randomised trial. *Lancet* 2002;359:2072-2077.

Chapter 3

Hyperglycemia and Tissue Damage

A lthough the molecular mechanisms involved in hyperglycemic tissue damage may differ by tissue type and stage of complication, they involve either direct toxic effects of hyperglycemia and its derivatives on tissues or sustained alteration in cellular signaling pathways induced by glucose metabolites.[1] Within these two main categories, several important damage-causing mechanisms have been identified, including increases in aldose reductase (AR) activity and polyol pathway flux, formation of advanced glycation end products (AGEs), oxidative stress caused by reactive oxygen intermediates (ROI), activation of protein kinase C (PKC) isoforms,[1] and flux through the hexosamine pathway[2] and other pathways sensitive to cellular stress.[3] Figure 3-1 illustrates how these mechanisms promote complications. All these mechanisms are closely interconnected, and they seem to stem from hyperglycemic overproduction of superoxide by the mitochondrial electron-transport chain.[2]

Aldose Reductase Activation and Increased Polyol Pathway Flux

AR is the enzyme responsible for the accumulation of sugar alcohols like sorbitol, a form of polyol, in tissues that develop diabetic complications.[4] Because AR activation only occurs at hyperglycemic intracellular glucose levels, hyperglycemia is strongly associated with

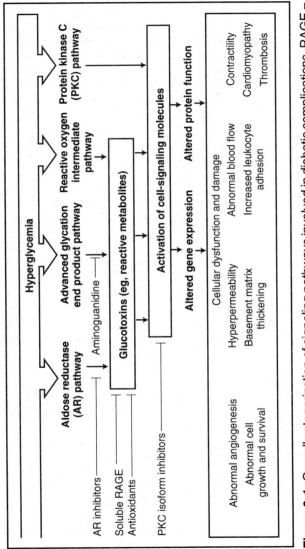

Figure 3-1: Overall categorization of signaling pathways involved in diabetic complications. RAGE = receptor for advanced glycation end products. Sheetz et al, *JAMA* 2002;288:2582, with permission.

33

increased glucose flux through the AR pathway. In this pathway, AR uses nicotinamide adenine dinucleotide phosphate (NADPH) to reduce glucose to fructose via sorbitol dehydrogenase, which uses oxidized nicotinamide adenine dinucleotide (NAD^+) as a cofactor[1] to produce reduced nicotinamide adenine dinucleotide (NADH). This process increases the ratio of NADH to NAD^+ in the cell, thereby increasing the formation of methylglyoxal, a precursor of AGEs, and diacylglycerol (DAG), an activator of PKC. It also decreases the level of NADPH in the cell. Because NADPH is needed to regenerate reduced glutathione (GSH), a potent antioxidant, decreased NADPH levels could induce or worsen cellular oxidative stress. This is the most probable means by which increased polyol pathway flux causes tissue damage. Several findings in animals support this assertion. For instance, GSH deficiency has been found in the ocular lenses of mice that overexpress AR, and genetic AR deficiency protects diabetic mice from GSH deficiency and decreased nerve conduction velocity.[2]

Sorbitol accumulation itself may directly lead to tissue damage and promote diabetic complications. Sorbitol is an inert organic osmolyte, and excess sorbitol in the cell may decrease intracellular levels of other, protective organic osmolytes. For example, the lenses of diabetic animals with cataracts contain decreased levels of taurine. Taurine's antioxidant effects have been observed in the retina and in the kidney, where they reverse inhibited mesangial cell growth caused by hyperglycemia and AGEs. Taurine may also be a free-radical scavenger. High levels of taurine and myoinositol are present in the normal retina and other tissues subject to sorbitol accumulation and oxidative stress. Aldose reductase inhibitors (ARIs) have been shown to restore levels of these osmolytes and prevent some diabetic complications.[5]

In some types of cells, the accumulation of sorbitol and depletion of alternative osmolytes such as taurine and myoinositol disrupt signal transduction and related cellular functions. For example, taurine protects against excess intracellular calcium ion flux and thereby inhibits calcium-ion-dependent PKC catalysis, and its depletion may promote diabetic complications by promoting PKC activation. PKC activation inhibits taurine's trophic effects on retinal ganglions and may thereby disrupt ocular nerve regeneration. Myoinositol depletion correlates with clinical neuropathy and impaired nerve fiber regeneration and may account for the decreased nerve conduction velocity found in experimental diabetes. By affecting signal transduction and fatty acid metabolism, myoinositol depletion may impair nitric oxide synthase (NOS) activity and lipoxygenase/COX pathways, disrupt NO and prostaglandin metabolism, and cause many metabolic and vascular defects in the sympathetic ganglia, peripheral nerves, and endoneurium. These effects can be corrected by γ-linolenic acid, acetyl-L-carnitine, and prostaglandin E_1 analogs.[5]

Another way in which sorbitol accumulation may promote retinopathy and neuropathy is by destroying pericytes, which regulate blood flow in retinal and neural tissue. Loss of pericytes in the retina and nerves increases capillary permeability and promotes endothelial cell proliferation, which leads to disturbed microcirculation and tissue-damaging ischemia. Endothelial dysfunction may also result as increased AR flux decreases NADPH levels in endothelial cells, thereby decreasing their ability to produce NO and altering their redox balance.[1] Intracellular NADPH depletion by AR may also increase levels of NO-quenching superoxide radicals. Low NO levels may be particularly important in neural tissue because NO inhibits acetylcholine release and thereby reduces sympathetic tone. NO also maintains the activity of sodium-potassium adenosine triphosphatase, which is vital to nerve energy metabolism and promotes impulse transmission by maintaining the Na^+ gradient, which is also required for myoinositol and taurine uptake. Thus, decreased NO from increased polyol pathway flux may slow

35

nerve conduction, deplete protective intracellular osmolytes, and decrease endoneurial blood flow.[5]

ARIs have been shown in animals to prevent microvascular pathologic changes[1] and preserve nerve conduction velocity,[6] but they have not been able to prevent or treat nephropathy or retinopathy in humans. Although they improved nerve conduction in patients with diabetic neuropathy, they did not relieve symptoms. This lack of efficacy may stem from insufficient length of treatment, poor penetration into tissues,[4] or use of an inadequate dose because of dose-limiting side effects. Alternatively, because increased AR pathway flux is only one of many mechanisms of hyperglycemic tissue damage, its suppression alone may be insufficient to prevent or treat complications.[1]

Advanced Glycation End Products

Another mechanism of hyperglycemic tissue damage involves the formation of AGE via the modification or glycation of proteins or lipoproteins by sugars.[1] One of the best examples of the effects of AGEs is glycated hemoglobin, whose measurement is widely used to monitor chronic glycemia.[4] Another example is glycated low-density lipoprotein (LDL). Levels of AGE on LDL are elevated in patients with diabetes relative to those without. Glycosylation of LDL components such as apolipoprotein B and phospholipids decreases LDL clearance and increases its susceptibility to modification by oxidation, enhancing its atherogenicity and accelerating atherosclerosis in diabetes. Glycated LDL is poorly recognized by the specific LDL receptor but preferentially recognized by the macrophage scavenger receptor. This shift stimulates foam cell formation and uptake of LDL by the intimal cells, which promotes accumulation of cholesteryl esters and atherosclerosis. Glycation in blood vessels also promotes atherosclerosis by inactivating complement regulatory protein CD59, which inhibits formation of the membrane attack complex of complement (MAC). MAC deposition stimulates the proliferation of fibroblasts and smooth muscle cells, and its disinhibition by glycation promotes endothelial hypertrophy. CD59 inactivation may further stimulate hypertrophy by sensitizing diabetic endothelium to the release of growth factors and cytokines by MAC.[7]

Intracellular hyperglycemia appears to be primary in the formation of extracellular and intracellular AGEs. The products of intracellular autoxidation of glucose to glyoxal, decomposition of Amadori product (glucose-derived 1-amino-1-deoxyfructose lysine adducts), or fragmentation of phosphate compounds into methylglyoxal react with the amino groups of cellular proteins to form AGEs.[2] Because AGE formation is virtually irreversible, these products accumulate with aging, and this accumulation is accelerated by diabetes.[7] Diabetic complications can thus be seen as the result of accelerated aging caused by covalent modification and cross-linkage of proteins by intracellular glucose, leading to impaired cellular function.[1] This impairment not only changes the function of intracellular proteins, but also causes abnormal interactions between extracellular matrix components and other matrix components or cellular receptors for matrix proteins. Abnormal matrix-matrix interactions decrease vascular elasticity and increase fluid filtration across arterial walls. Abnormal matrix-cell interactions decrease endothelial cell adhesion and reduce neurite outgrowth.[2] One sign of AGE-induced extracellular matrix impairment in patients with advanced diabetes is the 'prayer sign,' an inability to fully extend and appose the fingers, caused by thickening and stiffening of periarticular structures produced by changes in the physical characteristics of collagen and exacerbated by the 'shear stress' involved in many manual tasks. Such impairment may also explain the increased frequency of adhesive capsulitis and DuPuytren contracture in patients with diabetes.[4] In addition, modification of the extracellular matrix by AGEs increases the permeability of the glomerular basement membrane, which results in hyperfiltration of albumin,[6] a component of early diabetic nephropathy.[8]

AGEs also impair cellular function by binding to receptors such as the AGE receptor RAGE and the macrophage scavenger receptor. The results of such interactions include activation of mitogen activated protein (MAP) kinase or PKC and promotion of cellular dysfunction,[1] as well as production of ROI and activation of nuclear transcription factor (NF)-κ B,[6] a mediator of immune and inflammatory responses and apoptosis.[3] AGE binding to receptors on macrophages and mesangial cells stimulates production of tumor necrosis factor-α, interleukin-1, and insulin-like growth factor-1 at levels that increase smooth muscle cell proliferation and matrix production.[6] These molecular mechanisms may promote atherosclerosis and the renal basement membrane expansion found in diabetic nephropathy.[7]

In endothelial cells, AGE binding induces expression of procoagulant and proinflammatory molecules such as thrombomodulin, tissue factor, and vascular adhesion molecule-1. Ligand binding to endothelial AGE receptors promotes diabetic capillary hyperpermeability, probably by inducing vascular endothelial growth factor (VEGF).[2] These changes increase lipid entry into the subendothelium. They also enhance adhesion of monocytes to the endothelial surface and promote their migration across it. The importance of AGE binding in atherogenesis was confirmed by studies of atherosclerosis-prone mice, in which blockade of AGE binding largely arrested the development of atherosclerotic lesions at the fatty streak stage independent of glucose and lipid levels.[7]

AGE binding has also been implicated in suppressed wound healing and increased susceptibility to infection in diabetes. For example, RAGE blockade enhanced wound repair and inhibited periodontal disease in diabetic mice.[2] Furthermore, treatment of experimental animals with the AGE inhibitor aminoguanidine inhibited by 85% to 90% the abnormalities that characterize diabetic complications, including retinal acellular capillaries and microaneurysms, increased urinary albumin excretion and mesangial fraction volume, decreased nerve conduction velocity and amplitude, diminished arterial elasticity, and increased arterial fluid filtration.[6] Results of aminoguanidine therapy in humans have been inconclusive because of dose-limiting toxicity. Because aminoguanidine also inhibits oxidants and NOS, its primary effect may not be AGE-related.

Reactive Intermediates and Oxidative Stress

Tissue redox potential is an important determinant of AGE formation, which is greatly accelerated by a shift toward oxidative stress.[7] Oxidative stress results from a redox imbalance between the levels of reactive intermediates such as the reactive oxygen species (ROS) or reactive nitrogen species[3] commonly known as free radicals and the endogenous cellular defenses against them. Free radicals are molecular species that contain at least one unpaired electron and can exist independently. One such example is the superoxide radical, formed by the addition of a single electron to the outer shell of molecular oxygen. When combined with hydrogen, it forms the hydroxy radical, which initiates lipid peroxidation and thereby contributes to atherogenesis. When combined with NO, it forms peroxynitrite, which may nitrate tyrosine residues in proteins. The product thus formed, nitrotyrosine, has been associated with atherosclerosis, myocardial cell apoptosis,[9] and nerve damage.[10] Hyperglycemia increases the production of both nitrotyrosine and peroxidized lipids.[9]

Hyperglycemia produces harmful free radicals and increases oxidative stress through enzymatic and nonenzymatic processes. In mitochondria, glucose metabolism produces reducing equivalents that drive the synthesis of ATP by oxidative phosphorylation. The by-products of this process are free radicals. Glucose autoxidation also produces free radicals,[1] as does activation of the polyol pathway.[9] Unless neutralized by antioxidants such as GSH and vitamins C and E,[1] free radicals can damage cells directly by oxidizing their proteins, lipids, and mitochondrial DNA.[1,3] They can also damage cells indirectly by activating intracellular signaling pathways such as those dependent on PKC, MAP kinase, NF-κ B, and hexosamine. Activation of these pathways increases the expression of many gene products that greatly contribute to microvascular diabetic complications.[3]

Oxidative stress also helps to initiate diabetic vascular disease by reducing levels of bioavailable NO, promoting leukocyte adhesion to the endothelium, and inhibiting the endothelium's barrier function.[1] The role of oxidative stress in diabetic endothelial dysfunction is supported by the ability of GSH to reverse the increase in blood pressure induced by hyperglycemia. In addition, because hyperglycemia elevates prothrombin, and because GSH infusion reverses this elevation, oxidative stress seems to promote diabetic hypercoagulation.

Postprandial hyperglycemia may be an important determinant of the oxidative stress caused by eating foods high in AGEs and lipid peroxides. In one study, after patients consumed oxidized lipids, total radical-trapping activity decreased and lipid peroxidation levels increased with increasing postprandial hyperglycemia. This finding indicates that postprandial hyperglycemia may worsen the effect of toxic oxidation products in food.[9] The positive association between hyperglycemia and oxidative stress is further substantiated by the finding that, in patients with diabetes, levels of GSH and the antioxidant vitamins C and E are decreased and levels of oxidized LDL cholesterol and the oxidative stress marker isoprostane are increased.[1]

Many studies have shown that antioxidant therapy can inhibit diabetic complications. In diabetic animals, high-dose vitamin E and lipoic acid attenuated early hemodynamic perturbations in the kidney, retina, and peripheral nerves,[1] and feeding of several antioxidants in combination inhibited early diabetic retinopathy.[2] High-dose vitamin E (1,800 IU daily) reversed early retinal and renal hemodynamic changes in diabetic animals and patients, and vitamin C improved endothelium-dependent vasodilation in patients with type 2 diabetes. However, low-dose vitamin E (400 IU daily) did not prevent pathologic microvascular changes in the Heart Outcomes Prevention Evaluation trial[1] or decrease cardiovascular and renal disease risk in such patients.[2] This finding may indicate that large antioxidant doses are needed to counteract diabetes-related oxidant production or that high-dose vitamin E exerts its beneficial effects via a nonoxidative pathway such as PKC inhibition.[1]

Because conventional antioxidants scavenge superoxide stoichiometrically, they may not be able to counteract superoxide enough to prevent tissue damage.[2] Counteracting the oxidative stress promoted by increased levels of superoxide and other free radicals is crucial because this stress stimulates other hyperglycemia-related mechanisms of tissue damage. For example, some AGEs are produced only by glycation plus oxidation, and a strong correlation exists between levels of these glycoxidation products in skin collagen and severity of complications.[7]

Protein Kinase C Activation

The PKC family of signaling molecules[1] is a group of phospholipid-dependent protein kinases that mediate cellular responses to growth factors, neurotransmitters, and hormones.[11] These kinases regulate many vascular functions, including permeability, vasodilator release, endothelial activation, and growth factor signaling. PKC is activated in response to activation of phospholipase C and increased levels of calcium and DAG, whose vascular effects are similar to those of PKC. Hyperglycemia can activate PKC to pathologic levels by increasing DAG levels, and hyperglycemia-induced AGE and ROI can activate DAG and PKC directly. As a result, diabetic tissue contains high levels of DAG and PKC.[1]

PKC exerts proinflammatory effects by activating NF-κ B[1,2] and induces the transcription of growth factors and signal transduction.[7] These growth factors include VEGF, which enhances endothelial permeability; transforming growth factor (TGF)-β, which promotes matrix expansion; endothelin-1 (ET1), which causes vasoconstriction;[1] and platelet derived growth factor-β, which stimulates vascular wall growth.[7] PKC activation also inhibits insulin-stimulated production of endothelial NOS.[2] These mechanisms enable PKC to modulate growth rate, DNA synthesis, and turnover of growth factor receptors in blood vessels,[7] and they account for the ability of PKC overactivation to induce vascular hyperpermeability, increase adhesion of leukocytes, dysregulate NO, and alter blood flow.[1] PKC activation by hyperglycemia may also contribute to cardiovascular disease by inducing vascular occlusion via overexpression of the fibrinolysis inhibitor plasminogen activator inhibitor-1 (PAI-1) and by promoting oxidation via activation of NADPH-dependent oxidases associated with cell membranes.[2]

The PKC-β isoform is particularly active in the vasculature, retina,[1] and glomeruli.[7] In animals, inhibition of this isoform by ruboxistaurin mesylate blocks several vascular abnormalities caused by endothelial and contractile tissue dysfunction[1] and prevents or reverses many of the early hemodynamic changes that occur in diabetic retinopathy, nephropathy, and neuropathy. Ruboxistaurin is being studied in humans. PKC-β inhibition seems to counteract increased expression of TGF-β, one of the most important regulators of extracellular matrix production. TGF-β not only activates expression of proteoglycans and collagen, but also decreases synthesis of matrix-protein degrading enzymes. By promoting the accumulation of microvascular matrix protein, increased TGF-β expression causes thickened capillary basement membrane, an early structural abnormality that is widespread in diabetic tissue. PKC-β inhibition attenuates this abnormality. For example, in the kidney of diabetic animals, the PKC inhibitor LY333531 decreases glomerular expression of TGF-β as well as the extracellular matrix proteins fibronectin and type IV collagen,[7] possibly by reversing PKC-inhibited NO production.[2] LY333531 also normalized mean glomerular filtration rate and albumin excretion rate after they had been elevated by experimental diabetes.[6] In the retina of diabetic animals, LY333531 has been found to normalize PKC levels[11] and reverse some of the early retinopathic changes caused by hyperglycemia, such as increased retinal circulation time.[2,11] PKC inhibitors may also prevent or reverse impaired angiogenesis in late-stage diabetic retinopathy by reducing elevated levels of TGF-β, collagen, and fibronectin, which promote capillary occlusion,[2] and of VEGF, which promotes vascular permeability and angiogenesis.[6] However, because the importance of PKC activation and other mechanisms of glucose toxicity may vary by patient, the benefits of specific PKC inhibitors may vary depending on the patient's genetic background.[11]

Increased Hexosamine Pathway Flux

Shunting of excess intracellular glucose through the hexosamine pathway is an important contributor to diabetic tissue damage and complications. In this pathway, fructose phosphate is diverted from glycolysis to provide substrates for reactions that include synthesis of proteoglycans and formation of O-linked glycoproteins. Inhibiting the rate-limiting enzyme that converts glucose to glucosamine blocks hyperglycemic increases in TGF-β and PAI-1. In aortic endothelial cells, hyperglycemia roughly doubled hexosamine pathway activity. Glucosamine itself can activate the PAI-1 promoter via transcription factor sites in mesangial cells and can also activate PKC isoforms. Because glucosamine may increase renal PAI-1 levels and exert other tissue-damaging effects via these mechanisms, patients with diabetes should be warned against using this popular supplement to self-treat arthritis and joint pain.

By inducing oxidative stress, activation of the hexosamine pathway also damages pancreatic β cells, which have low antioxidant enzyme levels. Hexosamine pathway activation therefore helps to initiate diabetes by promoting β-cell dysfunction and decreased insulin release. In addition, the glucosamine generated by this pathway may act as a toxic ROS in β cells by increasing their hydrogen peroxide levels. Treatment with the antioxidant *N*-acetyl-L-cysteine suppresses many of the pathologic changes associated with hexosamine pathway activation.[12]

Activation of Other Signaling Pathways

One of the best-studied cellular signaling pathways targeted by hyperglycemia and oxidative stress is the NF-κ B pathway, which regulates numerous genes, including those that express VEGF and RAGE. Many gene products regulated by NF-κ B in turn activate the NF-κ B pathway, establishing a vicious cycle of dysregulation. Studies of hyperglycemia in bovine endothelial cells indicate that NF-κ B activation may be the initial activator of other mechanisms of tissue damage.[3] Aberrant NF-κ B regulation is associated with diabetes and atherosclerosis.

Other signaling pathways implicated in hyperglycemic tissue damage include the p38 MAP-kinase pathway, which is activated by hyperglycemia in smooth muscle, glomeruli, and nerve tissue, and the stress-activated Jun terminal MAP-kinase pathway, which promotes endothelial apoptosis via hyperglycemic oxidative stress.[3] Poly(adenosine diphosphate-ribose) polymerase (PARP) also mediates hyperglycemic vascular dysfunction, and PARP inhibitors reverse endothelial dysfunction in diabetic animals.[1]

Kinase pathways promote insulin resistance, hyperglycemia, and related tissue damage. ROS-mediated inhibition of insulin-stimulated glucose transport has been shown to activate p38 MAP kinase. This effect was reversed by the antioxidant α-lipoic acid. Although the effectiveness of lipoic acid may be limited by its rapid breakdown, oral therapy with a controlled-release formulation lowered plasma fructosamine levels in patients with type 2 diabetes in 6 weeks.[3]

Superoxide Overproduction by the Electron-Transport Chain

Although there are many mechanisms whereby hyperglycemia causes tissue damage, it is possible that a central mechanism underlies them. Hyperglycemia-induced overproduction of superoxide by the mitochondrial electron-transport chain may be this central mechanism. In endothelial cells, inhibition of mitochondrial superoxide overproduction by manganese superoxide dismutase (SOD) or uncoupling protein-1 completely prevented increases in polyol pathway flux, AGE formation, PKC activation, and hexosamine pathway activity. Such inhibition also completely blocked hyperglycemia-induced monocyte adhesion and inhibition of antiatherogenic prostacyclin synthetase and peroxisome proliferator-activated receptor-γ activation in these cells. Because this central mechanism may induce mitochondrial DNA mutations, it may explain the phenomenon of 'hyperglycemic memory,' in which hyperglycemia continues to promote retinopathy long after normoglycemia has been reestablished.[6] Defective electron-transport subunits created by mutations could increase superoxide production and continue to activate submechanisms of hyperglycemic tissue damage at normal glucose levels. These findings may lead to the development of new SOD-mimicking agents that can scavenge ROS continuously, are nearly as efficient as endogenous enzymes, and may be uniquely effective in preventing hyperglycemic tissue damage and diabetic complications.[2]

References

1. Sheetz MJ, King GL: Molecular understanding of hyperglycemia's adverse effects for diabetic complications. *JAMA* 2002;288:2579-2588.

2. Brownlee M: Biochemistry and molecular cell biology of diabetic complications. *Nature* 2001;414:813-820.

3. Evans JL, Goldfine ID, Maddux BA, et al: Are oxidative stress-activated signaling pathways mediators of insulin resistance and beta-cell dysfunction? *Diabetes* 2003;52:1-8.

4. Nathan DM: The pathophysiology of diabetic complications: how much does the glucose hypothesis explain? *Ann Intern Med* 1996;124(1 Pt 2):86-89.

5. Stevens MJ, Obrosova I, Feldman EL, et al: The sorbitol-osmotic and sorbitol-redox hypotheses. In: LeRoith D, Taylor SI, and Olefsky JM, eds. *Diabetes Mellitus: A Fundamental and Clinical Text*, 2nd ed. Philadelphia: Lippincott Williams & Wilkins, 2000. pp. 972-983.

6. Nishikawa T, Edelstein D, Brownlee M: The missing link: a single unifying mechanism for diabetic complications. *Kidney Int* 2000;58(suppl 77):S26-S30.

7. Aronson D, Rayfield EJ: How hyperglycemia promotes atherosclerosis: molecular mechanisms. *Cardiovasc Diabetol* 2002; 1:1-10.

8. Vora JP, Ibrahim HA, Bakris GL: Responding to the challenge of diabetic nephropathy: the historic evolution of detection, prevention and management. *J Hum Hypertens* 2000;14:667-685.

9. Ceriello A: Mechanisms of tissue damage in the postprandial state. *Int J Clin Pract Suppl* 2001;123:7-12.

11. Vinik AI: New developments in the treatment of neuropathy. Diabetes and Endocrinology Homepage. Medscape conference coverage of the 62nd Scientific Sessions of the American Diabetes Association. WebMD, 2002. Available from: http://www.medscape.com/viewarticle/438361. Accessed August 3, 2002.

11. Dutour A: Mechanisms of glucose toxicity. New hope for prevention of diabetic complications? *Eur J Endocrinol* 1997;136:39-40.

12. Kaneto H, Xu G, Song KH, et al: Activation of the hexosamine pathway leads to deterioration of pancreatic beta-cell function through the induction of oxidative stress. *J Biol Chem* 2001;276:31099-31104.

Chapter 4

Goals of Therapy

T he treatment goals in diabetes are: (1) to alleviate symptoms (eg, polyuria, polydipsia, blurry vision), (2) to rectify glucose toxicity, and (3) to prevent chronic complications. These aims focus largely on improvement and near normalization of glucose control, but importantly, with regard to chronic complications, include aggressive control of hypertension, dyslipidemia, thrombosis, and other cardiovascular risk factors. Thus, an important question when considering antihyperglycemic approaches is what is the advantage regarding the impact on long-term complications (ie, direct vascular effects). Similarly, when choosing an antihypertensive agent or lipid-lowering agent, an important consideration is its impact on glucose control or insulin sensitivity. With these considerations in mind and with results of clinical trials that have allowed establishment of critical therapeutic targets, we can develop rational treatment plans for the needs of each patient.

Glycemia

The American Diabetes Association (ADA) and American College of Endocrinology have established criteria for glucose therapy based on levels of circulating glucose and glycated hemoglobin (Hb A_{1c}) associated with minimal risk of microvascular complications (Tables 4-1 and 4-2).[1,2] The Diabetes Control and Complications Trial (DCCT) identified an exponential relationship between development and progression of retinopathy, development

Table 4-1: ADA Goals for Glycemic Control

Hemoglobin A_{1c}	<7.0%
Preprandial plasma glucose	90-130 mg/dL
Peak postprandial plasma glucose	<180 mg/dL

ADA = American Diabetes Association

and progression of nephropathy, and progression of neuropathy and Hb A_{1c} level over 4 years in patients with type 1 diabetes, as shown in Figure 4-1. These results clearly established a role for hyperglycemia in contributing to the small vessel and neurologic complications of diabetes and led to a reexamination of glycemic goals.[3] A small study in Japan, the Kumamoto study, demonstrated similar results in patients with type 2 diabetes. Tight glucose control, or Hb A_{1c} 7% vs 9.5%, not only improved microvascular complications, but decreased macrovascular complications by 52% during a 3-year period.[4] Although the United Kingdom Prospective Diabetes Study (UKPDS) found less difference in Hb A_{1c}, 7% vs 7.9%, over 15 years, it also demonstrated a strong relationship between glucose control and microvascular complications and, to a lesser extent, glucose control and macrovascular complications, as shown in Figure 4-2.[5] Thus, the goal for glycemic control is near normalization of glucose and Hb A_{1c}.

Blood Pressure

Hypertension substantially contributes to development and progression of all vascular complications of diabetes. These complications include renal disease, coronary artery disease (CAD), stroke, peripheral vascular disease (PVD), lower extremity amputations, and retinopathy. Clinical

Table 4-2: ACE Goals for Glycemic Control

Hemoglobin A_{1c}	<6.5%
Preprandial plasma glucose	<110 mg/dL
2-hour postprandial plasma glucose	<140 mg/dL

ACE = American College of Endocrinology

trials have demonstrated a linear relationship between blood pressure and diabetic nephropathy, as well as cardiovascular events and mortality. In fact, the Hypertension Optimal Treatment (HOT) trial did not find a 'J-curve' in patients with diabetes at high risk for cardiovascular disease.[6] Additionally, hypertension is known to accelerate the development and progression of diabetic cardiomyopathy, which is characterized by left ventricular hypertrophy (LVH) and extensive interstitial fibrosis. Diabetic cardiomyopathy and LVH markedly enhance the risk of ischemic events and heart failure in diabetes. Thus, in addition to achieving glycemic goals, an emphasis should be placed on achieving blood pressure goals.

Evidence now suggests that elevated systolic blood pressure is more significant than diastolic blood pressure or mean arterial pressure as a risk factor for cardiovascular disease and renal disease. The *Sixth Report of the Joint National Committee on Prevention, Detection, Evaluation, and Treatment of High Blood Pressure* (JNC VI) recognized diabetes as a state that confers a high risk of cardiovascular disease and recommended a blood pressure goal of 130/85 mm Hg for diabetic patients. For patients without diabetes but with essential hypertension, the recommended goal is 140/90 mm Hg.[7] Subsequently, four additional long-term clinical trial results became available and, based on these additional data, the National Kidney Foun-

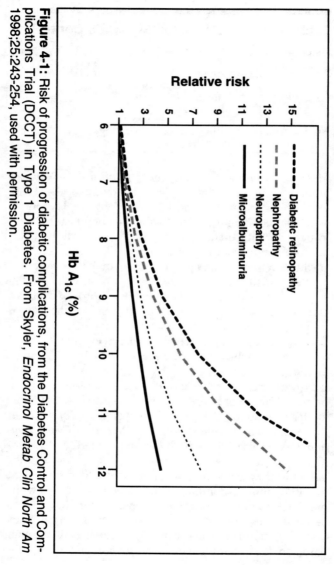

Figure 4-1: Risk of progression of diabetic complications, from the Diabetes Control and Complications Trial (DCCT) in Type 1 Diabetes. From Skyler, *Endocrinol Metab Clin North Am* 1998;25:243-254, used with permission.

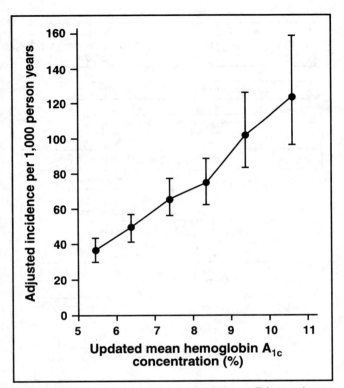

Figure 4-2: Incidence rate and 95% confidence intervals for any end point related to diabetes by category of updated mean hemoglobin A_{1c} concentration, adjusted for age, sex, and ethnic group, expressed for men 50 to 54 years of age at diagnosis and with mean duration of diabetes of 10 years. *Lancet* 1998;352:837-853, with permission from Elsevier.

dation (NKF) recommended a target blood pressure of 130/80 mm Hg in patients with diabetes. These trials included the HOT, UKPDS,[8] the Heart Outcomes Prevention Evaluation (HOPE) study,[9] and the Modification of Diet in Re-

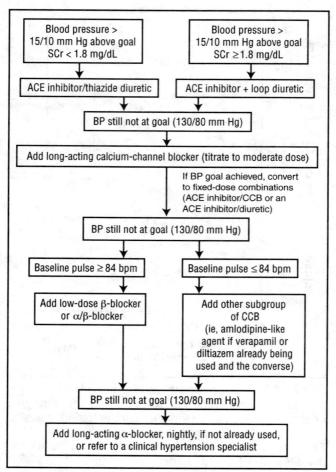

Figure 4-3: A suggested paradigm by which blood pressure goals in people with renal insufficiency and/or diabetes can be achieved by the least intrusive means possible. SCr = serum creatinine level; ACE = angiotensin-converting enzyme; BP = blood pressure; CCB = calcium-channel blocker. Bakris et al, *Am J Kid Dis* 2000;36:646-661.

nal Disease (MDRD) study.[10] The HOT trial not only demonstrated a direct correlation between blood pressure and cardiovascular events and mortality, but also showed that to achieve target blood pressure goals, most patients with diabetes require at least three different antihypertensive medications.[6] The UKPDS demonstrated that lower blood pressure (144/82 mm Hg vs 154/87 mm Hg) over 8.4 years resulted in not only improved cardiovascular and renal end points, but also in less diabetic retinopathy and loss of vision.[8] In the MDRD study, which included patients with a variety of renal diseases, the lower the blood pressure, the better the inhibition of the progressive loss in glomerular filtration rate (GFR). In particular, patients with >1g per day of proteinuria and renal insufficiency have slower rates of renal disease progression when the blood pressure is <125/75 mm Hg.[10]

The Captopril Trial was the first to clearly demonstrate that inhibition of the renin-angiotensin system provides renal protection in patients with type 1 diabetes.[11] Smaller studies suggested similar renal protection in patients with type 2 diabetes, and results of two major trials using angiotensin II AT_1 receptor blockers demonstrated decreased doubling of serum creatinine or end-stage renal disease with losartan (Cozaar®) compared with conventional therapy or irbesartan (Avapro®) compared with amlodipine (Norvasc®) or placebo.[12,13] Recently, a number of small studies have suggested that when compared with dihydropyridine calcium-channel blockers, angiotensin-converting enzyme inhibitors (ACEIs) are associated with fewer cardiovascular events and lower mortality. These findings were underscored by the HOPE trial, which demonstrated that in patients with diabetes and patients without diabetes at high risk for cardiovascular disease, ACEIs were associated with less myocardial infarction (MI), stroke, or cardiovascular death compared with placebo. In patients with diabetes in this study, ACEI treatment was associated with less progression of microvascular complications, as well as less diagnosis of new onset diabetes than treatment with antihypertensive agents that do not inhibit ACE.[9] Thus, increasing clinical evidence suggests that angiotensin II is an important cardiovascular and microvascular culprit in diabetes. Therefore, first-line therapy of hypertension in diabetes should be aimed at inhibiting the renin-angiotensin system.

The treatment algorithm suggested by the NKF special report is depicted in Figure 4-3. Patients with diabetes and hypertension should adopt lifestyle modifications as described in JNC VI. If blood pressure is less than 5/10 mm Hg above the goal of 130/80 mm Hg, then ACEIs alone may be used. If blood pressure is greater than 5/10 mm Hg above goal, then two different antihypertensive agents will be needed to achieve the goal. Details of the algorithm are further examined in the hypertension and diabetes chapter.

Lipids

Elevation in low-density lipoprotein cholesterol (LDL-C) and triglyceride and decreases in high-density lipoprotein cholesterol (HDL-C) accelerate the risk of atherosclerosis in diabetic patients. The risk is so dependent on lipid levels that the recommended goal of lipid therapy was designed to achieve a low level of cardiovascular risk in patients with diabetes (Table 4-3). Recommendations are now based on large clinical trials that have had relatively small numbers of patients with diabetes. In a secondary prevention study of more than 4,400 subjects, the Scandinavian Simvastatin Survival Study (4S), more than 1,000 patients with diabetes or impaired glucose tolerance were treated with either simvastatin (Zocor®) or placebo. In subjects with diabetes or with impaired glucose tolerance, the treated group had decreased cardiovascular mortality, MI, stroke, and need for revascularization. Patients with glucose intol-

Table 4-3: Category of Risk Based on Lipoprotein Levels in Adults With Diabetes

Risk	LDL Cholesterol	HDL Cholesterol*	Triglycerides
High	≥130	<35	≥400
Borderline	100-129	35-45	200-399
Low	<100	>45	<200

Data are given in mg/dL.

*For women, the HDL cholesterol values should be increased by 10 mg/dL.

erance had more events than patients with normal glucose tolerance in the placebo group; there was a suggestion that risk reduction with treatment was greater in the group with diabetes compared with those without diabetes. This study underscored the need for aggressive LDL-C lowering in patients with glucose intolerance.[14]

In another secondary prevention study, the Cholesterol and Recurrent Events (CARE) study, patients with and without diabetes and with lower levels of LDL-C compared with patients in the 4S study had similar risk reduction when treated with pravastatin (Pravachol®) compared with placebo.[15] In the Veteran Affairs High Density Lipoprotein Cholesterol Intervention Trial (VA-HIT), gemfibrozil (Lopid®) was used to increase HDL-C by 3 mg/dL, which was not associated with a change in LDL-C. Patients with diabetes had a 24% decrease in cardiovascular events.[16]

The optimal LDL-C level for adults with diabetes is <100 mg/dL with or without CAD or PVD. The National Cholesterol Education Program (NCEP) report now suggests that patients with or without diabetes who manifest clinical CAD should have a target LDL-C level of <100 mg/dL.[17] In the East-West Study, more than 1,000 patients with diabetes and more than 1,000 patients without diabetes were followed prospectively to determine the incidence of MI during a 7-year period. Patients with diabetes without a history of myocardial disease had the same rate of MI as patients without diabetes who had documented CAD, suggesting that diabetes confers the same risk of having an MI as a diagnosis of known CAD.[18] Additionally, a large portion of patients with diabetes who suffer an MI die before they ever reach the hospital, indicating that secondary prevention may be too late.

Low HDL-C is a known risk factor for CAD. The optimal HDL-C level is >40 mg/dL, as recommended by the ADA and NCEP. Triglyceride goals are now recommended to be <150 mg/dL.[1] The level of small, dense LDL-C indicates the available LDL-C for oxidation; oxidized LDL-C is more atherogenic and may emerge as an independent risk factor for CAD. Small, dense LDL-C correlates directly with triglyceride levels. Although it is not clear whether triglyceride itself is a risk factor for CAD, even lower levels of triglycerides may be recommended.

References

1.   Standards of medical care for patients with diabetes mellitus. *Diabetes Care* 2003;26(suppl 1):S33-S50.

2.   American College of Endocrinology: Consensus statement on guidelines for glycemic control. *Endocr Pract* 2002;8(suppl 1):6-11.

3.   The effect of intensive treatment of diabetes on the development and progression of long-term complications in insulin-dependent diabetes mellitus. The Diabetes Control and Complications Trial Research Group. *N Engl J Med* 1993;329:977-986.

4.   Ohkubo Y, Kishikawa H, Araki E, et al: Intensive insulin therapy prevents the progression of diabetic microvascular complications in Japanese patients with non-insulin-dependent diabetes mellitus: a randomized prospective 6-year study. *Diabetes Res Clin Pract* 1995;28:103-117.

5.   Intensive blood-glucose control with sulphonylureas or insulin compared with conventional treatment and risk of complications in patients with type 2 diabetes (UKPDS 33). UK Prospective Diabetes Study (UKPDS) Group. *Lancet* 1998;352:837-853.

6.   Hansson L, Zanchetti A, Carruthers SG, et al: Effects of intensive blood-pressure lowering and low-dose aspirin in patients with hypertension: principal results of the Hypertension Optimal Treatment (HOT) randomised trial. HOT Study Group. *Lancet* 1998;351:1755-1762.

7.   The sixth report of the Joint National Committee on Prevention, Detection, Evaluation, and Treatment of High Blood Pressure. *Arch Intern Med* 1997;157:2413-2446.

8.   Tight blood pressure control and risk of macrovascular and microvascular complications in type 2 diabetes: UKPDS 38. UK Prospective Diabetes Study Group. *BMJ* 1998;317:703-713.

9.   Yusuf S, Sleight P, Pogue J, et al: Effects of an angiotensin-converting-enzyme inhibitor, ramipril, on cardiovascular events in high-risk patients. The Heart Outcomes Prevention Evaluation Study Investigators. *N Engl J Med* 2000;342:145-153.

10.   Lazarus JM, Bourgoignie JJ, Buckalew VM, et al: Achievement and safety of a low blood pressure goal in chronic renal disease. The Modification of Diet in Renal Disease Study Group. *Hypertension* 1997;29:641-650.

11.   Lewis EJ, Hunsicker LG, Bain RP, et al: The effect of angiotensin-converting-enzyme inhibition on diabetic nephropathy. The Collaborative Study Group. *N Engl J Med* 1993;329:1456-1462.

12.   Brenner BM, Cooper ME, de Zeeuw D, et al: Effects of losartan on renal and cardiovascular outcomes in patients with type 2 diabetes and nephropathy. *N Engl J Med* 2001;345:861-869.

13.   Lewis EJ, Hunsicker LG, Clarke WR, et al: Renoprotective effect of the angiotensin-receptor antagonist irbesartan in patients with nephropathy due to type 2 diabetes. *N Engl J Med* 2001; 345:851-860.

14.   Randomised trial of cholesterol lowering in 4,444 patients with coronary heart disease: the Scandinavian Simvastatin Survival Study (4S). *Lancet* 1994;344:1383-1389.

15.   Sacks FM, Pfeffer MA, Moye LA, et al: The effect of pravastatin on coronary events after myocardial infarction in patients with average cholesterol levels. Cholesterol and Recurrent Events Trial investigators. *N Engl J Med* 1996;335:1001-1009.

16. Rubins HB, Robins SJ, Collins D, et al: Gemfibrozil for the secondary prevention of coronary heart disease in men with low levels of high-density lipoprotein cholesterol. Veterans Affairs High-Density Lipoprotein Cholesterol Intervention Trial Study Group. *N Engl J Med* 1999;341:410-418.

17. Executive Summary of The Third Report of The National Cholesterol Education Program (NCEP) Expert Panel on Detection, Evaluation, And Treatment of High Blood Cholesterol In Adults (Adult Treatment Panel III). *JAMA* 2001;285:2486-2497.

18. Haffner SM, Lehto S, Ronnemaa T, et al: Mortality from coronary heart disease in subjects with type 2 diabetes and in nondiabetic subjects with and without prior myocardial infarction. *N Engl J Med* 1998;339:229-234.

Chapter 5

Glucose Control

Diet plus exercise should be emphasized as the primary form of treatment for type 2 diabetes and may be sufficient to control symptoms and to reach target serum glucose levels. Diet and exercise must be tailored to the needs of each patient. However, in most patients, pharmacologic therapy will be necessary. This chapter also examines insulin treatment and the various classes of oral antidiabetic drug therapy.

Diet Therapy

The goals of diet therapy are to maintain blood glucose levels as close to normal as possible; to balance food intake with activity levels, oral glucose-lowering agents, and/or insulin; to provide enough calories to maintain or attain a reasonable weight; to prevent and treat both short-term (eg, hypoglycemia) and long-term (eg, cardiovascular) complications of diabetes; and to improve overall health. Nutritional training is a proven means of reaching many of these goals. For example, in a randomized study, type 2 diabetes patients who received either a prepared meal program or instruction in selecting food servings from exchange lists for 10 weeks showed significant weight loss and reduction in glycated hemoglobin (Hb A_{1c}). When dietitians provided basic or practice-guideline-based care to patients with type 2 diabetes over 6 months, Hb A_{1c} improved significantly compared with that of a control group that did not have contact with dietitians.[1] In addition, weight-loss meal plans plus thrice-weekly exercise was twice as likely to produce a one-unit decrease in Hb A_{1c} as usual care in older African-American patients with type 2^2 diabetes. Common features of these successful interventions include individualized programs, close contact with educators, education in self-management skills, use of behavioral change techniques, and frequent follow-up.[3]

Strategies for Achieving Nutrition Goals

Providing a brochure such as the American Diabetes Association's (ADA's) 'First Step in Diabetes Meal Planning' and endorsing behavior change are simple but effective ways to introduce the type 2 diabetes patient to diet therapy. Office-based computer-assisted nutrition assessment has also proven effective as a first step toward diet therapy.[3] However, successful diet therapy requires a coordinated team effort that involves the patient as well as ongoing education in nutrition self-management. Patients should be referred to a registered dietitian with appropriate expertise in nutrition care and education. To maximize adherence, the approach must be tailored to the patient's lifestyle, goals, and cultural, ethnic, and financial considerations. As a first step, an assessment must be made to determine the nutrition prescription, which is based on therapeutic goals and what the patient is able and willing to do. To evaluate outcomes, adequate monitoring is required, including measurement of serum glucose and Hb A_{1c}. If results indicate that goals are not being met, the nutrition prescription must be changed to better meet these goals.[4]

Tactics for Achieving Nutrition Goals

Low-calorie diets and weight loss usually improve glycemic levels in the short term and may improve long-term metabolic control. Independent of weight loss, a low-calorie diet is associated with increased sensitivity to insulin and improved blood glucose levels, and even moderate weight loss (as little as 5 lb) can reduce hyperglycemia. Traditional diets have usually not produced long-term weight loss, even when based on low numbers of calories. The best approach is moderate calorie restriction (250 to 500 calories less than average daily intake) within an adequate meal plan featuring reduced fat (especially saturated fat) intake. Meal planning often includes fat-gram and calorie counting and portion control. Spacing smaller meals throughout the day can help promote weight loss if total caloric intake does not increase.[4] However, achieving and maintaining near-normal blood glucose levels should be emphasized more than weight loss. Three evenly spaced meals a day are generally recommended to help stabilize blood glucose levels. Timing of meals and amount of food intake at each meal should be consistent. Meal planning for patients with type 2 diabetes usually involves combining servings of foods or items from food category exchange lists. These systems are based on the recommended percentages of macronutrient components that should make up total calories.

Dietary Components
Macronutrients

Evidence is insufficient to support a protein intake for diabetic patients that is higher or lower than the average for the general population. Most patients with diabetes should obtain 10% to 20% of their daily caloric intake from protein. The contribution of protein to the glucose pool is minimal, and no reason exists to restrict the amount of protein consumed, even in patients who have microalbuminuria.[4] Diet therapy for patients with type 2 diabetes emphasizes the type of protein that should be consumed rather than the amount: changing from a diet containing animal-based protein to one containing plant-based protein may improve glucose and lipid control and prevent complications.[3]

The other 80% to 90% of total calories should be derived from dietary fats and carbohydrates. Patients at a healthy weight with normal lipid levels should follow the National Cholesterol Education Program recommendations: total fat intake should be no more than 30% of total calories, and obese patients should consider restricting dietary fat intake to less than 30%. Foods that incorporate fat replacers can help control fat intake if patients avoid overconsumption of these foods. Overconsumption of fat replacers may hamper reduction in fat consumption and/or increase carbohydrate intake and adversely affect glycemic control.[4]

Little scientific evidence supports the notion, based on the assumption that simple sugars are more rapidly digested and thereby worsen hyperglycemia, that diabetic patients should avoid simple sugars and replace them with starches. On the contrary, fruits and milk produce a lower glycemic response than most starches, and sucrose produces a glycemic response similar to that of bread, rice, and potatoes. Learning the glycemic index (a ranking of foods based on their potential to raise blood glucose) of common foods and using foods with a low index can be important means of stabilizing blood sugar for type 2 diabetes patients.

Patients should also pay attention to the total amount of carbohydrates they consume. The percentage of calories recommended as total carbohydrates in the diabetic meal plan ranges from about 45% to 60%. Within this range, the percentage should be tailored to reach individual treatment goals. Patients should learn how to limit carbohydrate consumption by either calculating the carbohydrate content of meals based on grams of carbohydrate in commonly consumed foods or exchanging servings of foods based on carbohydrate unit equivalents from exchange lists. Although use of sucrose does not impair blood glucose control in patients with type 2 diabetes, sucrose or foods containing it must be substituted for other carbohydrates and not simply added to the diet.

Fructose produces a smaller increase in plasma glucose than isocaloric amounts of sucrose and most starches. Despite this apparent advantage, fructose may have no overall advantage as a sweetening agent in the diabetic diet because doubling the intake of calories from fructose adversely affects serum cholesterol and low-density lipoprotein (LDL) levels. As a result, people with dyslipidemia should avoid consuming large amounts of fructose. However, no reason exists to recommend that diabetic patients avoid consumption of fruits and vegetables or moderate amounts of fructose-sweetened foods. Sweetening foods with corn syrup, fruit juice or fruit juice concentrate, honey, molasses, dextrose, or maltose instead of with sucrose or fructose does not decrease calorie consumption or dietary carbohydrate content or improve glycemic control. Although the common sugar alcohols sorbitol, mannitol, and xylitol result in a lower glycemic response than sucrose and other carbohydrates, evidence suggesting that they can reduce the total calorie or carbohydrate content of the diet is limited. Moreover, excessive consumption of sugar alcohols may cause diarrhea, and sorbitol buildup in cells may contribute to microvascular complications.

Pregnant patients, patients with a history of alcohol abuse, and patients with pancreatitis, dyslipidemia, or neuropathy should avoid consuming alcohol. However, in general, patients with diabetes should follow the same precautions in using alcohol as the general public: no more than two daily drinks for men and no more than one for women. Alcohol is not metabolized into sugar, and it inhibits gluconeogenesis. Therefore, if patients who are taking insulin or oral glucose inhibitors consume alcohol without eating, hypoglycemia can result, even at low blood alcohol levels that result in only mild intoxication. However, if alcohol is used in moderation with food by patients whose diabetes is well controlled, blood glucose levels are not affected. Calories from alcohol are best substituted for fat calories.

Patients with diabetes should consume the amount of fiber recommended for the general population, 20 to 35 g daily.[4] Dietary fiber provides a feeling of fullness, which can aid in weight loss or maintenance. Some fiber can inhibit glucose absorption from the small intestine, but its effect on blood glucose levels is probably insignificant. However, soluble fiber rich in β-glucans, such as oat bran, may reduce postprandial hyperglycemia.

Micronutrients

Use of moderate to high doses of antioxidants such as vitamin E may reduce risk of diabetic complications. However, no formal recommendations in this area have been made. A Chinese study found that high levels of supplemental chromium improved glucose and insulin levels in patients with type 2 diabetes. However, because the Mainland Chinese diet is low in chromium, these patients were probably chromium deficient. Most US diabetic patients are not chromium deficient. As a result, chromium supplementation is not routinely recommended for patients with diabetes.[3] Nevertheless, in patients who are chromium deficient from parenteral nutrition, glycemic control may improve with chromium replacement.

Magnesium deficiency may play a role in insulin resistance, carbohydrate intolerance, hypertension, and excess cardiovascular morbidity. However, serum magnesium levels determined with widely available technology are relatively insensitive indicators of deficiency, and evidence to support magnesium supplementation in patients with diabetes is lacking. Routine evaluation of serum magnesium levels is recommended only in patients at high risk for magnesium deficiency. These include patients with congestive heart failure or acute myocardial infarction (AMI), ketoacidosis, or potassium or calcium deficiency; patients on long-term parenteral nutrition; patients who abuse alcohol; pregnant patients; and chronic users of diuretics, aminoglycosides, or digoxin. The use of sensitive magnesium assays that measure intracellular magnesium may be indicated for such patients. Patients with documented hypomagnesemia should receive potent, bioavailable oral magnesium chloride until the serum magnesium level normalizes or the precipitating condition is reversed.[4]

Exercise

Exercise can be a therapeutic tool for a variety of patients with type 2 diabetes. The challenge is to get patients to start an exercise or physical activity program and make it a lifelong behavior. For many, walking for at least 20 to 30 minutes at least three times weekly is the first step. As with any treatment, the effects of exercise must be thoroughly understood so that the benefits and risks can be analyzed for each patient and an exercise program can be tailored accordingly.

Benefits

One exercise session often causes an acute decrease in plasma glucose level in type 2 diabetes patients. Postexercise enhancement of glucose metabolism, possibly from increased insulin sensitivity in muscle, may last for hours or even days. Better glycemic control may result from the additive effects of many exercise sessions and not from increased fitness.[5] Long-term studies have shown that regular exercise training consistently improves carbohydrate metabolism and insulin sensitivity and can maintain this effect for at least 5 years. In these studies, exercise intensity was 50% to 80% of maximum oxygen consumption ($\dot{V}O_2$max), frequency was three to four times a week, and duration was 30 to 60 minutes per session. Hb A_{1c} decreased 10% to 20%, and improvement was greatest in patients with mild disease and in the most insulin-resistant patients. This finding is consistent with the observation that exercise reverses insulin resistance.[6]

In patients with type 2 diabetes, most excess morbidity and mortality can be attributed to coronary artery disease (CAD), stroke, and peripheral vascular disease (PVD); all are caused by accelerated atherosclerosis. Reducing atherogenesis is therefore particularly crucial in these patients.[5] Hyperinsulinemia, hyperglycemia, and the insulin resistance syndrome are also increasingly being viewed as important risk factors for premature coronary disease in type 2 diabetes patients. The benefits of exercise in lowering cardiovascular risk are likely related to improved insulin sensitivity.[6] In patients with type 2 diabetes, decreases in adiposity frequently increase insulin sensitivity and glycemic control and reduce risk factors for coronary heart disease. Weight loss and its maintenance are enhanced by combining exercise with diet therapy, and exercise disproportionately decreases intra-abdominal fat, which is the type of fat most closely associated with metabolic abnormalities. Moreover, exercise training is associated with decreased anxiety, better mood, higher self-esteem, and increased sense of well-being, which may improve compliance with other therapies that enhance glycemic control.[5] However, exercise may cause or worsen hypoglycemia in some patients, particularly those taking sulfonylureas or insulin.[5]

Recommendations and Precautions

Use of exercise to treat type 2 diabetes is only appropriate if the benefits outweigh the risks. Although this is almost always the case, appropriate guidelines must be followed to avoid any potential adverse effects. Preexercise evaluation of all patients is required. The clinician should obtain a complete history and perform an extensive physical examination, paying special attention to identifying macrovascular, microvascular, and neurologic complications that may put the patient at greater risk from exercise. Recommendations on the appropriate tests to pursue and precautions to follow for specific diabetic complications can be found in the ADA position statement on diabetes mellitus and exercise.[6]

If there are no contraindications to certain types of exercise, exercise type is a matter of patient preference. Rhythmic aerobic exercises such as swimming and walking are generally preferred. Resistance exercises like weight lifting may improve glucose disposal but may also result in orthopedic and vascular problems. However, studies have shown that properly designed resistance exercise programs may be safer and more effective than assumed. High-resistance exercise using weights may be safe for young, healthy diabetic patients, but not for older patients or those with long-standing disease. Moderate weight training programs using light weights and high numbers of repetitions can be used to maintain or enhance upper body strength in almost all diabetic patients. Studies indicate that elderly patients benefit from exercise at least as much as the general population and that the incidence of complications in this group is acceptable. Optimum cardiovascular benefits result from exercise at 50% to 70% of $\dot{V}o_2$max. This intensity is usually prescribed if diabetic complications permit and blood pressure does not change excessively during or after exercise. Prolonged exercise at less than 50% of $\dot{V}o_2$max (eg, walking, dancing) may also improve cardiovascular fitness. Exercise intensity should be limited so that systolic blood pressure does not exceed 180 mm Hg. Optimal exercise intensity is best estimated from maximal heart rate (HR) before rising in the morning by using the equation:

$$ME_{50} = 0.5(HR_{max} - HR_{rest}) = HR_{rest}$$

where HR_{max} is maximum heart rate, HR_{rest} is resting heart rate, and ME is maximal effort. If the true HR_{max} is unknown, it can be estimated by the equation:

$$HR_{max} = 220 - \text{patient's age}$$

but this formula may greatly overestimate HR_{max} in autonomic neuropathy.

Sessions at 50% to 70% of $\dot{V}o_2$max should last 20 to 45 minutes. Shorter sessions do not affect metabolism, and longer ones cause more musculoskeletal trauma.[5] In patients taking insulin, exercise should be scheduled to avoid coinciding with periods of peak insulin absorption. Patients should exercise at least 3 days a week or every other day to improve insulin sensitivity and glycemic control. For weight reduction, at least 5 days of exercise is needed weekly, and exercise should result in a weekly energy expenditure of 700 to 2,000 calories.[3]

Sufficient fluid should be taken early and frequently during the exercise session to compensate for losses in sweat, particularly during hot spells; consuming the maximal amount of fluid tolerated is optimal. Patients taking insulin or sulfonylureas should self-monitor blood glucose before, during, and after exercise and follow hypoglycemia prevention guidelines.[6]

Quantitative measurements of progress should be used to provide the patient with feedback on the effectiveness of exercise efforts, but unrealistic performance goals should be avoided.[6] A formal program is not required for exercise to be successful; a randomized trial showed that obese women who increased their level of common daily activities such as housework regained less weight after 1 year than those in a formal aerobics program.[7] More detailed exercise recommendations for patients with type 2 diabetes can be found in *The Health Professional's Guide to Diabetes and Exercise* by the ADA.

Even if oral antidiabetic agents are required, the patient should be warned against abandoning diet plus exercise as a failed strategy or viewing medication as a means of avoiding dietary restrictions and exercise sessions. Instead, the patient should be taught that continuing these efforts is important to maintain the effectiveness of drug therapy and to avoid diabetic complications.

Pharmacotherapy

Oral Agents

The long-term goal in the treatment of type 2 diabetes is to avoid chronic complications. Because the mean serum glucose level determines the incidence of complications, the ideal treatment target is the lowest serum glucose level reachable while avoiding hypoglycemia.[8] Practically speaking, this target is an Hb A_{1c} less than 6.5% to 7.0% or a fasting serum glucose level less than 110 mg/dL. New therapeutic agents based on a better understanding of the pathophysiology of type 2 diabetes have

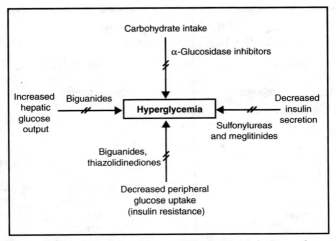

Figure 5-1: Causes of hyperglycemia and sites of action of oral antidiabetic agents. Adapted from *Am Fam Physician* 1999;59:2841.

put these targets within the reach of more patients. However, the clinical advantages and disadvantages of these agents must be fully understood to ensure their appropriate use.[8] Oral agents target the main physiologic determinants of blood glucose levels: carbohydrate intake, insulin supply, and glucose production and uptake by tissues (Figure 5-1). They fall into two categories: those that increase insulin supply and those that boost insulin's effect.[8] Tables 5-1 and 5-2 summarize the action, dosing, and effects of oral hypoglycemic agents,[9-11] and Figure 5-2 includes an algorithm for their use.

General contraindications

Oral agents are not suitable for every patient. Because most oral agents are metabolized by the liver and excreted by the kidney, they are generally contraindicated for patients with severe liver or kidney disease. The exception is the thiazolidinediones (TZDs), which can be used in pa-

Table 5-1: Insulin Secretagogues
for Type 2 Diabetes

Drug Class, Oral Agent, and Brand Name(s)	Duration of Action	Approved Daily Dosage Range; Usual Effective Dosage
*Sulfonylureas**		
First Generation		
acetohexamide (Dymelor®)	12-18 h	250-1,500 mg; 500-750 mg q.d.
chlorpropamide (Diabinese®)	48+ h	100-500 mg; 250-500 mg q.d.
tolazamide (Tolinase®)	12-24 h	100-1,000 mg; 250-500 mg q.d.
tolbutamide (Orinase®)	6-12 h	250-3,000 mg; 500-1,000 mg b.i.d.
Second Generation		
glyburide		
Micronase®	12-24 h	1.25-20 mg; 5 mg b.i.d.
Glynase® (micronized)	12-24 h	0.75-12 mg; 3 mg b.i.d.
glipizide		
Glucotrol®	12-18 h	2.5-40 mg; 10 mg b.i.d.
Glucotrol XL®	24 h	5-20 mg; 5-10 mg q.d.
glimepiride (Amaryl®)	24 h	1-8 mg; 1-4 mg q.d.
*Meglitinides***		
nateglinide (Starlix®)	2-4 h	180-360 mg; 120 mg t.i.d.
repaglinide (Prandin®)	2-6 h	1.5-16 mg; 1-2 mg t.i.d.

* The mean decrease in fasting plasma glucose level for these agents is 60 to 70 mg/dL; the mean decrease in hemoglobin A_{1c} is 0.8% to 2%.

Clearance	Titration/Side Effects
Renal	Take 15-30 min before meals (except for Glucotrol XL®);
Hepatic, renal	begin with lowest effective dose and titrate upward every
Hepatic	couple of weeks. Increased risk of hypoglycemia, weight gain.
Renal	
Hepatic, renal	
Hepatic, renal	
Hepatic	
Hepatic	
Hepatic, renal	
Hepatic	Take 15 minutes before meals; skip dose if meal is missed; add
Hepatic	dose if meal is added. Hypoglycemia; weight gain.

** The mean decrease in fasting plasma glucose level for these agents is 65 to 75 mg/dL; the mean decrease in hemoglobin A_{1c} is 0.5% to 2%.

Table data were obtained from references 9, 10, and 11 and from package inserts for agents listed.

Table 5-2: Other Classes of Oral Agents for Type 2 Diabetes

Drug Class, Oral Agent, and Brand Name(s)	Mode of Action	Duration of Action
Biguanides		
metformin	Insulin	>3-4 wk
Glucophage®	sensitizers	>3-4 wk
Glucophage® XR		
Thiazolidinediones		
pioglitazone (Actos®)	Insulin	>3-4 wk
rosiglitazone (Avandia®)	sensitizers	>3-4 wk
α-Glucosidase Inhibitors		
acarbose (Precose®)	Delay	<4 h
miglitol (Glyset®)	carbohydrate absorption	<4 h

tients with advanced renal disease. However, these patients, like pregnant patients, should be treated with insulin. Oral agents are contraindicated in pregnancy because safety data in this setting are sparse. Patients with severe, symptomatic hyperglycemia are also usually treated with insulin. However, once their condition stabilizes enough to allow switching to oral agents, the choice of treatment for these patients should be reconsidered. Children and adolescents with type 2 diabetes are usually treated with sulfonylureas and metformin, the oral agents with which there is clinical experience in this age group.[8]

Monotherapy
Sulfonylureas

For a list of agents in this class that are available in the United States, see Table 5-1.

Approved Daily Dosage Range; Usual Effective Dosage	Clearance
850-2,550 mg; 1,000 mg b.i.d.	Renal
500-2,000 mg; 1,000 mg q.d.	Renal
15-45 mg; 45 mg q.d.	Hepatic
4-8 mg; 4 mg b.i.d.	Hepatic
75-300 mg; 50 mg t.i.d.	Renal
75-300 mg; 50 mg t.i.d.	Renal

(continued on next page)

Indications. Sulfonylureas are indicated as adjuncts to diet and exercise to lower blood glucose levels in patients with type 2 diabetes whose hyperglycemia cannot be controlled by diet and exercise alone.[12]

Mechanism of action. Sulfonylureas bind to a specific receptor on pancreatic β cells (Figure 5-3). This binding augments the effect of glucose by closing a potassium-dependent adenosine triphosphate (K_{ATP}) channel. Most sulfonylureas bind to a 140-kDa protein at the potassium channel. Glimepiride (Amaryl®) binds to a 65-kDa protein at the same site. No difference in effects attributed to differential binding is apparent.[8] Sulfonylureas may also enhance tissue sensitivity to insulin, but most investigators believe the improved insulin action they cause results from decreased glucose toxicity.[9]

Table 5-2: Other Classes of Oral Agents for Type 2 Diabetes *(continued)*

Drug Class, Oral Agent, and Brand Name(s)	Titration/Side Effects
Biguanides	
metformin	Take with the largest meal or meals of the day. Gastrointestinal, rare lactic acidosis (?)
Thiazolidinediones	
pioglitazone rosiglitazone	Monitor AST/ALT levels before initiating therapy, every 2 months in first year, then periodically. Edema, weight gain, increased LDL cholesterol level, potential hepatotoxicity
α-Glucosidase Inhibitors	
acarbose miglitol	Take with meals; initiate at 25 mg q.d. with supper; increase dose 25 mg daily every 2-4 wk for 6-8 wk; for acarbose, monitor AST/ALT every 3 months in first year then periodically. Gastrointestinal.

AST/ALT = serum transaminases; FPG = fasting plasma glucose level; Hb A_{1c} = glycated hemoglobin.

Mean FPG Decrease (mg/dL)	Mean Hb A_{1c} Decrease (%)
50-70	1.5-2
25-50	0.5-1.5
35-40	0.7-1

Table data were obtained from references 9, 10, and 11 and from package inserts for agents listed.

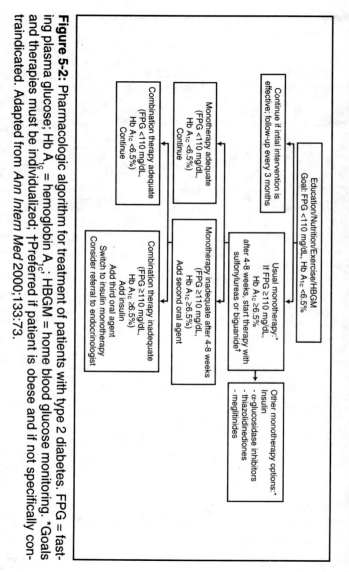

Figure 5-2: Pharmacologic algorithm for treatment of patients with type 2 diabetes. FPG = fasting plasma glucose; Hb A$_{1c}$ = hemoglobin A$_{1c}$; HBGM = home blood glucose monitoring. *Goals and therapies must be individualized; †Preferred if patient is obese and if not specifically contraindicated. Adapted from *Ann Intern Med* 2000;133:73.

Education/Nutrition/Exercise/HBGM
Goal: FPG <110 mg/dL, Hb A$_{1c}$ <6.5%

Continue if initial intervention is
effective; follow-up every 3 months

Usual monotherapy:*
If FPG ≥110 mg/dL,
Hb A$_{1c}$ ≥6.5%
after 4-8 weeks, start therapy with
sulfonylureas or biguanide†

Other monotherapy options:*
Insulin
- α-glucosidase inhibitors
- thiazolidinediones
- meglitinides

Monotherapy adequate
(FPG <110 mg/dL,
Hb A$_{1c}$ <6.5%)
Continue

Monotherapy inadequate after 4-8 weeks
(FPG ≥110 mg/dL,
Hb A$_{1c}$ ≥6.5%)
Add second oral agent

Combination therapy adequate
(FPG <110 mg/dL,
Hb A$_{1c}$ <6.5%)
Continue

Combination therapy inadequate
(FPG ≥110 mg/dL,
Hb A$_{1c}$ ≥6.5%)
Add insulin
Add third oral agent
Switch to insulin monotherapy
Consider referral to endocrinologist

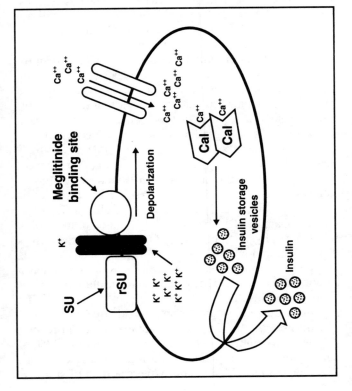

Figure 5-3: Sulfonylureas (SU) bind to the sulfonylurea receptor (rSU) at the ATP-dependent potassium channel, while meglitinides bind at a distinct site that is as yet uncharacterized. Both contacts inhibit potassium efflux, resulting in maintained membrane depolarization and calcium influx. The calcium-calmodulin (Cal) complex acts as a second messenger, signaling the release of insulin from insulin storage vesicles by way of exocytosis. Adapted from Luna et al, *Diabetes* 1999;26:895.

Effectiveness. All sulfonylureas are essentially equally effective in reducing hyperglycemia.[8] Patients with an initial mean Hb A_{1c} of about 10% who respond to initial therapy with sulfonylureas have shown a 1.5% to 2.0% decrease in Hb A_{1c} in most studies. The potency of sulfonylureas is directly related to the starting fasting plasma glucose level (FPG): the higher the FPG at baseline, the greater its decrease after treatment. Factors associated with a good response to sulfonylurea therapy include recently diagnosed diabetes, mild to moderate fasting hyperglycemia, good β-cell function as indicated by a high fasting C-peptide level, and no islet cell or glutamic acid decarboxylase antibodies. Many patients (up to 75%) with type 2 diabetes will not reach the desired FPG during sulfonylurea treatment and will require a second oral agent or insulin.

After showing an initially adequate response to sulfonylureas, about 5% to 10% of patients per year will begin to respond inadequately (secondary failure) and require a second oral agent. Secondary treatment failure may be related to patient-associated factors such as weight gain, lack of exercise, poor compliance, or coexisting conditions; therapy-associated factors such as use of other medications that interfere with insulin action or secretion, β-cell desensitization from long-term sulfonylurea therapy, and insufficient drug dosage; and disease-associated factors such as increasing insulin resistance and/or insulin deficiency.[9] Chlorpropamide (Diabinese®), like glipizide (Glucotrol®), has a more physiologic pattern of insulin release as well as a significantly lower secondary failure rate than glyburide (Diaβeta®, Glynase® PresTab®, Micronase®), which has a prolonged, exaggerated secondary-phase insulin-release pattern. Fasting insulin levels are significantly higher during glyburide treatment than during glipizide treatment.[13]

Adverse effects. These are generally mild and reversible with discontinuation of therapy.[9] Fewer than 2% of sulfonylurea-treated patients discontinue therapy because of adverse effects.[8] The major adverse effect of sulfonylurea therapy is hypoglycemia, which is more common with agents with a longer duration of action, such as chlorpropamide and glyburide. Both drugs have long half-lives, and both depend on renal excretion, which increases risk of hypoglycemia in patients with renal impairment.[13] Increased hypoglycemia with glyburide may result because glyburide suppresses hepatic glucose production more than other agents do.[9] However, the association between longer duration of action and greater incidence of hypoglycemia does not hold true for glimepiride and extended-release glipizide.[8]

Severe hypoglycemia requiring hospital admission has been reported at a frequency of 0.2 to 0.4 case per 1,000 treatment-years for sulfonylurea therapy,[14,15] but the United Kingdom Prospective Diabetes Study (UKPDS) reported a much higher incidence.[16] Short-acting agents may therefore be preferred in patients at high risk for hypoglycemia, such as those with mild fasting hyperglycemia (less than 140 mg/dL), those with a reduced glomerular filtration rate, and those older than 80 years.[9] Patients who are taking several drugs simultaneously, such as patients with concomitant conditions or the elderly, are also at increased risk of hypoglycemia.[13] However, no long-term prospective studies have compared short-acting and long-acting sulfonylureas in elderly patients with type 2 diabetes. One small, short-term study found no difference between glyburide and glipizide in occurrence of hypoglycemia in these patients.[9]

Hypoglycemia is most likely to occur during initiation of therapy. Therapy initiation requires small doses and frequent blood glucose monitoring in patients at high risk for hypoglycemia. Additionally, patients must be warned about increased risk of hypoglycemia from skipping or delaying meals or drinking alcohol.[8]

Animal studies have suggested that sulfonylureas may block cellular K_{ATP} channels that may protect the heart from the effects of ischemia or metabolic impairment,[13] and the University Group Diabetes Program (UGDP) study, which was conducted in the 1970s, found that patients treated with tolbutamide (Orinase®) had increased mortality from ischemic heart disease.[17] However, subsequent studies found that patients treated with tolbutamide had a lower mortality from ischemic heart disease.[13] ADA policy opposes formal restrictions on the use of sulfonylureas based on UGDP findings.[9] Also, the UKPDS showed that after 10 years of therapy, use of sulfonylureas was associated with fewer chronic complications without increased incidence of cardiovascular events. Sulfonylurea-treated UKPDS patients even showed a trend toward reduction in myocardial infarction. The beneficial glucose-lowering effects of sulfonylureas may thus outweigh potential adverse effects on vascular reactivity.[8]

Sulfonylureas may have adverse cardiovascular events in patients who have already had an AMI. In the Diabetes Mellitus Insulin-Glucose Infusion in AMI (DIGAMI) comparative study of diabetes therapies for postinfarct patients, the difference in mortality between the insulin-treated group and the sulfonylurea-treated group mainly resulted from a difference in incidence of sudden death and fatal reinfarction. The UKPDS excluded patients with clinically relevant CAD and thus was unable to disprove the possibility that sulfonylureas have a detrimental effect on postinfarct patients.[18]

No published clinical study has shown a cardiovascular advantage of one sulfonylurea over another.[9] Based on preliminary findings, glimepiride was proposed to have cardiovascular advantages over glyburide and possibly other sulfonylureas, but these claims are unsubstantiated.[8] Because placebo-treated patients had a beneficial reduction in ST segment depression during coronary angioplasty that did not occur in patients taking glyburide, glyburide was proposed to adversely effect cardiac ischemic preconditioning.[13] However, another study showed that glyburide reduced abnormal arrhythmias in patients with type 2 diabetes.[13]

Sulfonylurea therapy is often associated with weight gain, especially if glycemic control improves substantially, although in one study, long-acting glipizide caused no weight gain.[9] Other adverse effects of sulfonylureas include rash, nausea, indigestion, and abnormalities in liver enzymes.[8] Chlorpropamide and tolbutamide have been associated with hyponatremia. Elderly patients, women, and those treated with diuretics are most at risk for this complication. Chlorpropamide also causes flushing during alcohol consumption.[13]

Drug interactions. Protein-binding competition between sulfonylureas and common drugs (nonsteroidal antiinflammatory agents, warfarin, salicylates, β-blockers) may exacerbate hypoglycemia. Because second-generation sulfonylureas are nonionically bound to plasma proteins, they pose less risk of drug interaction than first-generation sulfonylureas.[8]

Contraindications and precautions. Use of sulfonylureas is contraindicated in patients with allergies to sulfa drugs.[8]

Cost. Sulfonylureas are the least expensive oral agents for type 2 diabetes, and generic (first-generation) agents are the least expensive sulfonylureas. If cost is of major concern, sulfonylureas are preferred.[9]

Meglitinides

Like sulfonylureas, meglitinides stimulate insulin secretion. However, meglitinides were specifically developed to reduce the risk of hypoglycemia associated with sulfonylurea therapy and to decrease the likelihood of secondary treatment failure from exhausted β cells. Meglitinides are a novel group of rapid-acting agents designed to stimulate insulin secretion when needed at mealtimes and to return insulin levels to the basal baseline between meals.[19] Because they are rapidly absorbed and eliminated, they cause a fast but brief release of insulin.[9] The temporal relation between dosing with these agents and their action with meal consumption provides an inherent advantage in type 2 diabetes.[8] As a result, meglitinides could become the preferred treatment for the large group of newly diagnosed type 2 diabetes patients with postprandial hyperglycemia but normal FPG.[19] In the United States, two agents are available in this drug class. They are repaglinide (Prandin®), a carbamoyl methyl benzoic acid derivative that was approved by the FDA in 1998, and nateglinide (Starlix®), which is derived from the amino acid D-phenylalanine and was approved by the FDA in December 2000.

Indications. Repaglinide was approved for use as initial monotherapy for the treatment of type 2 diabetes.[8] Nateglinide was approved for use as monotherapy as an adjunct to diet and exercise to improve glycemic control in adult patients with type 2 diabetes who have not been taking other diabetic medicines regularly.[20]

Mechanism of action. Like sulfonylureas, meglitinides stimulate insulin secretion. However, this insulin release occurs only in the presence of glucose.[21] Because nateglinide has a more rapid interaction with the potassium channel, it produces a faster release of insulin than other insulin secretagogues.[22] Nateglinide also has the shortest duration of action of all the insulin secretagogues. These features result in more physiologic insulin secretion at mealtimes, lower insulin levels, and less risk of hypoglycemia. Moreover, unlike sulfonylureas, nateglinide does not inhibit the counterregulatory glucagon response to hypoglycemia, so repeated administration for 2 weeks enhances insulin secretion in the same manner as a single dose. This feature provides a consistent effect with less risk of hypoglycemia.[19]

Effectiveness. Studies indicate that, when used alone, repaglinide is as effective as sulfonylureas in reducing Hb A_{1c}.[8] Moreover, in diet-treated, drug-naïve patients, 1 year of repaglinide treatment decreased Hb A_{1c} as much as 1 year of glyburide treatment.[9] In patients with an Hb A_{1c} of about 8% after diet therapy, nateglinide reduced mean Hb A_{1c} by 0.5 percentage point. Unlike repaglinide, nateglinide was found to increase Hb A_{1c} in patients previously treated with sulfonylureas.[20] Secondary failure rates are not yet available.[8]

Adverse effects. The most common adverse effect from meglitinide therapy is hypoglycemia. Mild hypoglycemia was reported in 1.3% of patients who received the recommended dose of nateglinide.[19] Frequency of hypoglycemic episodes with repaglinide appears to be comparable with that for sulfonylureas. In one study, patients receiving repaglinide did not experience more episodes of hypoglycemia than those taking sulfonylureas.[9] Administering meglitinides only before meals and avoiding them before strenuous exercise can minimize hypoglycemia.[8,19]

Both meglitinides cause weight gain. However, patients switched from sulfonylurea to repaglinide therapy experienced no weight gain.[9]

Cardiovascular toxicity has not appeared in meglitinide-treated patients, although this association has not been ruled out by large, long-term clinical studies.[8] Patients who receive nateglinide alone have not shown clinically significant changes in liver enzyme levels.[19]

Drug interactions. Interactions between repaglinide and common drugs such as warfarin, digoxin, or cimetidine have not been found. Metabolism of repaglinide is inhibited by ketoconazole and erythromycin and may be enhanced by drugs that induce the CYP 3A4 isoenzyme.[8] Like repaglinide, nateglinide is highly bound to plasma proteins (98%). Nonsteroidal anti-inflammatory agents, salicylates, monoamine oxidase inhibitors, and nonselective β-blockers may potentiate the hypoglycemic action of meglitinides; thiazides, corticosteroids, thyroid products, and sympathomimetics may reduce it. When these agents are coadministered or withdrawn, patients taking meglitinides should be watched for changes in glycemic control.[20]

Contraindications and precautions. Repaglinide and nateglinide are contraindicated in patients with type 1 diabetes and in patients with a known hypersensitivity to these agents or any of their ingredients.[20,23] Geriatric or malnourished patients and those with adrenal or pituitary insufficiency are more susceptible to hypoglycemia as a side effect. Risk of hypoglycemia increases with strenuous physical exercise, alcohol ingestion, insufficient caloric intake, and combination treatment with other oral antidiabetic agents.[20] Because meglitinides are not sulfa based, they are not contraindicated for patients who are allergic to sulfa drugs.[8] Repaglinide therapy is not contraindicated in patients with renal insufficiency[9] and may be safe for patients with renal failure. Nateglinide and repaglinide should be used cautiously in patients with liver disease.[8] Initiation of therapy should proceed on a slower titration schedule for these patients than that recommended for patients with normal liver function.[9] Patients who skip meals should also skip any scheduled dose of meglitinide to reduce the risk of hypoglycemia. Transient loss of glycemic control may occur with fever, infection, trauma, or surgery, during which times insulin therapy may be needed.[20]

Cost. Meglitinides are about 2.5 times more expensive than brand-name sulfonylureas and slightly more expensive than brand-name metformin.[9]

Biguanides

Metformin (Glucophage®) is the sole available member of the biguanide drug class, which has been used in Europe since the 1950s. Metformin was approved for use in the United States in 1995. Another biguanide, phenformin, was withdrawn from the US market in the 1970s because of its association with lactic acidosis.[8] Metformin recently became available in a generic version; however, the extended-release version is still available only as a brand-name product.

Indications. Metformin is indicated as an adjunct to diet and exercise to improve glycemic control in patients with type 2 diabetes. Regular metformin is indicated for use in patients at least 10 years old, and the extended-release version is indicated for use in patients at least 17 years old.[24] Therapy should be initiated when Hb A_{1c} is 7.5% to 8% or less. Use of metformin may be associated with reduced progression of macrovascular complications.[25] Because of its ability to cause weight loss, metformin is indicated for the treatment of obese patients with diabetes and is usually the first-line agent for this patient population.[26]

Mechanism of action. Metformin enhances the sensitivity of hepatic tissue and, to a lesser degree, of peripheral tissue to insulin. Metformin also inhibits hepatic gluconeogenesis and glycogenolysis, increases insulin receptor tyrosine kinase activity, augments GLUT4 glucose transporter number and activity, enhances glycogen sensitivity, and augments glycogen synthesis. The primary receptor responsible for these effects is undetermined, but metformin has no direct effect on β-cell function.[9] Metformin may also have a mild effect on glucose absorption. It often reduces insulin secretion as glucose levels decline and therefore poses no risk of hypoglycemia.[8] This effect reflects the normal pancreatic compensatory response to enhanced insulin sensitivity.[9] Metformin's ability to inhibit fatty acid oxidation also contributes to its antihyperglycemic effect.[27]

Effectiveness. Metformin consistently decreases FPG by 60 to 70 mg/dL and Hb A_{1c} by 1.5 to 2.0 percentage points in patients with poorly controlled diabetes independent of duration of diabetes, body mass index (BMI), fasting or glucose-stimulated plasma insulin levels, or C-peptide levels. About 25% of patients receiving metformin monotherapy achieve an FPG of 140 mg/dL or lower and an Hb A_{1c} less than 7%.[28] The effects of metformin in reducing FPG and Hb A_{1c} are equivalent to those of sulfonylureas;[9] frequencies of adequate initial response are also similar.[8] As with sulfonylureas, the decrease in FPG with metformin strongly correlates with initial FPG. However, the hypoglycemic action of metformin increases linearly even at high FPGs (>300 mg/dL).

Patients with secondary sulfonylurea treatment failure seldom respond well to substitution with metformin.[9] In the UKPDS, the secondary treatment failure rate for metformin was similar to that for sulfonylureas in general. However, because metformin improves insulin sensitivity and decreases plasma insulin levels, metformin was expected to preserve β-cell function. This study finding indicates that once the FPG exceeds 140 to 160 mg/dL, β-cell failure may progress no matter which agent is used.[9]

Adverse effects. Gastrointestinal side effects (nausea, anorexia, abdominal bloating/cramping, diarrhea) are common and occur in 20% to 30% of patients. They are usually mild and transient and can be minimized by slow dosage titration[9] and dosage with food. Only about 5% to 10% of patients cannot tolerate metformin because of gastrointestinal effects.[8] Other clinically significant adverse side effects of metformin include metallic taste, which tends to dissipate over time, and decreased vitamin B_{12} levels, which can be corrected with supplementation.[29] Figure 5-4 weighs the benefits of metformin treatment of type 2 diabetes against its risks of adverse effects.

Lactic acidosis is a rare, often catastrophic metformin side effect[8] whose mortality ranges from 30% to 50%.[29] The frequency of lactic acidosis in patients taking metformin has been reported to be three cases per 100,000 patient-years. However, no metformin-treatment-related cases of lactic acidosis were seen in the UKPDS or in several US surveillance studies. At therapeutic doses, metformin does not interfere with lactate metabolism or increase basal plasma lactate levels. Lactic acidosis in metformin-treated patients is rare in the absence of the serious medical disorders listed under *Contraindications and precautions*, below. In patients with these conditions, discerning whether lactic acidosis results from the medical disorder or the metformin is difficult.[9] Retrospective analysis of study results for metformin-treated patients with lactic acidosis indicates that mortality is linked to the underlying disease rather than to metformin accumulation. The lowest mortality

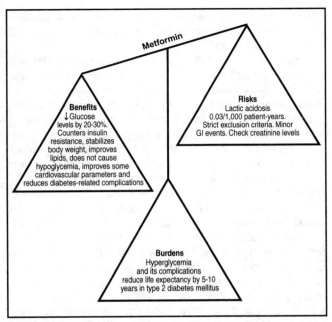

Figure 5-4: Key elements in the risk-benefit assessment of metformin against the burdens of type 2 diabetes. Reprinted with permission from Howlett et al, *Drug Safety* 1999;20:489-503.

was seen in patients with the highest plasma concentrations of metformin, suggesting that metformin may actually benefit these patients by increasing vasomotility. In summary, no known cases of fatal lactic acidosis caused by metformin treatment alone exist.[30]

Drug interactions. Any drug that decreases metformin's renal clearance theoretically increases the risk of metformin-associated lactic acidosis, but cimetidine is the only drug shown to reduce renal clearance of metformin. Other drugs that could decrease renal excretion of metformin include vancomycin, procainamide, digoxin, quinidine, quinine, ranitidine, morphine, and amiloride, but scientific evidence against coadministration of these agents with metformin is lacking.[29]

Contraindications and precautions. Because of its possible association with lactic acidosis, metformin is contraindicated in patients with renal and hepatic disease; alcohol abuse syndrome; congestive heart failure requiring drug treatment; peripheral vascular disease; respiratory insufficiency; severe infection; any condition associated with hypoxemia, dehydration, or sepsis; or any acute illness that may be associated with hypotension and hypoperfusion. Metformin treatment is contraindicated by serum creatinine concentrations of more than 1.4 mg/dL in women or 1.5 mg/dL in men. Elderly patients require determination of creatinine clearance; if it is less than 1 to 1.17 mL/s, metformin is contraindicated. Because diabetic patients are at increased risk for renal failure after receiving radiocontrast dye, continuation of metformin treatment during unrecognized dye-induced renal failure may result in lactic acidosis. Patients receiving metformin who need a radiocontrast dye study should have metformin withheld until normal renal function is documented by serum creatinine level 48 hours after the study.[9,24]

Cost. Brand-name metformin costs twice as much as second-generation sulfonylureas, slightly less than acarbose and repaglinide, and about a third of the cost of TZDs.[9]

Thiazolidinediones (PPAR-γ ligands)

These agents, which many consider the best examples of true insulin sensitizers,[8] bind to peroxisome proliferator-activated receptor (PPAR)-γ, a transcription cofactor that modifies the expression of genes that encode proteins involved in glucose and lipid homeostasis (Figure 5-5).[31] In the United States, available agents in this drug class include pioglitazone (Actos®), which received FDA approval in July 1999, and rosiglitazone (Avandia®), which was approved by the FDA in May 1999. Troglitazone

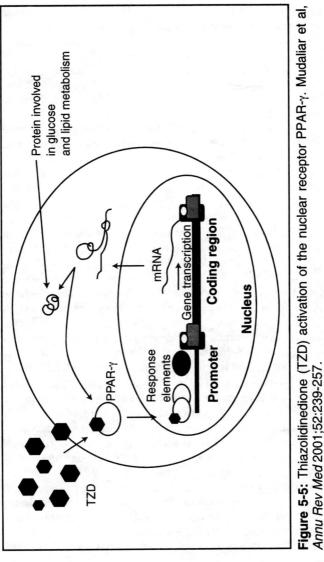

Figure 5-5: Thiazolidinedione (TZD) activation of the nuclear receptor PPAR-γ. Mudaliar et al, *Annu Rev Med* 2001;52:239-257.

(Rezulin®), the first TZD approved by the FDA for type 2 diabetes, was marketed in the United States from March 1997 to March 2000, when it was withdrawn because it caused severe idiosyncratic liver injury.[32]

Indications. Rosiglitazone and pioglitazone are approved for the treatment of type 2 diabetes as monotherapy and in combination with a sulfonylurea, metformin, or insulin.[23]

Mechanism of action. TZDs decrease hepatic glucose output and increase glucose uptake in skeletal muscle and adipose tissue, thereby enhancing the effectiveness of insulin.[33] They thus improve glycemic control without stimulating insulin secretion.[34] For example, they stimulate glucose transporter gene expression on cell membranes, thereby enhancing glucose uptake (Figure 5-6). Rosiglitazone increases the level of a major component of insulin action in adipocytes, which may improve insulin sensitivity and lower triglyceride and free fatty acid levels.[35]

The global effects of TZDs on gene expression appear to promote the net transfer of triglycerides and fatty acids from muscle and liver into storage by adipocytes, thereby improving glucose utilization.[31] In muscle, TZDs may enhance insulin sensitivity by reducing levels of tumor necrosis factor (TNF)-α, interleukin-6 (IL-6), resistin, and leptin, which are associated with insulin resistance.[31,35] TZDs also exert direct beneficial effects on vascular smooth muscle by causing the PPAR-γ receptor to inhibit cellular proliferation and migration, thereby limiting atherogenesis.[35] They may also reduce cholesterol in atherosclerotic lesions by causing the PPAR-γ receptor to induce the expression of cholesterol transport proteins.[31]

Effectiveness. As monotherapy, pioglitazone and rosiglitazone approach metformin and sulfonylureas in effectiveness. Patients with considerable endogenous insulin secretion but significant insulin resistance, including obese patients, respond best.[8] Clinical trials of rosiglitazone

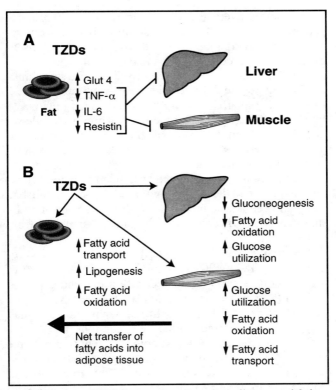

Figure 5-6: PPAR-γ promotes insulin sensitivity. Noncompeting models of the mechanisms by which PPAR-γ activation by thiazolidinedione (TZD) drugs ameliorates insulin resistance are shown. In *A*, TZDs act on PPAR-γ in adipose tissue to increase the glucose transporter Glut 4 and to decrease levels of cytokines that induce insulin resistance in liver and muscle. In *B*, TZDs act directly on multiple tissues to redistribute fatty acids away from muscle and liver and into fat, resulting in improved glucose utilization in the periphery. Reprinted with permission from Rosen et al, *J Biol Chem* 2001;276:37731-37734.

have reported average decreases in Hb A_{1c} of 0.3 to 1.6 percentage points.[36] In a 26-week study, rosiglitazone reduced FPG by as much as 76 mg/dL and Hb A_{1c} by as much as 1.54 percentage points in patients in whom previous treatment failed.[34] However, in a short-term study, full-dose rosiglitazone did not reduce Hb A_{1c} after 8 weeks.[33] In a direct comparison, rosiglitazone reduced FPG by 25 to 41 mg/dL depending on the dose, while glyburide reduced it by 30 mg/dL, and rosiglitazone maintained improved glycemic control through week 52 of the study.[35] After 1 year of treatment, patients taking the maximum dose of rosiglitazone achieved statistically greater reductions in FPG than those taking glyburide.[34] An unpublished study showed a sustained loss of glycemic control and a sharp rise in LDL cholesterol in patients switched from metformin to rosiglitazone.[33]

Depending on the dose, pioglitazone was found to reduce mean FPG by 30 to 56 mg/dL and Hb A_{1c} by 0.3 to 0.9 percentage point compared with a placebo group in which FPG rose by 9 mg/dL and Hb A_{1c} increased by 0.7 percentage point.[35] Like meglitinides, pioglitazone may help control postprandial glucose excursions.[37]

Adverse effects. The most common reported adverse effects of TZDs are upper respiratory tract infection and headache. These effects are mostly mild to moderate and do not require treatment discontinuation.[34] In contrast to experience with troglitazone, only two reports of hepatotoxicity have been associated with rosiglitazone.[35] One case report indicated that ischemic hepatitis was a more likely explanation for the reported hepatocellular injury than a rosiglitazone-induced adverse event.[34] There are no reports of hepatotoxicity associated with pioglitazone.[35]

TZDs increase plasma volume by 6% to 7%, and hematocrit may fall by a modest amount. Peripheral edema may occur in about 5% of patients. The decreases in hematocrit tend to occur during the first 4 to 12 weeks of treatment. Rosiglitazone-treated patients also experienced slight decreases in white blood cell counts, possibly related to increased plasma volume.[35]

TZDs are also associated with weight gain. Mean weight gain in patients taking rosiglitazone ranged from 0.7 to 3.5 kg depending on the dose vs a mean weight loss of 1 kg in placebo-treated patients.[34] Pioglitazone-treated patients had a weight gain of 0.5 to 2.8 kg in monotherapy trials vs a weight loss of 1.3 to 1.9 kg for placebo-treated patients.[35] In one study, 16 weeks of pioglitazone treatment was associated with a weight gain of 3.6 kg.[37] Finally, because TZDs showed tumor-inducing effects in a murine model of colon cancer, they are not recommended for patients with familial adenomatous polyposis.[35]

Drug interactions. Because pioglitazone induces the cytochrome P-450 isoform CYP 3A4, its safety and efficacy could be affected when given with other drugs metabolized by this enzyme. Common agents of concern include alprazolam, carbamazepine, some corticosteroids, cyclosporine, diazepam, diltiazem, erythromycin, felodipine, fexofenadine, lidocaine, lovastatin, midazolam, nifedipine, quinidine, some retroviral agents, simvastatin, tacrolimus, terfenadine, triazolam, and verapamil. By inducing CYP 3A4, pioglitazone may also reduce the effectiveness of oral contraceptives containing ethinyl estradiol and norethindrone. Patients taking pioglitazone may therefore need higher dosages of oral contraceptives or alternate forms of contraception.

In contrast, rosiglitazone is predominantly metabolized by CYP 2C8 and has no drug interactions with any of the drugs metabolized by the CYP 3A4 enzyme system.[35] However, the potential for drug interactions between rosiglitazone and other drugs inhibited or induced by CYP 2C8 or CYP 2C9 should be considered. These agents include phenobarbital, primidone, omeprazole, rifampin, amiodarone, cimetidine, fluconazole, fluvoxamine, isoniazid, and zafirlukast. The high plasma-protein binding of the TZDs also suggests a potential for interactions with other highly protein-bound drugs.[34]

Contraindications and precautions. TZDs should be used cautiously in patients with liver disease. Liver transaminases should be checked before initiation of treatment, and treatment should not be initiated in patients with transaminases more than 2.5 times the upper limit of normal. Alanine aminotransferase (ALT) should be monitored every 2 months for the first year and periodically thereafter.[35] Patients with mildly elevated liver enzymes (ALT = 1 to 2.5 times the upper limit of normal) should be evaluated to determine the cause, and TZD therapy should proceed with caution and include close follow-up and more frequent monitoring of liver-enzyme levels. If ALT levels increase to more than three times the upper limit of normal on two occasions 2 weeks apart, TZD therapy should be discontinued. Patients should be encouraged to report symptoms of liver dysfunction, such as unexplained nausea, vomiting, abdominal pain, fatigue, anorexia, or dark urine, to their physician, who should check liver enzyme levels in response to these symptoms. TZDs should be discontinued if jaundice is observed, and they should not be used in patients who experienced any form of troglitazone-related hepatotoxicity. Because they require long-term monitoring of liver enzyme levels, TZDs are inappropriate for patients who may not comply with follow-up testing.

TZDs should be used cautiously in patients with peripheral edema or congestive heart failure. Patients with severe congestive heart failure (New York Heart Association Functional Class III and IV) should not receive TZDs. TZD therapy may cause premenopausal, anovulatory, insulin-resistant women to resume ovulation, putting them at risk of pregnancy. TZDs are contraindicated in pregnancy[38] and during lactation because human data are lacking. In animals, rosiglitazone produces fetal death or growth retardation.[35]

Cost. The TZDs are the most expensive oral antidiabetic agents on the US market. They cost about two to three times more than brand-name metformin and at least two to four times more than brand-name sulfonylureas.[9]

α-Glucosidase inhibitors

α-Glucosidase inhibitors are the only nonsystemic agents that have been shown to be effective for the treatment of type 2 diabetes. They can be used as initial monotherapy in any patient with type 2 diabetes. Because they do not induce hypoglycemia when used as monotherapy, these agents are useful in patients who are sensitive to hypoglycemia or who respond to it poorly.[39] Acarbose (Precose®) and miglitol (Glyset®) are the two agents in this class on the US market. Acarbose was approved for use in the United States by the FDA in September 1995; miglitol was approved in December 1996.[23]

Indications. As monotherapy, both α-glucosidase inhibitors are indicated for use as an adjunct to diet to improve glycemic control in patients with type 2 diabetes whose hyperglycemia cannot be managed with diet alone.[23]

Mechanism of action. These agents competitively inhibit the ability of α-glucosidase enzymes in the small intestinal brush border to break down polysaccharides and disaccharides (Figure 5-7), delaying the hydrolysis of these carbohydrates into absorbable glucose. As a result, the glucose is absorbed over a larger area and more distal parts of the bowel.[8,9] The overall absorption of carbohydrates is not reduced,[39] and therefore, they are weight-neutral but produce a smaller peak in serum glucose concentration after meals and a smoother, more prolonged carbohydrate absorption curve. This delay provides the β cells, which, in type 2 diabetes, respond sluggishly to the appearance of nutrients, with greater opportunity to match insulin response to glucose demand.[38] It also allows the available insulin to metabolize circulating glucose better after a meal, stems the increase in postprandial plasma insulin,[8] reduces insulin requirements, enhances deposition of glucose in tissue, and decreases Hb A_{1c}.[39]

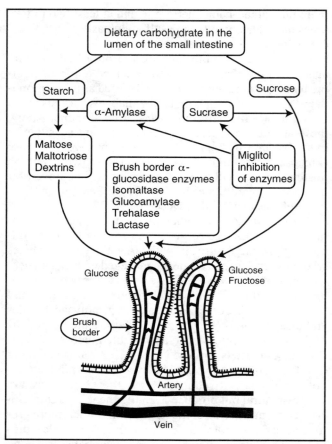

Figure 5-7: Schematic representation of the enzymatic degradation of carbohydrates by glucosidases and their competitive inhibition by miglitol. The bold arrows indicate the points at which miglitol delays carbohydrate degradation and, as a consequence, inhibits the uptake of glucose in the small intestine and reduces the increase in postprandial plasma glucose levels. Scott et al, *Drugs* 2000;50:521-549, with permission.

Effectiveness. The α-glucosidase inhibitors are modestly effective in treating diabetes[8] and less effective than sulfonylureas and metformin in reducing FPG.[9] However, although the α-glucosidase inhibitors only decrease FPG by 20 to 30 mg/dL,[39] they decrease postprandial glucose level (PPG) as well as or better than sulfonylureas (by 40 to 60 mg/dL) while slightly decreasing or maintaining the insulin level.[9,39] These agents reduce Hb A_{1c} by 0.5 to 1.0 percentage point compared with 1.5 to 2.0 percentage points for other agents.[39] Patients consuming more than 50% of daily calories from carbohydrate have the greatest reductions in Hb A_{1c}.[8] α-Glucosidase inhibitors are most useful in patients with new-onset type 2 diabetes who have mild fasting hyperglycemia and in patients with predominant postprandial hyperglycemia.[9] Both agents are about equally effective.[39]

Adverse effects. Gastrointestinal side effects include bloating, abdominal pain or discomfort, diarrhea, and flatulence[8] from the delivery of carbohydrates to the intestine, where they attract fluid and ferment.[39] As many as 70% of patients report flatulence.[8] Although these effects tend to dissipate in 4 to 6 weeks as the bowel adjusts to treatment, initial treatment acceptance by patients has been poor.[8] The stool-softening effect of these agents may in fact be helpful in patients with constipation. Initiating treatment with a low dose and slow titration minimizes the adverse gastrointestinal effects of these agents.[39]

High doses of acarbose (200 to 300 mg three times daily) may, rarely, result in elevated serum aminotransferase levels that resolve when treatment is discontinued.[9] Miglitol may have fewer side effects than acarbose at equally effective doses.[39]

Drug interactions. Miglitol roughly halves the bioavailability of ranitidine and propranolol in healthy volunteers. Intestinal adsorbents and digestive enzyme preparations containing carbohydrate-splitting enzymes may reduce the effects of α-glucosidase inhibitors and should not be taken concomitantly with them.[40]

Contraindications and precautions. Use of acarbose, which may disrupt liver function, is contraindicated by cirrhosis. This is not the case for miglitol. However, use of either agent is contraindicated in patients allergic to it and in those with severe renal insufficiency. Moreover, they are also contraindicated in patients with bowel disease because they may exacerbate preexisting diarrhea and because their efficacy is uncertain when bowel motility or absorption is aberrant.[8,39]

Cost. The cost of an average daily dose of an α-glucosidase inhibitor is about twice that of a brand-name sulfonylurea, slightly less than that of brand-name metformin, and considerably less than that of TZDs and meglitinides.[9]

Combinations of Oral Agents

Most patients with type 2 diabetes require combination therapy to achieve good glycemic control. Moreover, most patients who initially respond well to oral agents will require a second or even a third medication.[9] The UKPDS found that intensive monotherapy resulted in a deterioration in glycemic control and β-cell function over time regardless of the therapeutic agent used, although TZDs were not used in the study.[41] About 60% of UKPDS patients required a second agent for symptomatic hyperglycemia or had an FPG of more than 270 mg/dL by 6 years after randomization to monotherapy.[8] Moreover, because Hb A_{1c} increased by a mean 0.2% to 0.3% annually in the UKPDS, monotherapy often failed to keep Hb A_{1c} at or below target levels.[41] Therefore, substitution therapy provides no significant benefit.[8] Patients with an FPG greater than 200 mg/dL at diagnosis may not be adequately controlled with monotherapy even initially.[41] Because tight initial glycemic control significantly delays or prevents complications, combination therapy can be started whenever monotherapy is unable to keep Hb A_{1c} below target values or to address multiple defects simultaneously before response to monotherapy declines. The two defects that characterize type 2 diabetes, insulin resistance and de-

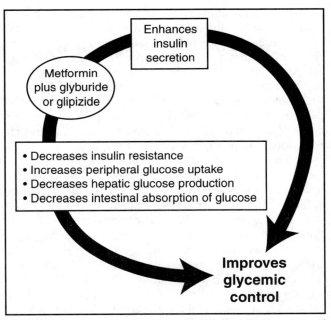

Figure 5-8: Complementary mechanisms of action of sulfonylurea and metformin combination preparations. Adapted from Singh, A new approach to the management of type 2 diabetes and its chronic complications.

fective β-cell function, can be treated synergistically by oral agents with different mechanisms of action (Figure 5-8).

Combination therapy has several advantages. For many drugs, dose and benefit are not directly proportional; therefore half the maximum dosage produces more than half the maximum therapeutic effect, with fewer side effects. Thus, when agents are combined, lower doses of each can be used to enhance outcomes and, often, to reduce costs.[41] Benefits of various combinations have not been measured in head-to-head studies in the same group under the same conditions. However, combinations of an insulin secretagogue and an insulin sensitizer produce the greatest decrease in blood glucose levels,[8] and patients with an Hb A_{1c} of more than 8.5% to 9% often benefit from receiving this combination as initial therapy.[25] Failure to achieve an Hb A_{1c} of less than 7% while taking an insulin sensitizer suggests more advanced disease with β-cell failure and the need for addition of an insulin secretagogue.[25] Most patients avoid or postpone insulin therapy if possible because of the discomfort and inconvenience of the required injections.[41] In one retrospective study, after monotherapy failure, combination therapy with sulfonylurea and metformin was shown to maintain glycemic control (Hb A_{1c} less than 8%) and to avoid addition or substitution of insulin or addition of a TZD for a mean of 7.9 years. Moreover, oral agents control PPG better than therapy with most types of insulin alone while causing less weight gain.[42] Although research has focused on adding insulin-sensitizing drugs to the sulfonylureas, the oldest and most widely used insulin augmenters,[43] other possible combinations have also been explored. Details of selected clinical studies of combinations of oral antidiabetic agents are presented in Table 5-3.

Double Oral Agent Therapy
Sulfonylurea plus metformin

Sulfonylurea plus metformin is the most extensively studied FDA-approved oral agent combination.[43] Metformin is available in combination with glyburide (Glucovance®) or glipizide (Metaglip®).[10] Clinical trials have shown these agents to have significant additive glucose- and lipid-lowering effects and no more adverse effects together than alone.[41] Reductions in FPG of up to 70 mg/dL and in Hb A_{1c} of 1.7 percentage points from baseline have been reported.[44] Reported reduction in PPG has been modest.[44] In one study, patients were randomly assigned to receive metformin, glyburide, or both. All patients initially treated with monotherapy required a second oral agent. Half the combination group achieved an FPG less than 112 mg/dL, all patients had an Hb A_{1c} less than 7%, and no weight was gained.[41] In the Multicenter Metformin Group study, patients whose blood glucose levels were poorly controlled by full-dose glyburide either continued to receive this therapy or were switched to full-dose metformin or to therapy with both agents. Continued glyburide treatment was associated with poor glycemic control, and switching agents produced no advantage. However, combination therapy reduced Hb A_{1c} by 1.5 to 2.0 percentage points below baseline to near the 7% target level.

In a Swedish trial in recently diagnosed patients, sulfonylurea plus metformin was as effective as monotherapy but produced less hypoglycemia and weight gain than glyburide alone and fewer gastrointestinal symptoms than metformin alone.[41] Despite these positive findings, a UKPDS substudy found that although patients receiving metformin plus sulfonylurea showed significant reduction in Hb A_{1c} initially, their mean Hb A_{1c} (7.7%) approached that of the sulfonylurea monotherapy group (8.2%) after 4 years.[44]

A 96% increase in risk of diabetes-related death and a 60% increase in risk of death from any cause was found when combination therapy was compared with sulfonylurea monotherapy. However, meta-analysis of results for all patients taking a sulfonylurea plus metformin in the UKPDS showed significant reductions in all diabetes-related end points and in myocardial infarction.[9] Additionally, the relative increase in mortality in the substudy resulted from a mortality decrease in the sulfonylurea monotherapy group and not a mortality increase in the combination group.[44]

Sulfonylurea plus a meglitinide

In a 12-week study of patients whose hyperglycemia was inadequately controlled by glyburide, adding nateglinide conferred no benefit. Nateglinide is not indicated in addition to or instead of glyburide or other insulin secretagogues in patients whose hyperglycemia is not adequately controlled by these agents.[20]

Table 5-3: Results of Selected Studies of Combinations of Oral Antidiabetic Agents

Treatment	Change in FPG (mg/dL)	Change in Hb A_{1c}
Sulfonylurea plus metformin	-70	-1.7
Sulfonylurea plus metformin	—	-1.5 to -2.0
Sulfonylurea plus metformin	-8.5 (vs +7.9)	-0.6
Sulfonylurea plus nateglinide	0	0
Sulfonylurea plus rosiglitazone	-37.7	-0.9
Sulfonylurea plus pioglitazone	-57.9	-1.3
Sulfonylurea plus an α-glucosidase inhibitor	-10 to -50	-2.2
Sulfonylurea plus acarbose	-25 (between-group difference)	-0.9
Repaglinide plus rosiglitazone	-91 (vs -58 or -62)	-1.4 (vs -0.2 or -0.5)

Qualifications or Other Clinical Benefits/Disadvantages	Study Length	Reference
Values cited are maximums.	Various	44
Patients initially had poor glycemic control with glyburide alone.	6 months	41
Patients initially had poor glycemic control with sulfonylurea alone.	3 years	41
Patients initially had poor glycemic control with 10 mg/d glyburide alone.	12 weeks	20
Patients had initially been taking a sulfonylurea for at least 6 months.	6 months	34
Triglycerides decreased by 27% (vs 1% for sulfonylurea alone), and the LDL/HDL ratio decreased by 3.5% (vs an increase for sulfonylurea alone).	16 weeks	21
Less likely to compound risk of hypoglycemia than other combinations.	Various	41, 44
Effect was maximal in 6 months and lasted for 1 year.	1 year	41
Not yet FDA approved.	24 weeks	45

(continued on next page)

Table 5-3: Results of Selected Studies of Combinations of Oral Antidiabetic Agents *(continued)*

Treatment	Change in FPG (mg/dL)	Change in Hb A$_{1c}$
Repaglinide plus pioglitazone	-86 (vs -28 or -25)	-1.8 (vs -0.2 or +0.2)
Metformin plus repaglinide	-39.2 (vs -4.5 or +8.8)	-1.4 (vs -0.3 or -0.4)
Metformin plus nateglinide	-50.4	-1.9
Metformin plus nateglinide	-9 or -12.6	-0.4 or -0.6 (depending on dose of nateglinide)
Metformin plus rosiglitazone	—	-0.8 (vs +0.5)
Metformin plus pioglitazone	-37.7	-0.8
Metformin plus acarbose	—	-0.6

FDA = US Food and Drug Administration
FPG = fasting plasma glucose level
Hb A$_{1c}$ = glycated hemoglobin

Qualifications or Other Clinical Benefits/Disadvantages	Study Length	Reference
Not yet FDA approved.	24 weeks	46
Patients initially had poor glycemic control from metformin alone; body weight increased with repaglinide.	3 months	44
Patients initially had poor glycemic control with diet and exercise; body weight increased 0.2 kg during therapy.	24 weeks	19
Mild hypoglycemia was >3 times more frequent in the high-dose (120 mg t.i.d.) nateglinide plus metformin group.	24 weeks	19
28% reached an Hb A_{1c} of less than 7%.	26 weeks	34
Triglyceride levels decreased 21%, and LDL/HDL level was unchanged.	16 weeks	21
Patients were obese and had poor glycemic control with metformin alone.	—	41

LDL = low-density lipoprotein cholesterol
HDL = high-density lipoprotein cholesterol
— = not given in review article cited

Sulfonylurea plus a thiazolidinedione

Unlike sulfonylureas, TZDs do not stimulate insulin release or cause hypoglycemia. This advantage, combined with their direct insulin-sensitizing effect, makes their combination with an insulin secretagogue a logical approach[41] whose benefits are supported by the results of clinical studies detailed in Table 5-3. Moreover, pioglitazone combined with a sulfonylurea has received FDA approval for use when diet and exercise plus monotherapy does not result in adequate glycemic control.[23]

Sulfonylurea plus an α-glucosidase inhibitor

This combination has been formally approved by the FDA.[39] Numerous studies have shown that acarbose and sulfonylureas have additive effects.[9] When given in combination, α-glucosidase inhibitors and sulfonylureas improve control of FPG by 10 to 50 mg/dL and PPG by as much as 95 mg/dL.[41,44] Although significant reductions in Hb A_{1c} of up to 2.2 percentage points have been observed,[44] adding an α-glucosidase inhibitor typically produces modest benefit. However, this may be sufficient in patients with mild fasting hyperglycemia.[9] However, patients should be advised that orange juice with sugar will not resolve symptoms of hypoglycemia during therapy with this combination because the α-glucosidase inhibitor will block sucrose absorption. Instant glucose or milk products should be used instead.[39]

Meglitinide plus a thiazolidinedione

The combination of repaglinide and a TZD has received FDA approval after several trials showed that it improved Hb A_{1c} more than monotherapy with either agent.

Metformin plus a meglitinide

Repaglinide or nateglinide plus metformin has been approved by the FDA for use in treating type 2 diabetes in patients whose hyperglycemia cannot be controlled by exercise, diet, and either repaglinide, nateglinide, or metformin alone.[47,48] Repaglinide's glucose-lowering effect is completely additive to metformin's,[9] and administration of metformin with nateglinide does not affect the pharmacokinetics of either drug.[19]

Metformin plus a thiazolidinedione

Use of either TZD with metformin has received FDA approval, has resulted in an Hb A_{1c} reduction of at least 1 percentage point relative to monotherapy in obese patients, and, although relatively new, is becoming commonplace.[8] A tablet that combines metformin and rosiglitazone (Avandamet®) is available. However, an increased incidence of edema and reduced hemoglobin and hematocrit has been reported in a small percentage of patients taking metformin plus rosiglitazone.

Metformin plus an α-glucosidase inhibitor

This combination has been approved by the FDA. Adding acarbose to metformin significantly lowered peak PPG, resulting in corresponding decreases in Hb A_{1c}.

Triple Oral Agent Therapy

Although triple oral agent therapy is a reasonable approach, few data are available on optimal combinations, dosages, and outcomes. Adding an α-glucosidase inhibitor to an insulin secretagogue plus metformin should provide complementary benefits but has not been adequately studied.[41] Adding a TZD to sulfonylurea plus metformin confers additional benefit and has been approved by the FDA for use in patients in whom blood glucose control cannot be achieved with glyburide plus metformin. Before proceeding with triple oral therapy, careful consideration of its cost relative to that of insulin therapy is required.[8] Less-challenging insulin delivery systems may make triple oral therapy less attractive.

Insulin

Insulin is the best studied and ultimately the most effective agent for treating type 2 diabetes. Its use reduces microvascular events by 20% to 30% per 1% absolute reduction in Hb A_{1c}, and its complications are modest. In key studies, clinically significant adverse events were mild to moderate or rare. Many patients will eventually require insulin therapy because oral agents eventually fail to adequately control progressive hyperglycemia.[49] The UKPDS showed that about 30% of newly diagnosed patients taking sulfonylureas and 22% of those taking metformin required insulin within 6 years because the oral agents failed to maintain control.[43]

Patients may find the fear of injection initially daunting; however, they soon learn that the improved sense of well-being insulin therapy provides is worth the effort and minor discomfort and inconvenience.[50]

Available agents

The many different types of insulin available and their chief characteristics, brand names, and manufacturers are listed in Table 5-4.[51] All commercially available insulin is now made by recombinant DNA technology and is identical to human insulin unless specifically modified to be otherwise (analog insulin). Insulin is categorized on the basis of its speed of action and is available in rapid-, short-, intermediate-, and long-acting forms.[52] In rapid-acting insulin analogs, the change in amino acid sequence decreases molecular self-association, enabling the molecule to dissociate and diffuse into the blood stream more rapidly and resulting in more rapid onset of action than regular insulin. Rapid-acting insulin analogs are also eliminated more rapidly than regular insulin and therefore have a shorter duration of action. These differences provide better plasma insulin levels in the absorptive period, better control of postprandial hyperglycemia, and fewer hypoglycemic episodes between meals and at night compared with regular insulin.[53] One rapid-acting analog, insulin lispro (Humalog®), was approved by the FDA in 1996. Another insulin analog, insulin aspart (NovoLog®) was approved by the FDA in June 2000.[23]

In contrast to rapid-acting analogs, some insulins are mixed with zinc and/or protamine to delay absorption from the subcutis.[54] Prompt insulin zinc suspension, or Semilente®, consists of regular insulin modified by zinc chloride to produce a suspension of amorphous (noncrystalline) insulin. The intermediate-acting insulin Lente® is a stable mixture of Semilente® and extended insulin zinc suspension, Semilente®'s long-acting, crystalline counterpart, that yields a 7:3 ratio of crystalline to amorphous insulin. Another intermediate-acting insulin, isophane, or neutral protamine Hagedorn (NPH) insulin, consists of insulin reacted with zinc chloride and protamine to form a protein complex. NPH's action therefore lies between that of regular insulin and long-acting protamine zinc insulin. Long-acting insulins include Ultralente®, which consists of insulin in the form of large zinc-insulin crystals,[55] and the long-acting insulin analog glargine (Lantus®), which was approved by the FDA in April 2000 for once-daily use by adults with type 2 diabetes who need basal insulin for glycemic control.[23] The action of a bolus of insulin glargine plateaus in 6 to 8 hours at a concentration one-third that of NPH and remains virtually unchanged for 24 hours. A bolus injection of NPH has its peak effect in 6 to 10 hours and returns to baseline levels in 16 hours.[54] A single 9:00 p.m. injection of NPH has its greatest effect on blood glucose between 4:00 and 8:00 a.m. and has no effect by 3:00 p.m., increasing the risk of nocturnal hypoglycemia and high dinnertime blood glucose levels.[56] In contrast, insulin glargine is 'peakless' and therefore poses less risk of hypoglycemia. In a comparison in patients with type 2 diabetes, bedtime insulin glargine resulted in a much lower frequency of nocturnal hypoglycemia but similar glycemic control and similar or less weight gain than bedtime NPH.[54] Moreover, insulin glargine plus oral agents resulted in 56% fewer episodes of nocturnal hypoglycemia and significantly lower dinnertime blood glucose levels than NPH plus oral agents.[56]

Using insulin glargine at bedtime and insulin lispro or insulin aspart at mealtimes is probably the closest means of reproducing normal physiologic insulin profiles by subcutaneous injection apart from pump therapy. However, insulin glargine cannot be mixed with neutral insu-

Table 5-4: Types of Insulin and Their Chief Characteristics

Type	Onset of Action	Peak of Action
Rapid-acting		
Lispro	<15 min	30-90 min
Aspart	5-10 min	1-3 hr
Short-acting		
Regular or soluble, human	30 min-1 hr	2-3 hr

lin formulations because it precipitates instantly in them.[54] Mixing regular insulin with zinc-containing insulin such as Lente® or Ultralente® is also not recommended because zinc ions may bind to the short-acting regular component and delay its onset of action. Nevertheless, many other forms of insulin and its analogs can be mixed in the same syringe. Premixed insulin preparations are also available.[51] Most commonly, short-acting regular insulin is mixed with intermediate-acting NPH insulin to meet basal metabolic needs, boost insulin levels at mealtimes, and minimize the number of injections.[57] In fact, about half of all US patients with type 2 diabetes who use NPH combine it with regular insulin.[43] However, the use of fixed insulin combinations

Usual Effective Duration of Action	Brands and Manufacturers
2-4 hr	Humalog® (Eli Lilly) Humalog® Cartridge (Eli Lilly) Humalog® Prefilled Pen (Eli Lilly)
3-5 hr	NovoLog® (Novo Nordisk) NovoLog® Cartridge (Novo Nordisk)
3-6 hr	Humulin® R (Eli Lilly) Novolin® R (Novo Nordisk) ReliOn®/Novolin® R (Wal-Mart Pharmacies/Novo Nordisk) Novolin® R Prefilled (Novo Nordisk) Novolin® R PenFill (Novo Nordisk) Velosulin® BR (Novo Nordisk)

(continued on next page)

limits flexibility because the short-acting and long-acting components cannot be adjusted independently. They should not, therefore, be used indiscriminately.

In the United States, the most commonly used premixture is 70% NPH:30% regular, or 70/30.[57] Brand names include Humulin® 70/30, Novolin® 70/30, Novolin® 70/30 Prefilled, Novolin® 70/30 PenFill, and ReliOn®/Novolin® 70/30. Additionally, insulin lispro is available in a mixture with its intermediate-acting counterpart (NPL) in a 75:25 ratio of NPL to insulin lispro (Humalog® Mix 75/25 and Humalog® Mix 75/25 Pen).[51] This formulation has been shown to reduce postprandial hyperglycemia in patients with type 2 diabetes more than 70/30 NPH/regular insulin; how-

Table 5-4: Types of Insulin and Their Chief Characteristics *(continued)*

Type	Onset of Action	Peak of Action
Intermediate-acting		
Isophane, or neutral protamine Hagedorn (NPH), human	2-4 hr	4-10 hr
Lente®, human	3-4 hr	4-12 hr
Long-acting		
Ultralente®	6-10 hr	8-12 hr
Glargine	1 hr	None

Onset, peak, and duration of action are approximate for each type of insulin because of variability caused by differences in patients and their injection sites and exercise programs. Adapted from *Diabetes Forecast* 2002;55:42-48.

ever, Hb A_{1c} did not differ by mixture used.[57] Other than these mixtures, the 50/50 mixture of regular to NPH insulin (Humulin® 50/50) accounts for about 2% of the US market for premixed insulin.[51,57] Premixtures increase accuracy, effectiveness, and convenience of insulin dosing, which may improve compliance, long-term control, and outcome.[52,57]

Indications

Generally, insulin is approved for use in treating type 2 diabetes that cannot be properly controlled by diet, ex-

Usual Effective Duration of Action	Brands and Manufacturers
10-16 hr	Humulin® N (Eli Lilly) Humulin® N Prefilled Pen (Eli Lilly) Novolin® N (Novo Nordisk) Novolin® N Prefilled (Novo Nordisk) Novolin® N PenFill (Novo Nordisk) ReliOn®/Novolin® N (Wal-Mart Pharmacies/Novo Nordisk)
12-18 hr	Humulin® L (Eli Lilly) Lente® L (Novo Nordisk) Novolin® L (Novo Nordisk)
18-20 hr	Humulin® U (Eli Lilly)
24 hr	Lantus® (Aventis Pharmaceuticals)

ercise, and weight reduction.[23] Insulin can be given to almost all patients regardless of stage of disease.[49] However, by convention, the principal indication for the use of insulin in type 2 diabetes is the failure of oral agents even when given in combination to sustain glycemic control.[49] Insulin is also the treatment of choice in many special circumstances. Insulin therapy is indicated as initial therapy in any patient with ketonuria, ketonemia, or marked hyperglycemia associated with electrolyte, acid-base, or hemodynamic abnormalities. When diabetes cannot be controlled by diet and exercise alone, insulin is the only approved treatment in pregnancy at this time. Severe sepsis or acute myocardial failure often dictates use of insulin because of stress hormone response. Renally impaired and presurgical patients or those with major trauma are usually given insulin because of risk of severe hypoglycemia from sulfonylureas and lactic acidosis from metformin. Hepatically impaired or alcoholic patients are usually given insulin because all oral agents are relatively or absolutely contraindicated.[49]

Mechanism of action

Insulin helps glucose, amino acids, fatty acids, and various ions to enter cells; promotes glycogen, protein, and lipid synthesis; and inhibits gluconeogenesis, glycogen and protein degradation, and lipolysis.[55]

Dosage, dosing schedule, and administration

Dosages must be tailored to the individual needs of each patient. During adolescent growth spurts, 0.8 to 1.2 U/kg/d is recommended,[58] but for most children and adults, 0.5 to 1.0 U/kg/d has near-maximal effects on glucose levels.[18] Although failure to reach target blood glucose levels is more likely to result from insufficient insulin dose than from an insufficiently complex regimen,[59] insulin type and timing and number of daily doses should be considered for each patient to enhance outcomes. Almost half of patients with type 2 diabetes in the United States now inject insulin twice daily, and more than 10% inject it three to four times daily.[43] Once-daily NPH is typically unable to adequately control postprandial glycemia[56] and rarely exerts satisfactory 24-hour control. Increasing a single daily dose enough to adequately suppress nighttime glucose production by the liver and thereby control fasting hyperglycemia risks hypoglycemia at other times, especially in lean patients, who are less insulin resistant than obese patients.[49] In general, basal insulin needs are best met by single-dose insulin glargine, two doses of NPH or Lente®, or one to two doses of Ultralente®.[49]

Home monitoring of blood glucose levels is essential to safe and effective insulin dose titration. The goal is an FPG of 70 to 110 mg/dL and pre-meal and post-meal glucose targets of <130 mg/dL and <160 mg/dL, respectively. If patients can learn to adapt insulin dosages to self-monitoring results, timing and carbohydrate content of meals can be kept flexible.[18] However, only 20% of patients or fewer take regular insulin 30 minutes before a meal as recommended to adequately control postprandial blood glucose levels. Rapid-acting insulin analogs can overcome this common failing because they can be given 5 to 15 minutes before a meal.[54] Dosing immediately after a meal is occasionally useful when food intake is uncertain.[60]

Effectiveness

The Veterans Administration Cooperative Study of Diabetes Mellitus (VACSDM) showed that although near-normoglycemia can be achieved in most patients, large doses of insulin (about 1 to 2 U/kg/d) may be needed.[61] However, obesity predicts a poor response to any type of insulin therapy, especially if insufficient doses of insulin are used.[56]

Adverse effects

The most-feared adverse consequence of insulin therapy is hypoglycemia, which may cause incapacity, seizures, or injury and is particularly problematic in the elderly, who have a high probability of clinically significant atherosclerosis, social isolation, and/or cognitive impairment. Hypoglycemia was reported in more than 70% of middle-aged patients taking insulin in the UKPDS, and major hypoglycemia (requiring third-party assistance or hospital stay) occurred in 11% of these patients over 6 years.[62] In the intensive treatment arm, annual incidence of severe hypoglycemia was about 3%,[16] which was the same figure reported in the VACSDM[61] and much lower than that suggested by previous smaller, retrospective studies.[63]

Hypoglycemia limits insulin therapy's ability to sustain target blood glucose levels.[49] Although rapid-acting insulin analogs have been reported to reduce the number of hypoglycemic episodes, particularly severe and nocturnal ones,[53,54] when all relevant studies were analyzed as a whole, findings were inconsistent. Further research is therefore necessary.[64]

Both lean body mass and adipose tissue mass predictably increase during insulin therapy. Table 5-5 lists reported gains in mean body weight from several key studies by duration of insulin therapy. A study of intensive insulin therapy found that weight gain directly correlated with mean day-long serum insulin level and total insulin dose.[72] Weight gain also seems to be proportional to the number of insulin injections used. Three injections of regular insulin resulted in the same glycemic control but significantly greater weight gain than a single injection of bedtime insulin.[56] Patients whose glycemic control is poor before insulin therapy but who respond well to treatment are at greatest risk of weight gain.[56]

Based on data obtained in a study of type 1 diabetic patients, caloric intake may need to be reduced by up to 20% to achieve thermodynamic balance after insulin therapy is commenced in patients with type 2 diabetes.[72] Increased appetite probably indicates hypoglycemia from overinsulinization. Most data indicate that when hyperinsulinemia does not induce hypoglycemia, it actually decreases appetite and food intake.[72] Theoretically, weight gain from insulin therapy could worsen insulin resistance and increase macrovascular disease risk. However, weight gain from insulin therapy is accompanied by improved glycemic control, blood pressure, and plasma lipid levels. No data suggest that atherogenesis accelerates when improved glycemic control produces weight gain.[72] Untreated hyperglycemia is clearly a more serious risk factor for atherosclerosis.[49] Proper patient education, counseling, and weight maintenance interventions can minimize weight gain with insulin therapy, even when multiple daily injections are used. In the VACSDM, which incorporated continuous dietary counseling,

Table 5-5: Mean Body Weight Gain Reported During Insulin Therapy by Study

Increase in Mean Body Weight[*]	Study (duration)	Reference
9.9 kg	UKPDS 23 (—)	65
7 kg	UKPDS 17 (9 yr)	66
4.6 kg (intensive therapy)	DCCT (5 yr)	67
5 kg (for a decrease of 90 mg/dL from a baseline FPG of 270 mg/dL or of 2.5% in Hb A_{1c}) 2 kg (for a decrease of 1.0% in Hb A_{1c} from same)	Finnish trials/ Yki-Jarvinen et al (1 yr)	62
4.5 kg (obese patients) 5.1 kg (nonobese patients)	Finnish Multicenter Insulin Therapy Study (1 yr)/ Yki-Jarvinen et al (1 yr)	68
8.7 kg (intensive therapy)	Henry et al (6 mo)	69
4 kg (intensive therapy in elderly patients)	Wolffenbuttel et al (6 mo)	70
2.9 kg (intensive therapy)	Yki-Jarvinen et al (3 mo)	71

* Type of insulin therapy in terms of number of injections per day (ie, once daily vs multiple daily or intensive) was not specified in reference cited unless otherwise noted.
DCCT = Diabetes Control and Complications Trial; FPG = fasting plasma glucose level; Hb A_{1c} = glycated hemoglobin; UKPDS = United Kingdom Prospective Diabetes Study; — = not given.

weight gain from intensive insulin therapy was similar to that from standard insulin therapy,[50] and no change in BMI occurred in the intensively treated patients in more than 30 months of follow-up.[61]

Controversy exists regarding whether insulin therapy increases blood pressure by causing proliferation of endothelial smooth muscle cells, increasing adrenergic sympathetic tone, and altering renal tubular reabsorption of sodium. However, physiologic increases in plasma insulin levels in obese, insulin-resistant patients do not increase blood pressure,[73] and the increases in blood pressure seen in patients taking insulin are probably related to increased body weight. The literature does not support the hypothesis that insulin therapy increases blood pressure independent of weight gain.[72]

Other adverse effects of insulin therapy include injection-site reactions such as redness, pain, itching, hives, and swelling, which can be minimized by good injection technique. Lipohypertrophy or lipoatrophy may appear at the injection site; rotating the site can prevent such changes in fat tissue.[52] Few or no differences have been found between insulin lispro, insulin aspart, and human insulin in receptor binding and mitogenic and metabolic potency.[54]

Drug interactions

Insulin requirements may be increased by hyperglycemia-inducing medications such as corticosteroids, oral contraceptives, sympathomimetic agents, thiazide diuretics, and thyroid hormone and decreased by hypoglycemia-inducing medications such as some ACE inhibitors, fibrates, salicylates, pentamidine, oral hypoglycemic agents, and sulfa antibiotics. β-Blockers and clonidine may either potentiate or weaken the blood-glucose-lowering effect of insulin, as do alcohol and lithium salts, and may mask hypoglycemic symptoms.[23]

Contraindications and precautions

Insulin should not be administered during episodes of hypoglycemia or to patients sensitive to any ingredient in the product. Patients with renal or hepatic failure may have increased levels of circulating insulin, and careful glucose monitoring and dose adjustment may be necessary.[58] Analogs should be used with caution in pregnant patients because of two reports of deformities in infants born to pregnant patients taking insulin lispro and because of lack of data.[23,60]

Combinations of Insulin and Oral Agents

Insulin and oral agents may be combined to improve the glycemic control exerted by significant but ineffective doses of either or to reduce the dose or eliminate the need for the original therapy (most commonly insulin) while reducing side effects or using properties of the other agent.[50] If large doses of insulin do not produce adequate control, the addition of an oral agent to insulin therapy can be considered.[8] Such combination therapy improves glycemic control and reduces the required insulin dosage and weight gain associated with insulin therapy. Metformin, in particular, as well as sulfonylureas and acarbose, may help to offset the weight gain associated with insulin therapy.[43] No study has reported worse glycemic control with combination therapy than with insulin alone,[56] and randomized, prospective clinical trial data support combining insulin therapy with metformin and TZDs for enhanced glycemic control. More modest improvement in glycemic control has been documented from combining insulin therapy with acarbose or sulfonylureas.

Sulfonylureas, metformin, TZDs, and to a lesser extent, acarbose can help reduce the required insulin dosage.[43] The need for fewer insulin injections that results from lower insulin requirements may ease dose titration and enhance compliance.[56]

The results of selected studies of insulin combined with oral antidiabetic agents are listed in Table 5-6. Some aspects of clinical decision making lack an adequate foundation in terms of long-term outcome data. The combination of oral agents with insulin has not been linked with a significant increase in the rate or severity of any adverse effects except weight gain and hypoglycemia.[41] However, data on the effects of insulin combination therapy vs insulin alone on the development of diabetic complications are nonexistent.[56]

If oral agents are working but not producing the desired hypoglycemic effect, their residual effect can be amplified by adding insulin. Continuing oral agents may allow a simpler insulin regimen to succeed in controlling blood glucose levels.[41] Insulin should be added in the manner in which it appears necessary to obtain better glycemic control. For example, if glucose is high in the morning, a single nighttime injection of long-acting or intermediate-acting insulin may suffice. If it is high at bedtime, short-acting insulin with supper is indicated. Giving insulin based on specific needs that tailors therapy to the individual patient is preferable to algorithmic approaches such as adding 'bedtime' or 'breakfast-time' insulin.

Double Combinations

Insulin plus a sulfonylurea

This combination has been studied for decades.[43] Both glimepiride and extended-release glipizide have received FDA approval for use with insulin,[43] but combinations of insulin with other sulfonylureas are equally well studied and can be expected to provide similar effects.[50]

Insulin plus sulfonylurea therapy has been associated with less weight gain and risk of daytime hypoglycemia than insulin monotherapy.[50] Studies indicate that insulin plus sulfonylureas can improve Hb A_{1c} by about 0.5 to 1.0 percentage point or reduce the insulin dose required to reach a target by 25%.[50] The Finnish Multicenter Insulin Study showed that, compared with sulfonylurea and morning NPH, among other regimens, sulfonylurea and bedtime (9:00 p.m.) NPH resulted in the greatest decline in Hb A_{1c}[43] and the least weight gain and halved the level of day-long serum free insulin.[9] Bedtime injection of intermediate-acting insulin in combination with oral sulfonylurea also results in fewer hypoglycemic episodes than morning injection.[56] It also serves as a gradual way to accustom reluctant patients to parenteral insulin therapy. As described in the preceding section, insulin should be added in the manner in which it is most likely to achieve glycemic control where it is needed (ie, where the sulfonylurea is failing). There is little point in adding more than one daily injection of insulin to sulfonylurea because this only serves to modestly reduce the amount of insulin being given by injection. In two studies, thrice-daily regular insulin or insulin lispro plus sulfonylurea produced the same glycemic control as bedtime NPH plus sulfonylurea.[56] Insulin plus a sulfonylurea is also relatively inexpensive.[43]

Insulin plus a meglitinide

In patients with sulfonylurea treatment failure, glycemic control was significantly better in patients taking repaglinide plus NPH than in those taking repaglinide or NPH alone. This improvement was associated with significantly more episodes of mild hypoglycemia but not with severe hypoglycemia.[43]

Insulin plus metformin

This combination has been approved by the FDA to improve glycemic control in patients with poorly controlled type 2 diabetes who are taking large doses of insulin. In patients with type 2 diabetes, metformin has been associated with an insulin-sparing effect of 15% to 32%,[43] and for patients with type 2 diabetes inadequately controlled with metformin alone, addition of bedtime insulin controlled blood glucose levels as well as a multiple-injection insulin regimen but required half the insulin and caused no weight gain.[9] A unique benefit is that combining metformin with insulin has been associated with less hypoglycemia than insulin alone.[56]

Insulin plus a thiazolidinedione

Combining insulin with an insulin-sensitizing agent is theoretically promising,[50] and VACSDM results suggest that when insulin dosages reach 1 to 2 U/kg daily without

Table 5-6: Results of Selected Studies of Insulin Plus Oral Antidiabetic Agents

Treatment	FPG	Reduction in Hb A$_{1c}$ (%)
Insulin plus sulfonylurea	—	1.1 (vs 0.25 for insulin alone)
NPH plus sulfonylurea	—	—
Pre-dinner 70/30 insulin plus 8 mg glimepiride b.i.d. for 24 weeks (twice the recommended maximum dosage)	Insulin dose was first titrated up to reach 140 mg/dL or less and then to reach 120 mg/dL or less	2.0 (for both groups)
Pre-meal lispro plus glyburide for 3 months	—	2.35 (vs 1.9 for glyburide plus metformin or bedtime NPH)
NPH plus repaglinide	Significantly better vs monotherapy with either agent	—

Reduction in Insulin Dose	Other Results	Reference(s)
25%	Results of meta-analysis; mean body weight increased 1.4 kg for combination therapy vs 0.8 kg for insulin alone	74
50% to 60% (vs regular insulin plus sulfonylurea)	Sulfonylurea and bedtime NPH produced less weight gain than sulfonylurea and morning NPH	71
40%	More patients on the combination regimen achieved their glycemic target and did so faster, but hypoglycemia was more common; a 4-mg dose of glimepiride could minimize risk of hypoglycemia and provide equal glycemic control	75
—	Multiple daily lispro injections caused greater weight gain than the comparison treatments	76
—	Mild hypoglycemia was more common with combination therapy than with monotherapy with either agent	77

(continued on next page)

Table 5-6: Results of Selected Studies of Insulin Plus Oral Antidiabetic Agents *(continued)*

Treatment	FPG	Reduction in Hb A$_{1c}$ (%)
Insulin plus metformin	92 mg/dL less than with insulin alone	1.8
Insulin plus metformin for 6 months	—	1.0
Insulin twice daily plus 4 mg rosiglitazone b.i.d. for 26 weeks	44.4 mg/dL	1.2
Insulin plus an α-glucosidase inhibitor	—	0.4 to 0.7

producing near-normoglycemia, insulin sensitizers should be added.[43] Preliminary studies indicate that use of insulin with the newer TZDs may provide additive benefits.[43] Rosiglitazone and pioglitazone have been approved by the FDA for use in combination with insulin and have shown a dose-dependent additive effect with insulin in reducing

Reduction in Insulin Dose	Other Results	Reference(s)
25%	Data for patients with poor glycemic control; combination therapy patients lost or maintained weight and had lower blood pressure, LDL, and total cholesterol levels and higher HDL cholesterol levels	78
25%	Patients initially had poor glycemic control	79
9.4%	Hypoglycemia was more frequent with this combination therapy, which may increase the the risk of serious heart problems	80
0% to 10%	Decreases postprandial glucose and triglyceride levels and body weight; data reflects combined results of two studies	81, 82

(continued on next page)

Hb A_{1c}.[43] When patients receiving insulin monotherapy were randomly assigned to receive placebo or pioglitazone, significant reduction in Hb A_{1c} and modestly decreased insulin requirements were observed in the pioglitazone-treated patients.[43] A greater than 25% decrease in total daily insulin dose was observed in 16% of patients in the

Table 5-6: Results of Selected Studies of Insulin Plus Oral Antidiabetic Agents *(continued)*

Treatment	FPG	Reduction in Hb A_{1c} (%)
Insulin plus metformin plus sulfonylurea for 1 year	—	1.3
Bedtime NPH plus metformin plus sulfonylurea for 1 year	—	1.9 (vs 2.5 for bedtime NPH plus metformin)

FDA = US Food and Drug Administration; FPG = fasting plasma glucose level; Hb A_{1c} = glycated hemoglobin; LDL = low-density lipoprotein cholesterol; NPH = neutral protamine Hagedorn insulin; — = not applicable to study or not given.

high-dose pioglitazone groups vs 2.1% of patients in the placebo group, indicating that pioglitazone may enhance insulin action enough to avoid the need for additional exogenous insulin.[21] Pioglitazone-treated patients had a slightly higher (5% to 8%) incidence of weight gain, hypoglycemia, and edema.[43]

Insulin plus an α-glucosidase inhibitor

Adding acarbose to insulin can modestly reduce both Hb A_{1c} and insulin requirements.[9] Acarbose has also been shown

Reduction in Insulin Dose	Other Results	Reference(s)
*	Patients initially had poor glycemic control with insulin alone; 76% of combination therapy patients were able to discontinue insulin therapy; mean body weight declined 2.3 kg	83
*	Patients initially had poor glycemic control with sulfonylurea, metformin, or both; weight gain in the triple-therapy group was 3.6 kg vs 0.9 kg for insulin plus metformin	84

* The weighted mean for the insulin-sparing effect of both oral agents when added to bedtime NPH in four studies in which no difference in glycemic control resulted was 62%.

to safely and effectively lower PPG and serum triglyceride levels in insulin-treated patients with type 2 diabetes.[81,82] In a 1-year randomized trial of acarbose with other agents, including insulin, long-term acarbose therapy was associated with slight weight loss.[85] In another study, acarbose was generally well tolerated by insulin-treated patients, despite more gastrointestinal side effects in the acarbose-treated group.[82]

Adding α-glucosidase inhibitors can minimize the weight gain associated with insulin therapy.[43] α-Glucosidase inhibitors also may be added to insulin therapy to slow the absorption of carbohydrates and thus minimize the risk of hypoglycemia between meals or during sleep.[50] However, patients treated with this combination should be warned that orange juice with sugar will not resolve symptoms of hypoglycemia because sucrose absorption will be blocked by the α-glucosidase inhibitor; instant glucose preparations should be kept on hand and used instead.[39]

Triple Combinations

Cost-effectiveness and risks of drug-drug interactions, hepatic effects, hypoglycemia, and weight gain are yet to be established by clinical trials of triple therapies, several of which are under way.

Insulin with a sulfonylurea plus metformin

When insulin-treated patients with poorly controlled type 2 diabetes were given metformin plus sulfonylurea in addition to insulin, 76% could be completely withdrawn from insulin therapy and, in 1 year, had a decrease in Hb A_{1c} of 1.3 percentage points and a decrease in body weight of 2.3 kg.[9] Nevertheless, because it may cause more hypoglycemia, this combination may be less beneficial than insulin plus metformin alone. In a study of type 2 diabetes patients with poor glycemic control from oral agents alone, patients who received bedtime insulin plus metformin had better control and fewer episodes of hypoglycemia than all other groups, including the group taking bedtime insulin, sulfonylurea, and metformin.[43] The superior performance of bedtime insulin plus metformin in terms of glycemic control was attributed to the relatively minor (0.9 kg) weight gain associated with it vs with the other regimens.[9] Triple combination therapy seems most successful in eliminating the need for exogenous insulin in patients with a lower BMI, a shorter duration of insulin therapy, or lower insulin requirements.[43]

Summary

The years since the mid-1990s have seen an explosion in new and effective oral agents and new types and preparations of insulin. Patients with type 2 diabetes can now use combination oral agent therapy to postpone use of exogenous insulin longer than before and can choose insulin preparations that minimize side effects and maximize convenience.

References

1.   Franz MJ, Monk A, Barry B, et al: Effectiveness of medical nutrition therapy provided by dietitians in the management of non-insulin-dependent diabetes mellitus: a randomized, controlled clinical trial. *J Am Diet Assoc* 1995;95:1009-1017.

2.   Agurs-Collins TD, Kumanyika SK, Ten Have TR, et al: A randomized controlled trial of weight reduction and exercise for diabetes management in older African-American subjects. *Diabetes Care* 1997;20:1503-1511.

3.   Wheeler ML: Nutrition management and physical activity as treatments for diabetes. *Prim Care* 1999;26:857-868.

4.   American Diabetes Association: Position statement: Nutrition recommendations and principles for people with diabetes mellitus. *Diabetes Care* 2001;24(suppl 1). Available at: http://www.diabetes.org/clinicalrecommentations/Supplement101/S44.htm.

5.   Exercise and NIDDM. *Diabetes Care* 1990;13:785-789.

6.   American Diabetes Association. Position statement: Diabetes mellitus and exercise. *Diabetes Care* 2001;24(suppl 1). Available at: http://www.diabetes.org/clinicalrecommentations/Supplement101/S51.htm.

7.   Andersen RE, Wadden TA, Bartlett SJ, et al: Effects of lifestyle activity vs structured aerobic exercise in obese women: a randomized trial. *JAMA* 1999;281:335-340.

8.   Ahmann AJ, Riddle MC: Oral pharmacological agents. In: Leahy J, Clark N, Cefalu W, eds. *Medical Management of Diabetes Mellitus*. New York, Marcel Dekker, 2000, pp 267-283.

9.   DeFronzo RA: Pharmacologic therapy for type 2 diabetes mellitus. *Ann Intern Med* 1999;131:281-303.

10.   Luna B, Feinglos MN: Oral agents in the management of type 2 diabetes mellitus. *Am Fam Physician* 2001;63:1747-1756.

11.   DeFronzo RA: Pharmacologic therapy for type 2 diabetes mellitus. *Ann Intern Med* 2000;133:73-74.

12. Sulfonylureas (Web page). Drug Facts Abridged. www.drugfacts.com. Facts and Comparisons, Lippincott Williams & Wilkins, Inc. Posted 2000; Accessed December 17, 2001.

13. Harrower AD: Comparative tolerability of sulphonylureas in diabetes mellitus. *Drug Saf* 2000;22:313-320.

14. Balodimos MC, Camerini-Davalos RA, Marble A: Nine years' experience with tolbutamide in the treatment of diabetes. *Metabolism* 1966;15:957-970.

15. Berger W, Caduff F, Pasquel M, et al: The relatively frequent incidence of severe sulfonylurea-induced hypoglycemia in the last 25 years in Switzerland. Results of 2 surveys in Switzerland in 1969 and 1984 [in German]. *Schweiz Med Wochenschr* 1986; 116:145-151.

16. Intensive blood-glucose control with sulphonylureas or insulin compared with conventional treatment and risk of complications in patients with type 2 diabetes (UKPDS 33). UK Prospective Diabetes Study (UKPDS) Group. *Lancet* 1998;352:837-853.

17. A study of the effects of hypoglycaemic agents on vascular complications in patients with adult-onset diabetes: sections I and II. *Diabetes* 1970;19(suppl 2):747-830.

18. Berger M, Jorgens V, Muhlhauser I: Rationale for the use of insulin therapy alone as the pharmacological treatment of type 2 diabetes. *Diabetes Care* 1999;22(suppl 3):C71-C75.

19. Dunn CJ, Faulds D: Nateglinide. *Drugs* 2000;60:607-617.

20. Starlix Package Insert. Novartis Pharmaceuticals Corp., Basel, Switzerland, 2001.

21. Fuchtenbusch M, Standl E, Schatz H: Clinical efficacy of new thiazolidinediones and glinides in the treatment of type 2 diabetes mellitus. *Exp Clin Endocrinol Diabetes* 2000;108:151-163.

22. Palumbo PJ: Glycemic control, mealtime glucose excursions, and diabetic complications in type 2 diabetes mellitus. *Mayo Clin Proc* 2001;76:609-618.

23. 2001 Mosby's GenRx. 11th ed. St. Louis, Mosby. 2001.

24. Glucophage Package Insert. Bristol-Myers Squibb Company, Princeton, NJ, 2001.

25. Reasner CA, DeFronzo RA: Treatment of type 2 diabetes mellitus: a rational approach based on its pathophysiology. *Am Fam Physician* 2001;63:1687-1688, 1691-1692, 1694.

26. Zimmet P, Collier G: Clinical efficacy of metformin against insulin resistance parameters: sinking the iceberg. *Drugs* 1999; 58(suppl 1):21-28.

27. Chan NN, Brain HP, Feher MD: Metformin-associated lactic acidosis: a rare or very rare clinical entity? *Diabet Med* 1999; 16:273-281.

28. DeFronzo RA, Goodman AM: Efficacy of metformin in patients with non-insulin-dependent diabetes mellitus. The Multicenter Metformin Study Group. *N Engl J Med* 1995;333:541-549.

29. Quillen DM, Samraj G, Kuritzky L: Improving management of type 2 diabetes mellitus: 2. Biguanides. *Hosp Pract (Off Ed)* 1999;34:41-44.

30. Lalau JD, Race JM: Lactic acidosis in metformin therapy. *Drugs* 1999;58(suppl 1):55-60.

31. Rosen ED, Spiegelman BM: PPARgamma: a nuclear regulator of metabolism, differentiation, and cell growth. *J Biol Chem* 2001;276:37731-37734.

32. Parulkar AA, Pendergrass ML, Granda-Ayala R, et al: Nonhypoglycemic effects of thiazolidinediones. *Ann Intern Med* 2001;134:61-71.

33. Gale EA: Lessons from the glitazones: a story of drug development. *Lancet* 2001;357:1870-1875.

34. Malinowski JM, Bolesta S: Rosiglitazone in the treatment of diabetes mellitus: a critical review. *Clin Ther* 2000;22:1151-1168.

35. Mudaliar S, Henry RR: New oral therapies for type 2 diabetes mellitus: The glitazones or insulin sensitizers. *Annu Rev Med* 2001;52:239-257.

36. Krische D: The glitazones: proceed with caution. *West J Med* 2000;173:54-57.

37. Miyazaki Y, Mahankali A, Matsuda M, et al: Improved glycemic control and enhanced insulin sensitivity in type 2 diabetic subjects treated with pioglitazone. *Diabetes Care* 2001;24:710-719.

38. Ghazeeri G, Kutteh WH, Bryer-Ash M, et al: Effect of rosiglitazone on spontaneous and clomiphene citrate-induced ovulation in women with polycystic ovary syndrome. *Fertil Steril* 2003;79:562-566.

39. Kuritzky L, Samraj G, Quillen DM: Improving management of type 2 diabetes mellitus: 1. alpha-Glucosidase inhibitors. *Hosp Pract (Off Ed)* 1999;34:43-46.

40. Glyset Package Insert. Pharmacia & Upjohn, Kalamazoo, MI, 2001.

41. Riddle M: Combining sulfonylureas and other oral agents. *Am J Med* 2000;108:15S-22S.

42. Bell DS, Ovalle F: How long can insulin therapy be avoided in the patient with type 2 diabetes mellitus by use of a combination of metformin and a sulfonylurea? *Endocr Pract* 2000;6:293-295.

43. Buse J: Combining insulin and oral agents. *Am J Med* 2000; 108(suppl 6a):23S-32S.

44. Luna B, Hughes AT, Feinglos MN: The use of insulin secretagogues in the treatment of type 2 diabetes. *Prim Care* 1999;26: 895-915.

45. Raskin P, McGill J, Hale P, et al: Repaglinide/rosiglitazone combination therapy of type 2 diabetes (presentation). Presented at the American Diabetes Association Annual Meeting, June 23, 2001, Philadelphia, PA.

46. Studies show combination therapy of oral antidiabetic drug repaglinide and insulin sensitizers improves blood glucose control (Web page). Novo Nordisk US Web site. Available at: http://www.novonordisk-us.com/view.asp?id=1279 &tID=232. Posted June 23, 2001; Accessed December 18, 2001.

47. Prandin Package Insert. Novo Nordisk Pharmaceuticals, Inc. Princeton, NJ, 1998.

48. Starlix (Nateglinide) Oral Tablets Indication (Web page). FDA Web site. Available at: http://www.fda.gov. Posted January 9, 2001; Accessed December 18, 2001.

49. Evans A, Krentz AJ: Benefits and risks of transfer from oral agents to insulin in type 2 diabetes mellitus. *Drug Saf* 1999;21:7-22.

50. Buse JB: The use of insulin alone and in combination with oral agents in type 2 diabetes. *Prim Care* 1999;26:931-950.

51. 'Insulin.' Resource Guide 2002. *Diabetes Forecast* 2002;55: 42-48.

52. American Diabetes Association. Position statement: insulin administration. *Diabetes Care* 2001;24(suppl 1). Available at: http://www.diabetes.org/clinicalrecommentations/Supplement101/S94.htm.

53. Hermans MP, Nobels FR, De Leeuw I: Insulin lispro (Humalog), a novel fast-acting insulin analogue for the treatment of diabetes mellitus: overview of pharmacological and clinical data. *Acta Clin Belg* 1999;54:233-240.

54. Owens DR, Zinman B, Bolli GB: Insulins today and beyond. *Lancet* 2001;358:739-746.

55. *Dorland's Illustrated Medical Dictionary.* 28th ed. Philadelphia, W.B. Saunders Co., 1994.

56. Yki-Jarvinen H: Combination therapies with insulin in type 2 diabetes. *Diabetes Care* 2001;24:758-767.

57. Turner HE, Matthews DR: The use of fixed-mixture insulins in clinical practice. *Eur J Clin Pharmacol* 2000;56:19-25.

58. Insulin (Web page). Drug Facts Abridged. Available at: http://www.drugfacts.com. Facts and Comparisons, Lippincott Williams & Wilkins, Inc. Posted 2000; Accessed December 17, 2001.

59. Dineen SF, Rand DA: Changing to insulin in type 2 diabetes. *Practitioner* 2000;244:986-989.

60. Nobels FR, Hermans MP, De Leeuw I: Insulin lispro (Humalog), a novel fast-acting insulin analogue: guidelines for its practical use. *Acta Clin Belg* 1999;54:246-254.

61. Abraira C, Colwell JA, Nuttall FQ, et al: Veterans Affairs Cooperative Study on glycemic control and complications in type II diabetes (VA CSDM). Results of the feasibility trial. Veterans Affairs Cooperative Study in Type II Diabetes. *Diabetes Care* 1995;18:1113-1123.

62. Turner R, Cull C, Holman R: United Kingdom Prospective Diabetes Study 17: a 9-year update of a randomized, controlled trial on the effect of improved metabolic control on complications in non-insulin-dependent diabetes mellitus. *Ann Intern Med* 1996;124(1 pt 2):136-145.

63. Hepburn DA, MacLeod KM, Pell AC, et al: Frequency and symptoms of hypoglycaemia experienced by patients with type 2 diabetes treated with insulin. *Diabet Med* 1993;10:231-237.

64. Heinemann L: Hypoglycemia and insulin analogues: is there a reduction in the incidence? *J Diabetes Complications* 1999;13:105-114.

65. Turner RC, Millns H, Neil HA, et al: Risk factors for coronary artery disease in non-insulin dependent diabetes mellitus: United Kingdom Prospective Diabetes Study (UKPDS: 23). *BMJ* 1998;316:823-828.

66. Mäkimattila S, Nikkilä K, Yki-Järvinen H: Causes of weight gain during insulin therapy with and without metformin in patients with type II diabetes mellitus. *Diabetologia* 1999;42:406-412.

67.   The effect of intensive treatment of diabetes on the development and progression of long-term complications in insulin-dependent diabetes mellitus. The Diabetes Control and Complications Trial Research Group. *N Engl J Med* 1993;329:977-986.

68.   Yki-Järvinen H, Ryysy L, Kauppila M, et al: Effect of obesity on the response to insulin therapy in noninsulin-dependent diabetes mellitus. *J Clin Endocrinol Metab* 1997;82:4037-4043.

69.   Henry RR, Gumbiner B, Ditzler T, et al: Intensive conventional insulin therapy for type II diabetes. Metabolic effects during a 6-mo outpatient trial. *Diabetes Care* 1993;16:21-31.

70.   Wolffenbuttel BH, Sels JP, Rondas-Colbers GJ, et al: Comparison of different insulin regimens in elderly patients with NIDDM. *Diabetes Care* 1996;19:1326-1332.

71.   Yki-Järvinen H, Kauppila M, Kujansuu E, et al: Comparison of insulin regimens in patients with non-insulin-dependent diabetes mellitus. *N Engl J Med* 1992;327:1426-1433.

72.   Boyne MS, Saudek CD: Effect of insulin therapy on macrovascular risk factors in type 2 diabetes. *Diabetes Care* 1999;22:C45-C53.

73.   Anderson EA, Mark AL: The vasodilator action of insulin. Implications for the insulin hypothesis of hypertension. *Hypertension* 1993;21:136-141.

74.   Johnson JL, Wolf SL, Kabadi UM: Efficacy of insulin and sulfonylurea combination therapy in type 2 diabetes. A meta-analysis of the randomized placebo-controlled trials. *Arch Intern Med* 1996;156:259-264.

75.   Riddle MC, Schneider J: Beginning insulin treatment of obese patients with evening 70/30 insulin plus glimepiride versus insulin alone. *Diabetes Care* 1998;21:1052-1057.

76.   Browdos R, Schwartz S, Stuart CA, et al: Combination of insulin lispro LP, metformin (MF), or bedtime NPH (NPH) with sulfonylurea (SU) following secondary SU failure. *Diabetes* 1999;48(suppl 1):A104. Abstract 0450.

77.   Landin-Olsson M, Brogard JM, Eriksson J, et al: The efficacy of repaglinide administered in combination with bedtime NPH-insulin in patients with type 2 diabetes: a randomized, semi-blinded, parallel-group, multi-center trial. *Diabetes* 1999;48(suppl 1):A117. Abstract 0450.

78.   Giugliano D, Quatraro A, Consoli G, et al: Metformin for obese, insulin-treated diabetic patients: improvement in glycaemic control

and reduction of metabolic risk factors. *Eur J Clin Pharmacol* 1993; 44:107-112.

79.   Aviles-Santa L, Sinding J, Raskin P: Effects of metformin in poorly controlled insulin-treated type 2 diabetes mellitus. A randomized, double-blind, placebo-controlled trial. *Ann Intern Med* 1999;131:182-188.

80.   Raskin P, Dole JF, Rappaport E: Rosiglitazone improves glycemic control in poorly controlled insulin-treated type 2 diabetes. *Diabetes* 1999;48(suppl 1):A94. Abstract 0404.

81.   Chiasson JL, Josse RG, Hunt JA, et al: The efficacy of acarbose in the treatment of patients with non-insulin-dependent diabetes mellitus. A multicenter controlled clinical trial. *Ann Intern Med* 1994;121:928-935.

82.   Kelley DE, Bidot P, Freedman Z, et al: Efficacy and safety of acarbose in insulin-treated patients with type 2 diabetes. *Diabetes Care* 1998;21:2056-2061.

83.   Bell DS, Mayo MS: Outcome of metformin-facilitated reinitiation of oral diabetic therapy in insulin-treated patients with non-insulin dependent diabetes mellitus. *Endocr Pract* 1997:373-376.

84.   Yki-Järvinen H, Ryysy L, Nikkilä K, et al: Comparison of bedtime insulin regimens in patients with type 2 diabetes mellitus. A randomized, controlled trial. *Ann Intern Med* 1999;130:389-396.

85.   Wolever TM, Chiasson JL, Josse RG, et al: Small weight loss on long-term acarbose therapy with no change in dietary pattern or nutrient intake of individuals with non-insulin-dependent diabetes. *Int J Obes Relat Metab Disord* 1997;21:756-763.

Chapter 6

Atherosclerosis: A Major Risk in Diabetes

Diabetes is a vascular disease as well as a metabolic disease.[1,2] Seventy-five percent of hospital admissions for diabetic complications are a result of atherosclerosis,[3] and 65% to 80% of deaths in North American diabetic patients are related to atherosclerosis, compared with 33% in the general population.[4] Cardiovascular complications are the main cause of death among patients with type 2 diabetes.[5]

One of the most life-threatening consequences of atherosclerosis, coronary artery disease (CAD), is the most common vascular complication of diabetes.[6] The age-adjusted prevalence of CAD in white Americans with type 2 diabetes is two to four times that in nondiabetic patients.[7] The manifestations of CAD, including angina pectoris, myocardial infarction (MI), and sudden death, are at least twice as common in patients with type 2 diabetes as in nondiabetic patients,[8] and, in certain studies, the incidence of some of these manifestations was nearly six times more common. For instance, in a large Finnish population study, the 7-year incidence of initial MI or death was 20% for patients with type 2 diabetes vs only 3.5% for nondiabetic patients.[2] This incidence for patients with diabetes was identical to that of nondiabetic subjects with known cardiovascular disease (CVD). Hence, the Adult Treatment Panel III (ATP III) considers diabetes as an atherosclerosis risk equivalent.[9] In the prospective Finnish study, patients with diabetes and known heart disease had a 45% incidence of recurrent MI.[10]

The presence of severe CAD in diabetic patients results from early development of atherosclerosis.[11] Accelerated atherogenesis and increased risk of CAD (generally twofold) are commonly found in prediabetic patients.[1] Patients with the metabolic syndrome as defined by the ATP III or World Health Organization (WHO) also have substantially increased risk of CVD and mortality, as well as increased all-cause mortality.[12]

CAD-related mortality is particularly elevated in patients with type 2 diabetes. According to Framingham study data, the risk of cardiac mortality is two to four times greater in diabetic patients than in nondiabetic patients.[13] In the Multiple Risk Factor Intervention Trial (MRFIT), even after adjustment for established risk factors, the absolute risk of CAD mortality was three times higher in diabetic men than in nondiabetic men.[4] Other studies have found that, compared with nondiabetic patients, patients with type 2 diabetes have up to six times the risk of death from cardiovascular causes.[7] Diabetic patients with end-stage renal disease have particularly high CAD mortality. CAD accounts for 40% of deaths in renal transplant patients, and the relative risk (RR) for age-specific death from MI among diabetic patients during the first year of dialysis is 89 times higher than that of the general population.[4]

Diabetic patients have a particularly poor outcome after MI.[13] In the first month after MI, mortality is 14% to 26% in diabetic men and 21% to 30% in diabetic women. Even since thrombolysis became available, death is statistically more likely to occur after MI among diabetic patients, particularly women, than among nondiabetic patients.[13] In the GISSI-2 trial (Gruppo Italiano per lo

Studio della Sopravvivenza nell'Infarto Miocardico-2), the age-adjusted RR of death was 1.4 for men and 1.9 for women, regardless of intervention. Another study found that diabetes increases mortality by 58% in men and by 160% in women in the first 28 days after MI. Five years after MI, mortality may be as high as 50% in diabetic patients, which is more than twice that in nondiabetic patients,[2] and 10 years after MI, mortality is 60% in diabetic men and as high as 80% in diabetic women. Even after adjustment for the effects of multivessel disease and infarct size, post-MI mortality in diabetic patients is still twice that in nondiabetic patients.[13] After MI, diabetes increases not only mortality, but also serious morbidity, including congestive heart failure and reinfarction.[2] The Finnish population study found that diabetic patients with a history of MI had an 18.5% annual rate of MI, stroke, or death, a rate that was twice as high as that of their nondiabetic counterparts.[5]

In addition to causing serious morbidity and excess mortality through CAD, atherosclerosis affects the extracranial carotid arteries and lower-extremity arteries of patients with diabetes.[2] The presence of diabetes in turn increases the risk of cerebrovascular artery disease and peripheral artery disease (PAD), which are strongly associated with CAD. Diabetic patients have 5 times the prevalence of calcified carotid atheroma and 1.5 to 4 times the stroke risk of nondiabetic patients. In patients younger than 55 years, diabetes confers a particularly high risk of stroke, increasing the odds ratio for stroke to 11.6 in general and to 23.1 for white men. Diabetes also doubles the risk of stroke recurrence and triples the rate of stroke-related dementia[2] and mortality.[4] The rate of PAD is two to four times higher in patients with diabetes than in nondiabetic patients, and diabetic patients are more likely to experience intermittent claudication and require amputation because of PAD. In the Framingham study, diabetes increased the risk of claudication 3.5-fold in men and 8.6-fold in women. In a Medicare population, the RR of lower extremity amputation was 23.5 in diabetic patients aged 65 to 74 years vs their nondiabetic counterparts.[2]

Women, Diabetes, and CVD

Diabetes not only erases the beneficial effect of female sex on CVD risk, but also increases the risk of MI, claudication, and stroke in women more than in men.[2] This increase may partly stem from increases in CVD risk factors such as obesity, dyslipidemia, and hypertension related to declining estrogen levels. Such abnormalities decrease the protection against CVD conferred by estrogen and may thus increase CVD risk in all diabetic women. Moreover, in one study, after adjustment for other unfavorable CVD risk factors, diabetic women, but not diabetic men, were found to have smaller, denser low-density lipoprotein (LDL) cholesterol, which is atherogenic. Diabetes also has a stronger effect in women than in men on several CVD risk factors such as waist-hip ratio and dyslipidemia,[6] and diabetic women have not fully shared in the improvement in CVD outcomes produced by recent advances in prevention and intervention. For example, although heart disease mortality decreased in diabetic men and nondiabetic patients in the 10-year follow-up to the first National Health and Nutrition Examination Survey (NHANES), it increased by 23% in diabetic women. Thus, aggressive management of CVD and its risk factors appears to be particularly crucial for women with type 2 diabetes.[6] Figure 6-1 depicts the multiple risk factor mechanisms that contribute to atherosclerosis in type 2 diabetes.

Risk Factors and Their Management

All the metabolic abnormalities of diabetes, including dyslipidemia, hypertension, and hypercoagulability, as well as hyperglycemia and hyperinsulinemia, contrib-

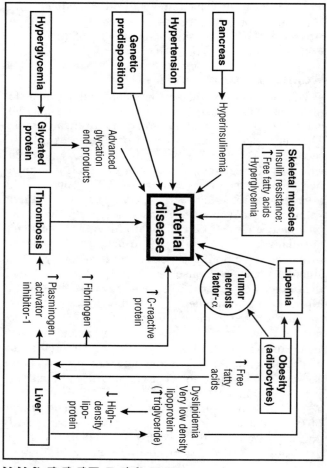

Figure 6-1: Multiple mechanisms contribute to arterial disease in patients with type 2 diabetes. Adapted from Libby et al, *Circulation* 2002;106:2760-2763.

140

ute to CVD, and therefore, all are appropriate therapeutic targets.[2] The presence of more than one risk factor exponentially increases CVD risk.[14] This finding, coupled with the heavy burden of CVD in patients with type 2 diabetes, has prompted the Joint National Committee, the American Diabetes Association (ADA), and the National Cholesterol Education Program to recommend aggressive, multifactorial risk factor modification in these patients.[5] In the Steno-2 study, this approach reduced the combined risk of death, nonfatal MI or stroke, revascularization, and amputation by 50% in patients with type 2 diabetes who were at particularly high CVD risk because of microalbuminuria.[7]

However, some CVD risk factors associated with diabetes increase risk more than others. For instance, the United Kingdom Prospective Diabetes Study (UKPDS) showed the most important MI risk factor to be elevated LDL cholesterol level, followed by elevated diastolic blood pressure (BP), cigarette smoking, a low high-density lipoprotein (HDL) cholesterol level, and a high level of glycated hemoglobin (Hb A_{1c}).[8] The American Heart Association has established hypertension, low HDL cholesterol, high total cholesterol, and smoking, as well as diabetes itself, as major CVD risk factors. Of these, hypertension and a low level of atheroprotective HDL cholesterol merit special attention in patients with diabetes. Total cholesterol levels in patients with type 2 diabetes are typically normal, but diabetic hypertriglyceridemia typically is associated with an increase in small, dense LDL particles that are high in triglyceride and more easily oxidized than normal LDL and thus are particularly atherogenic.[8] Together, the lipoprotein abnormalities that make up diabetic dyslipidemia confer a risk of CAD at least as great as that conferred by LDL cholesterol levels of 150 to 220 mg/dL.[15]

Although multifactorial intervention has been proven to reduce the burden of CVD in patients with type 2 diabetes, early recognition and management of the major CVD risk factors are the main priorities in the delivery of diabetes care. The importance of these risk factors may vary for each patient, but, in most cases, smoking cessation should be first. Other top priorities include control of BP, lipid, blood glucose levels, and coagulation. Because all elements of diabetic dyslipidemia appear to be independently atherogenic, efforts should focus on reaching established target levels for LDL, as well as HDL and triglyceride. The ability of improved glycemic control to reduce triglyceride levels indicates that aggressive antihyperglycemic therapy is also a critical aspect of CVD risk reduction.[3] Other established, modifiable CVD risk factors include hypercoagulability, obesity, and physical inactivity.[8] Emerging CVD risk factors such as hyperhomocysteinemia and increased oxidative stress and inflammation are receiving increasing attention as targets for modification and risk reduction.

Cigarette Smoking

Smoking doubles CVD risk in diabetic patients.[15] Cigarette smoke is a source of the advanced glycation end products that promote diabetic vascular complications,[6] and smoking reduces the benefits of modifying other CVD risk factors. Smoking cessation has therefore received high priority in reducing diabetes-related CVD risk. Synergy between smoking and hypercholesterolemia particularly promotes CVD risk, possibly by increasing the oxidation of LDL cholesterol[15] and its uptake by monocytes and vascular smooth muscle cells.[2]

Cigarette smoking is a particularly deadly habit for diabetic patients. In one report, the risk of early death in diabetic patients who smoked was 11 times that of nondiabetic patients who did not smoke. Other studies have consistently found an increased risk of morbidity and early death from macrovascular complications among diabetic patients who smoke.[16] If patients are unable to quit completely, cutting back may help to reduce risk. The MRFIT found that CAD mortality increased with the number of cigarettes smoked daily.[15] However, many diabetic patients remain unaware of the greatly increased CVD burden conferred by smoking. Moreover, although smoking cessation counseling has been proven effective in reducing tobacco use in these high-risk patients, only about half of all people with diabetes are advised to quit by their health care provider. Counseling by multiple providers, social support, and use of nicotine replacement therapy are crucial aspects of effective cessation programs. Nicotine replacement not only limits withdrawal symptoms, but also increases abstinence considerably when combined with counseling. Unless patients are pregnant or have serious diabetic complications, the benefits of nicotine replacement greatly exceed the risks.[16]

Hypertension

Hypertension not only worsens diabetes by promoting insulin resistance, but also, in the presence of diabetes, greatly accelerates atherogenesis.[14] As a result, the combination of diabetes and hypertension doubles CVD risk.[15] Moreover, aggressive hypertension treatment reduces CVD risk even more in diabetic patients than in nondiabetic patients.[1] Subgroup analyses of diabetic patients studied in large clinical trials have shown that major CVD events can be halved by reducing diastolic BP to 80 mm Hg or less.[11] Because of their substantial elevation in CVD risk, hypertensive patients with diabetes have been placed in the same risk category as hypertensive patients with clinical CVD, and even diabetic patients with high-normal BP (130-140/80-90 mm Hg) should receive prompt pharmacologic therapy.[4]

Hypertension is also a particularly important contributor to cerebrovascular disease and substantially reduces cognitive function in middle-aged patients.[5] In the UKPDS, tighter BP control reduced stroke risk by 44% despite a BP goal that was high by current standards and a between-group difference of only 10/5 mm Hg. Tighter control also reduced stroke risk more than other end points.[3] Current BP targets and an approach to reaching them are examined in Chapter 4, and a more in-depth examination of hypertension and the use of various antihypertensive agents to treat diabetic patients in specific circumstances is provided in Chapter 7.

Dyslipidemia

In animal models, hypertension alone does not cause atherosclerosis when cholesterol levels are low. Human populations with a high incidence of hypertension but low cholesterol levels also have a relatively low incidence of atherosclerotic complications. These findings suggest that the atherogenic changes in endothelium and vascular smooth muscle promoted by hypertension do not themselves lead to atherosclerotic fatty streaks and plaque. For atherosclerosis to develop, LDL or very low density lipoprotein (VLDL) cholesterol levels must be elevated as well as BP. Thus, although BP control is important, the antihypertensive agents used to achieve it should not promote dyslipidemia.[14]

Lipid-lowering therapy has been shown to reduce CVD risk more in diabetic patients than in nondiabetic patients.[3] The absolute benefit of lipid-lowering therapy may be greater in diabetic patients with CAD because these patients have a higher recurrence risk and case fatality rate and more atherogenic LDL cholesterol than nondiabetic patients with CAD.[4] Subgroup analyses of large clinical trials have shown a 25% reduction in major CVD events with statin therapy in patients with type 2 diabetes.[11] Statin therapy is effective in primary and secondary prevention of CAD in patients with type 2 diabetes;[8] however, the high cardiac event rates and poor prognosis in diabetic patients without evidence of CAD may make the distinction between these prevention categories in diabetic patients irrelevant.[4] Statins may be particularly useful in diabetic patients because of their ability to improve endothelial function and to reduce oxidation.[1]

Thiazolidinediones (TZDs) help to normalize lipid levels by improving glycemic control, as well as through direct effects that increase HDL and decrease triglyceride levels.[17] TZDs also decrease the level of small, dense, atherogenic LDL and thus increase LDL's resistance to oxidation.[2] Because low HDL levels decrease the outflow of lipids from the arterial wall and increase oxidative stress by decreasing the level of antioxidant enzymes,[18] the use of lipid-lowering agents and TZDs to increase HDL has been receiving increasing attention. Clinical trial data on the effectiveness of these agents in treating the various components of diabetic dyslipidemia, specific target levels for each component, and details on the relative benefits and use of the available lipid-lowering agents are provided in Chapter 8.

Hyperglycemia

Hyperglycemia promotes vascular dysfunction, dyslipidemia, and hypercoagulability.[2] Numerous epidemiologic studies have found an association between serum glucose level and increased risk of cardiovascular events among nondiabetic patients and diabetic patients.[5] For example, a meta-analysis of 20 studies that, together, included nearly 96,000 diabetic patients followed up for 12.4 years found a direct relation between increased CVD risk and plasma glucose level, beginning with levels in the nondiabetic range.[2,3] In the UKPDS, this increased risk began to appear at Hb A_{1c} values above 6.2%.[2] Thus, even prediabetic patients already have two to three times the CAD mortality of nondiabetic patients.[1] In addition, the degree of chronic hyperglycemia reflected by Hb A_{1c} measurement may be an independent risk factor for CAD, especially in women.[4] Nevertheless, poor glycemic control may not be a particularly strong CVD risk factor. In the Wisconsin Epidemiologic Study of Diabetic Retinopathy (WESDR), a 1% increase in Hb A_{1c} resulted in a 10% increase in CAD events vs a 20% increase in proteinuria and a 70% increase in proliferative retinopathy.[8] A Finnish study also showed that glycemic control is a weak, albeit significant, predictor of CAD in patients with type 2 diabetes.[19] Other studies have shown dyslipidemia to be a far more important determinant of CAD events than poor glycemic control.[8]

Although tight glycemic control can decrease levels of Hb A_{1c} and other glycated proteins that promote inflammation and atherogenesis, the ability of tight control to reduce CVD risk in patients with type 2 diabetes has been less clear-cut. The University Group Diabetes Program (UGDP) and UKPDS found a limited association between glycemic control and macrovascular complications.[18] In the UKPDS 33, tighter glucose control with chlorpropamide, glyburide, or insulin significantly reduced complications affecting the microcirculation (by 25%) compared with conventional control with diet therapy, but it did not have the same effect on the conduit muscular arteries.[2,8] However, the UKPDS did find a nonsignificant ($P = 0.052$, 16%) reduction in MI in the intensive control group, and this apparent trend toward event reduction with tighter control may indicate that the study lacked sufficient power to produce significant results. Alternatively, the interventions studied may have been initiated too late in the course of the atherogenic process or have been too brief to reduce CVD risk, and prevention of CVD may require lower glycemic levels than those targeted.[3] In the UKPDS 33, the intensive control group had an Hb A_{1c} of 7.0%, while the conventional control group treated with diet therapy alone had an Hb A_{1c} of 7.9%.[8]

The adverse cardiovascular effects of some glucose control agents may have counteracted the benefits of tighter glycemic control.[18] The phenformin and tolbutamide arms of the UGDP were halted because these agents appeared to increase cardiovascular mortality.[8] Moreover, agents that increase insulin levels seem less able to limit cardiovascular complications than agents that reduce insulin resistance. In the UKPDS 34, metformin (Glucophage®) monotherapy decreased the rate of MI by 39% ($P = 0.01$) in overweight patients with type 2 diabetes,[18] whereas metformin plus sulfonylureas or insulin neither decreased nor increased it.[3,18] The multifactorial nature of atherosclerosis in diabetes may attenuate the effect of tight glycemic control alone in reducing cardiovascular complications.[18]

Hypercoagulability

Elevated levels of plasminogen activator inhibitor-1 (PAI-1) in insulin-resistant patients increase the risk of acute cardiac events by inhibiting fibrinolysis[3] and clot dissolution.[19] Adipocytes can increase hepatic production of fibrinogen and PAI-1 and shift the hemostatic balance toward thrombosis,[18] which is a major determinant of the progression of atherosclerosis.[20] Thus, weight loss directly helps to reduce hypercoagulability in patients with type 2 diabetes. Weight loss and lipid-lowering therapy can also reduce hypercoagulability by decreasing triglyceride levels, which correlate with circulating PAI-1 levels.[21]

In addition to restricting caloric intake to promote weight loss, changing dietary composition may also be important for reducing the effects of PAI-1. A low-glycemic-index diet can halve elevated plasma PAI-1 activity, which is also decreased by soluble dietary fiber; consumption of fruit and vegetables has been associated with reduced PAI-1 levels;[21] and increased dietary magnesium attenuated the clotting tendency of platelets in a small study of diabetic patients.[19] Exercise increases fibrinolytic activity and decreases PAI-1 levels in nondiabetic patients and was shown to improve the impaired basal fibrinolytic response in type 2 diabetes in one study, although another study in similar patients reported no such change. Because hyperglycemia, hyperinsulinemia, and insulin resistance all contribute to hypercoagulability in type 2 diabetes, improving glycemic control is essential to reducing hypercoagulability.[20] Metformin reduces plasma PAI-1 levels and increases fibrinolysis in patients with type 2 diabetes. TZDs appear to have similar effects. Angiotensin-converting enzyme inhibitor (ACEI) therapy has been shown to decrease PAI-1 levels in diabetic patients and therefore helps to reduce hypercoagulability in these patients.[21] Moreover, because angiotensin II destabilizes plaque, thereby increasing the risk of plaque rupture and MI, ACEIs may help to prevent cardiac events.[1]

Aspirin rapidly and irreversibly inhibits synthesis of thromboxane, a potent platelet aggregant and vasoconstrictor. ADA guidelines therefore recommend the use of low-dose (75 to 325 mg/d), enteric-coated aspirin for virtually all patients with type 2 diabetes unless contraindicated by bleeding tendency, anticoagulant therapy, recent gastrointestinal bleeding, active liver disease, or aspirin allergy.[21,22] A 325-mg dose of aspirin every other day reduced MI risk in diabetic patients in the 5-year US Physician's Health Study, which found a RR of MI of 0.39 in treated patients. In the Hypertension Optimal Treatment (HOT) trial, 75 mg of aspirin per day reduced MI risk by 36% and reduced pooled CVD risk by 15% in about 4 years in a group of older diabetic patients with treated hypertension without increasing fatal bleeding. The Early Treatment of Diabetic Retinopathy Study, which produced similar results, found that even 650 mg of aspirin daily did not increase retinal bleeding. Meta-analysis has shown that aspirin reduces CVD events by 25% in diabetic patients who have had an MI or stroke and that low doses are as effective as higher doses but cause fewer severe bleeding episodes. However, the third National Health and Nutrition Examination Survey found that only about 13% of diabetic patients in whom aspirin therapy was indicated were receiving it, which indicates that this simple, inexpensive form of therapy is underused.[21] In patients with aspirin allergy, clopidogrel (Plavix®) may be substituted.[22] Clopidogrel 75 mg/d was about as effective as aspirin 325 mg/d in reducing the risk of MI, ischemic stroke, or vascular death (5.83% vs 5.32%; $P = 0.043$) in the Clopidogrel vs Aspirin in Patients at Risk of Ischemic Events (CAPRIE) trial.[21] Subgroup analysis of diabetic patients in CAPRIE found an annual combined vascular event rate of 15.6% for clopidogrel vs 17.7% for aspirin,[5] and clopidogrel was particularly beneficial in patients with PAD. Ticlopidine (Ticlid®), a thienopyridine, is another antiplatelet agent. However, the risk of neutropenia is much higher with ticlopidine than with clopidogrel, and both agents have been associated with rare cases of life-threatening aplastic anemia and thrombotic thrombocytopenic purpura.[21] No data support prophylactic use of anticoagulants or fibrinolytics in patients with type 2 diabetes.[20] Low-dose warfarin (Coumadin®) did not benefit diabetic patients in the Post Coronary Artery Bypass Graft Trial.[8]

Hyperinsulinemia and Insulin Resistance

Whether hyperinsulinemia or insulin resistance predicts macrovascular complications in patients with type 2 diabetes is controversial.[8] However, treatment with agents that increase insulin levels, such as sulfonylureas or insulin, did not increase CVD mortality in the UKPDS.[3] A prospective study of men in Quebec found an association between fasting insulin levels and ischemic heart disease after adjustment for other risk factors, and three similar studies found that insulin levels correlate with CAD in multivariate analysis, but smaller studies have found no significant association. A correlation between insulin levels and CAD has been found in middle-aged patients but not in the elderly. In the MRFIT, fasting hyperinsulinemia was a CAD risk factor only in men with an apolipoprotein abnormality, and another study found that hyperinsulinemia only affected CAD in the presence of hypertriglyceridemia. Thus, hyperinsulinemia may be a CAD risk factor only in certain age groups or in those with specific lipoprotein abnormalities. Alternatively, it may simply be a marker for insulin resistance, which also correlates with CAD.[19]

Insulin resistance is directly related to increased rates of MI, stroke, and PAD.[2] Furthermore, insulin resistance seems to independently increase atherogenesis, as indicated by the Insulin Resistance Atherosclerosis Study (IRAS). In that study, insulin resistance, determined by direct measurement of insulin action, correlated with carotid intima-media thickness in white non-Hispanics after adjustment for other risk factors.[19] A study of nondiabetic Mexican-Americans showed that endothelium-dependent vasodilation in insulin-resistant, obese subjects was half that in insulin-sensitive subjects,[1,9] which indicates that even nondiabetic obese patients require CVD risk factor management because of insulin resistance.

Insulin sensitizers such as TZDs and metformin decrease circulating insulin. TZDs improve insulin-mediated glucose uptake into skeletal muscle; metformin suppresses hepatic glucose production, which should also be suppressed by insulin.[23] Both agents suppress circulating PAI-1. TZDs improve the hypertriglyceridemia and low HDL associated with the metabolic syndrome and decrease small, dense LDL, while metformin decreases LDL. TZDs also are anti-inflammatory agents and decrease high-sensitivity C-reactive protein (hs-CRP) levels by 20% to 40% in diabetes.[24] Metformin decreases hs-CRP by 10%.[25] Results of clinical trials with rosiglitazone (Avandia®) and pioglitazone (Actos®) on CAD events and mortality in diabetes are pending.

Obesity and Physical Inactivity

Although obesity has not been independently associated with CAD or other CVD complications in patients with type 2 diabetes, it is an important determinant of insulin resistance. It is also associated with hypertension and dyslipidemia. Therefore, every effort should be made to restore obese patients to a more normal weight.[15] Weight reduction strategies that include decreasing fat consumption and increasing physical activity may help to decrease CVD risk. Consumption of a high level of saturated fat is a CVD risk factor,[6] and its decrease can promote weight loss even when total caloric intake is unrestricted.[26] Physical inactivity contributes to weight gain, is more common in patients with type 2 diabetes,[8] and is associated with increased mortality in these patients.[6] Moreover, inactivity predicts CVD in nondiabetic patients, although data on its ability to predict CVD in diabetic patients are limited.[8]

Oxidative Stress

In type 2 diabetes, oxygen-derived free radicals promote CAD by impairing endothelium-dependent relaxation (Figure 6-2), and scavengers of these free radicals, such as vitamins E and C, can reverse this impairment.[19] Although a prospective trial showed little effect on CVD events in a high-risk population after 4 to 6 years of high-dose vitamin E from natural sources, dietary antioxidant therapy may be useful because high antioxidant levels have been associated with lower rates of CAD and CVD mortality in population studies.[15] A daily supplement containing 250 mg of vitamin C and 100 mg of vitamin E was part of the CVD-reducing multifactorial intervention in the Steno-2 study of patients with type 2 diabetes.[7] ACEIs and angiotensin-receptor blockers (ARBs) may also be useful in reducing oxidative-stress-related CVD risk in type 2 diabetes. Oxidative stress shifts the balance between vasoactive agents toward vasoconstrictors. By reducing oxidative stress, ACEIs and ARBs increase nitric oxide levels and thereby shift this balance back toward vasodilators.[1]

Hyperhomocysteinemia

The methionine metabolite homocysteine is highly reactive at high levels and may damage the endothelium directly.[3] Hyperhomocysteinemia is an independent CVD risk factor,[15] and diabetic patients have been shown to have elevated homocysteine levels.[3] Five-year mortality in hyperhomocysteinemic patients with type 2 diabetes was almost twice as high as that in nondiabetic hyper-

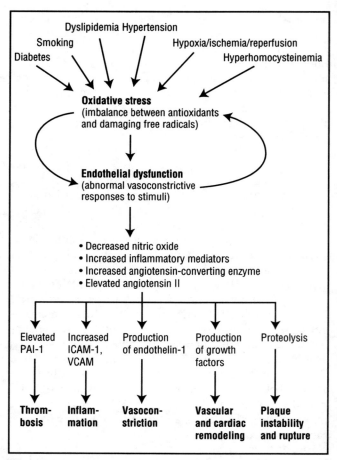

Figure 6-2: Schematic of how oxidative stress and endothelial dysfunction work synergistically to lead to heart disease in patients with diabetes. ICAM = intracellular adhesion molecule 1, PAI-1 = plasminogen activator inhibitor 1, VCAM = vascular cell adhesion molecule. Reprinted with permission from Hsueh WA, *Cleve Clin J Med* 2000;67:809.

homocysteinemic patients. Meta-analysis has found that folic acid 0.5 to 5 mg daily can decrease homocysteine levels by 15% to 40% in 6 weeks.[15] At-risk patients with homocysteine levels greater than 15 μmol/L benefit from folic acid 0.4 mg/d,[3] the dosage used in the multifactorial intervention that reduced CVD risk by 50% in patients with type 2 diabetes in the Steno-2 study.[7] If homocysteine levels do not revert to normal at this dosage, the elevation is probably caused by a genetic abnormality, and 1 mg or more of folic acid may be required daily. Vitamin B_{12} 1.2 μg/d should be used with folic acid to avoid the neurologic damage that folic acid can induce when vitamin B_{12} levels are deficient.[20]

Inflammation

In diabetes, oxidative stress, protein glycosylation, and obesity lead to chronic low-grade inflammation[3] that promotes atherosclerosis.[18] Endothelial damage further promotes inflammation and atherosclerosis by causing expression of adhesion molecules that attract platelets and leukocytes.[1] Hs-CRP levels are elevated in obesity and diabetes, and Hs-CRP has emerged as a marker of vascular risk.[18] CRP level was the best predictor of first MI in the Physicians' Health Study,[3] predicts long-term mortality in unstable CAD, and is associated with stroke risk.[6] CRP may also directly elevate CVD risk by promoting inflammation.[18] Inflammatory markers appear to contribute to CVD risk independently of other metabolic abnormalities of the insulin resistance syndrome. Women are much more likely to have elevated CRP levels than men, which may account for the relative increase in CVD risk in diabetic women compared with men even when the magnitude of other risk factors between them is equivalent.[6]

Statin therapy seems to reduce the vascular inflammatory response that promotes atherogenesis.[27] The mean reduction in CRP after long-term, full-dose statin therapy is about 20% to 40% from baseline.[28] TZDs reduce CRP by 30%.[27] Fibrates and metformin also decrease CRP. Further studies are in progress to determine whether reducing hs-CRP will reduce CAD events and mortality. The ability of fibrates to decrease elevated triglyceride levels may be particularly important in combating inflammation because lipoproteins that are rich in triglyceride, such as β-VLDL, activate transcription factor NF-κ B, which causes expression of atherogenic proinflammatory genes.[18]

Myocardial Infarction and Its Complications

Patients with diabetes are likely to have silent or unrecognized MI, possibly because of the effect of autonomic neuropathy on sensory nerves. As a result, in some studies, silent ischemia was more commonly detected with noninvasive techniques in diabetic patients than in nondiabetic patients. Diabetic patients are also much more likely to have atypical MI symptoms such as confusion, dyspnea, fatigue, or nausea and vomiting. Diabetic patients with MI have increased in-hospital mortality, largely related to a higher incidence of congestive heart failure, which may result from subclinical diabetic cardiomyopathy. Diabetic patients with CAD are also less able to form collateral vessels, which may explain their propensity toward infarct extension and angina after MI.[4]

Although patients with type 2 diabetes benefit as much as or more than nondiabetic patients from CVD risk factor management, the degree to which patients with type 2 diabetes benefit from pharmacotherapy and other interventions for established CVD is less clear.[8] One exception may relate to the use of β-blockers, which consistently reduces post-MI mortality in diabetic patients.[13] Some research indicates that β-blockers can reduce reinfarction and mortality in diabetic patients more than in matched controls.[2] In one study, β-blocker therapy reduced early mortality by 37% in diabetic patients with MI compared with 13% in the entire study group.[4] Although β-blockers may reduce insulin production and mask hypoglycemia,[2] these are seldom serious problems when cardioselective agents are used,[4] and a retrospective study of more than 45,000 patients showed that β-blockers reduced MI risk by 23% without increasing diabetic complications in patients with type 2 diabetes.[2]

Like β-blockers, ACEIs are also clearly beneficial in treating diabetic patients after MI, probably because they improve left ventricular dysfunction. This effect was convincingly demonstrated in the GISSI-2 trial of lisinopril (Prinivil®, Zestril®) therapy given soon after MI,[13] which reduced mortality dramatically more in diabetic patients than in nondiabetic patients after 6 weeks and 6 months.[4] This finding was supported by the Survival and Ventricular Enlargement (SAVE) study, in which ACEI therapy provided the greatest benefit in high-risk groups such as diabetic patients.[13] In the Trandolapril Cardiac Evaluation (TRACE) study of post-MI patients with left ventricular dysfunction, ACEI therapy not only reduced mortality by 36%, but also reduced progression to severe heart failure by 62%.[4] Although ramipril (Altace®) reduced BP by only 3 mm Hg in the Heart Outcomes Prevention Evaluation (HOPE) study, it significantly reduced (by 25%) the combined end point of MI, stroke, or CVD mortality in high-risk diabetic patients, which indicates that its cardiovascular benefit was greater than that attributable to its antihypertensive effect.[8] Intensive insulin therapy during acute MI has not proven useful;[4] however, the Diabetes and Insulin-Glucose Infusion in Acute MI (DIGAMI) study found a statistically significant 52% decrease in 1-year mortality when such therapy was used immediately after MI. This survival benefit persisted for at least 3.4 years post-MI.[13] The benefits of thrombolytic therapy in diabetic patients with acute MI have also been established. One meta-analysis found that the reduction in absolute mortality from thrombolysis in diabetic patients (3.7%) exceeded that in nondiabetic patients (2.1%) ($P > 0.01$).[2]

Angioplasty is at least as effective as thrombolysis in nondiabetic patients, but it is not clear whether this holds true for diabetic patients.[13] Although success rates immediately after angioplasty are comparable in both groups, diabetic patients tend to experience more in-stent thrombosis. Emergency surgery, late revascularization, MI, and death were more common in diabetic patients than in nondiabetic patients in some studies. For instance, an analysis of more than 25,000 cases found a twofold increase in in-hospital mortality after angioplasty in diabetic patients,[13] and the Bypass Angioplasty Revascularization Investigation (BARI) found significantly lower 5-year survival rates in diabetic patients (73.3%) than in nondiabetic patients (91.3%).[2] However, the Global Use of Strategies to Open Occluded Coronary Arteries IIB (GUSTO-IIB) study found a trend toward a better 30-day outcome in diabetic patients who received angioplasty than in those who received thrombolysis.[13]

Even with stent implantation, restenosis rates in diabetic patients range from 24% to 55%, although microalbuminuria may independently predict restenosis in these patients.[29] Diabetic patients also have a higher reinfarction rate and mortality than nondiabetic patients after stenting.[13] A substudy of the Evaluation of Platelet IIb/IIIa Inhibition for Stenting Trial (EPISTENT) indicated that combining stents with the glycoprotein inhibitor abciximab (ReoPro®) may enhance the results of angioplasty,[5] although greater need for target vessel revascularization and no significant difference in acute events was found in diabetic patients in the Evaluation of PTCA to Improve Long-Term Outcome with Abciximab GP IIa/IIIb Blockade (EPILOG) study of abciximab vs angioplasty alone.[4] The EPISTENT substudy found a significant reduction in the combined end point of death, MI, and target vessel revascularization after 6 months in diabetic patients treated with stent + abciximab + heparin compared with those treated with stent + heparin or angioplasty + abciximab + heparin. The rate of target vessel revascularization alone was also reduced by 8.1% in the diabetic stent + abciximab + heparin group compared with the other treatment groups in EPISTENT.[5] Pooled analysis of data from EPIC (Evaluation of c7E3 for the Prevention of Ischemic Complications), EPILOG, and EPISTENT indicates that abciximab significantly reduced 1-year mortality in diabetic patients ($P = 0.031$).[5]

Prognosis after surgical revascularization may be worse in diabetic patients than in nondiabetic patients,[2] and the same may hold true for nonacute revascularization. In the Thrombosis in Myocardial Infarction (phase 2) trial (TIMI 2), the mortality for diabetic patients undergoing nonacute angioplasty or coronary bypass surgery was substantially higher than that when such revascularization was done for acute MI only. This difference was not found in nondiabetic patients.[13] In contrast, in BARI, diabetic patients who required insulin had significantly higher survival rates after multivessel bypass surgery with internal mammary artery grafts (80.6%) than after percutaneous revascularization (65.5%).[2] However, when BARI was conducted, stents were not yet available, so the reported survival rate after angioplasty may underestimate that for angioplasty plus stenting.[8] Increased restenosis rates after stenting in diabetic patients may result in part from the greater intimal proliferative response in these patients.[2] Thus, pharmacologic stent-coating agents such as rapamycin (sirolimus) (Rapamune®) that decrease restenosis by inhibiting smooth muscle cell proliferation and migration may be of particular benefit in diabetic patients. In two small studies of stents that released this immunosuppressant macrolide, no patient had greater than 50% vessel narrowing.[30] However, no clear evidence yet exists that revascularization produces better outcomes than thrombolysis in diabetic patients with acute MI.[13]

In patients with unstable angina/non-Q-wave MI, low-molecular-weight heparin reduces the rate of cardiac events in diabetic patients as much as in nondiabetic patients. Moreover, a meta-analysis showed that glycoprotein inhibitors reduced the absolute event rate in diabetic patients twice as much as in nondiabetic patients.[2] However, because diabetic patients are already at increased risk of microvascular complications, any adverse effects of glycoprotein inhibitors on capillary function would tend to affect diabetic patients more than nondiabetic patients and could also adversely affect the course of PAD.

Peripheral Artery Disease

No evidence indicates that tight glycemic or BP control or antiplatelet therapy decreases the incidence of intermittent claudication or critical limb ischemia in diabetic patients with PAD,[2] who have a greater risk of progressing to ischemic ulceration than nondiabetic patients with PAD.[31] However, greater severity and duration of diabetes increases the incidence and extent of PAD.[2] Patients with PAD who receive intensive antihypertensive therapy have a lower cardiovascular event rate than those treated less intensively. In one study, the cardiovascular event rate was 13.6% in patients who reached a mean BP of 128/75 mm Hg compared to 38.7% in those who reached a mean BP of 137/81 mm Hg, and event rate reduction was similar regardless of whether enalapril or nisoldipine (Sular®) was used.[31] However, β-blockers may decrease walking distance in patients with intermittent claudication.[32]

A meta-analysis concluded that lipid-lowering therapy in PAD patients probably reduces mortality and that statins may also alter the clinical course of PAD.[32] Simvastatin (Zocor®) decreased the incidence of new or worsening claudication to a statistically significant degree in

CAD patients in the Scandinavian Simvastatin Survival Study.[32] Statin therapy has also been shown to enhance walking distance and speed in patients with lower-extremity PAD. This effect was slightly attenuated by adjustment for CRP levels but was independent of cholesterol levels, which suggests that the benefits of statins result partly from reduced inflammation but mostly from other mechanisms unrelated to their cholesterol-lowering effect, such as enhanced endothelial function, improved vasodilation, and inhibition of platelet function.[33] Subgroup analyses of the benefits of statins in diabetic patients with PAD are not available. Nevertheless, because cardiovascular events are the main cause of death in PAD patients, diabetic patients with PAD require intensive CVD risk factor management, including aggressive lipid lowering. Exercise aids in CVD risk management, and meta-analysis has shown that supervised walking programs increased walking distance by 122% in PAD patients.[32]

The phosphodiesterase type 3 inhibitor cilostazol (Pletal®) also increases walking distance in PAD patients by as much as 50% compared with placebo. Although cilostazol enhances lipid profile and antagonizes platelet activity, how it improves walking distance is not yet known.[2] The recommended cilostazol dose is 100 mg twice daily taken at least a half hour before or 2 hours after breakfast and dinner.[34] The xanthine pentoxifylline (Trental®) is also approved for intermittent claudication,[35] but it may affect blood rheology and decrease blood viscosity[2] and is seldom used. Recent placebo-controlled studies have failed to confirm the benefit found in earlier studies, and some studies indicate that pentoxifylline can be withdrawn without affecting walking ability.[35] Although antiplatelet therapy with aspirin or clopidogrel does not decrease symptom frequency or increase walking distance in patients with intermittent claudication, these agents improve the clinical course of PAD. Moreover, because the advantages of clopidogrel over aspirin are greatest in PAD patients, clopidogrel may be used instead of aspirin for secondary prevention in intermittent claudication.

The presence of severe, distal, and diffuse multivessel PAD makes lower-extremity revascularization less successful and restenosis more frequent in diabetic patients than in nondiabetic patients.[32] However, iliac artery stenting in diabetic patients has resulted in greater than 90% patency after 1 year in some studies. Angioplasty is preferred for short proximal stenosis of the aortoiliac vessels and may also be used for discrete lesions in the superficial femoral artery, but its results in treating more distal vessels such as the tibial arteries are poor.[32] In patients with severe claudication, surgery may be better than angioplasty in treating the femoral, popliteal, and infrapopliteal vessels. Although bypass surgery increases cardiovascular morbidity and mortality,[2] 5-year patency rates are high when distal runoff is good.[32]

Cerebrovascular Disease

Therapy with platelet antagonists, statins, and ACEIs is recommended in diabetic patients with cerebrovascular atherosclerosis. In patients with type 2 diabetes, enalapril halves the annual intima-media thickness rate in carotid arteries vs untreated controls ($P = 0.05$).[36] Antiplatelet agents produce similar results.[37] Cilostazol not only stabilized intima-media thickness after 3 years, but also prevented stroke and silent brain infarction.[38] Intensive BP reduction to a mean of 128/75 mm Hg decreased 5-year stroke risk vs moderate reduction to 137/81 mm Hg.[39] In diabetic patients, TZD therapy can prevent the progression of early carotid artery atherosclerosis,[40] and losartan (Cozaar®) can prevent stroke in hypertensive diabetes subjects with cardiac hypertrophy.[41] In diabetic patients with hemodynamically significant internal carotid artery atherosclerosis, combining medical therapy with surgical revascularization results in fewer strokes than medical therapy alone. However, after carotid endarterectomy, cardiovascular mortality (mainly from CAD events) is increased in diabetic patients compared with nondiabetic patients. Direct outcome data in diabetic patients after stenting for carotid atherosclerosis is sparse, but the available evidence suggests that outcomes may be similar to those of nondiabetic patients.[2]

References

1. Hsueh WA: In diabetes, treat hidden heart disease. *Cleve Clin J Med* 2000;67:807-813.

2. Beckman JA, Creager MA, Libby P: Diabetes and atherosclerosis: epidemiology, pathophysiology, and management. *JAMA* 2002;287:2570-2581.

3. Spanheimer RG: Reducing cardiovascular risk in diabetes. Which factors to modify first? *Postgrad Med* 2001;109:26-36.

4. Aronson D, Johnstone MT: Coronary artery disease in diabetes. In: Johnstone MT, Veves A, eds. *Contemporary Cardiology: Diabetes and Cardiovascular Disease.* Totowa, NJ: Humana Press, 2001, pp 123-129.

5. Marso SP: Optimizing the diabetic formulary: beyond aspirin and insulin. *J Am Coll Cardiol* 2002;40:652-661.

6. Resnick HE, Howard BV: Diabetes and cardiovascular disease. *Annu Rev Med* 2002;52:245-267.

7. Gaede P, Vedel P, Larsen N, et al: Multifactorial intervention and cardiovascular disease in patients with type 2 diabetes. *N Engl J Med* 2003;348:383-393.

8. Laakso M: Cardiovascular disease in type 2 diabetes: challenge for treatment and prevention. *J Intern Med* 2001;249:225-235.

9. Executive Summary of The Third Report of The National Cholesterol Education Program (NCEP) Expert Panel on Detection, Evaluation, And Treatment of High Blood Cholesterol In Adults (Adult Treatment Panel III). *JAMA* 2001;285:2486-2497.

10. Haffner SM: Coronary heart disease in patients with diabetes. *N Engl J Med* 2000;342:1040-1042.

11. Solomon CG: Reducing cardiovascular risk in type 2 diabetes. *N Engl J Med* 2003;348:457-459.

12. Lakka HM, Laaksonen DE, Lakka TA, et al: The metabolic syndrome and total and cardiovascular disease mortality in middle-aged men. *JAMA* 2002;288:2709-2716.

13. Paty BW: Managing myocardial infarction in the diabetic patient. *Endocrinol Metab Clin North Am* 2000;29:831-842.

14. Hsueh WA, Anderson PW: Hypertension, the endothelial cell, and the vascular complications of diabetes mellitus. *Hypertension* 1992;20:253-263.

15. Garber AJ: Attenuating cardiovascular risk factors in patients with type 2 diabetes. *Am Fam Physician* 2000;62:2633-2642, 2645-2646.

16. Haire-Joshu D, Glasgow RE, Tibbs TL: Position statement: smoking and diabetes. *Diabetes Care* 2003;26(suppl 1):S89-S90.

17. Mudaliar S, Henry RR. New oral therapies for type 2 diabetes mellitus: The glitazones or insulin sensitizers. *Annu Rev Med* 2001;52:239-257.

18. Libby P, Plutzky J: Diabetic macrovascular disease: the glucose paradox? *Circulation* 2002;106:2760-2763.

19. Hsueh WA, Law RE: Cardiovascular risk continuum: implications of insulin resistance and diabetes. *Am J Med* 1998;105: 4S-14S.

20. Schneider DJ, Sobel BE: Diabetes and thrombosis. In: Johnstone MT and Veves A, eds. *Contemporary Cardiology: Diabetes and Cardiovascular Disease*. Totowa, NJ: Humana Press, 2001, pp 149-167.

21. Colwell JA: Treatment for the procoagulant state in type 2 diabetes. *Endocrinol Metab Clin North Am* 2001;30:1011-1030.

22. Colwell JA: Position statement: aspirin therapy in diabetes. *Diabetes Care* 2003;26(suppl 1):S87-S88.

23. Shepherd PR, Kahn BB: Glucose transporters and insulin action–implications for insulin resistance and diabetes mellitus. *N Engl J Med* 1999;341:248-257.

24. Haffner SM, Greenberg AS, Weston WM, et al: Effect of rosiglitazone treatment on nontraditional markers of cardiovascular disease in patients with type 2 diabetes mellitus. *Circulation* 2002;106:679-684.

25. Chu NV, Kong AP, Kim DD, et al: Differential effects of metformin and troglitazone on cardiovascular risk factors in patients with type 2 diabetes. *Diabetes Care* 2002;25:542-549.

26. Weigle DS, Cummings DE, Newby PD, et al: Roles of leptin and ghrelin in the loss of body weight caused by a low fat, high carbohydrate diet. *J Clin Endocrinol Metab* 2003;88:1577-1586.

27. Dandona P, Aljada A: A rational approach to pathogenesis and treatment of type 2 diabetes mellitus, insulin resistance, inflammation, and atherosclerosis. *Am J Cardiol* 2002;90(suppl): 27G-33G.

28. Ridker PM, Buring JE, Cook NR, et al: C-reactive protein, the metabolic syndrome, and risk of cardiovascular events: an 8-year follow-up of 14,719 initially healthy American women. *Circulation* 2003;107:391-397.

29. Heper G, Durmaz T, Murat SN, et al: Clinical and angiographic outcomes of diabetic patients after coronary stenting: a comparison of native vessel stent restenosis rates in different diabetic subgroups. *Angiology* 2002;53:287-295.

30. Clowes A: Prevention of neointimal hyperplasia—taxol, rapamycin, and radiation. VascularWeb—the Global Network of Vascular Surgery Societies (Web site). Available at: http:// www.vascularweb.org/doc/140. Accessed March 10, 2003.

31. Mehler PS, Coll JR, Estacio R, et al: Intensive blood pressure control reduces the risk of cardiovascular events in patients with peripheral arterial disease and type 2 diabetes. *Circulation* 2003;107:753-756.

32. Donnelly R: Assessment and management of intermittent claudication: importance of secondary prevention. *Int J Clin Pract Suppl* 2001;119:2-9.

33. McDermott MM, Guralnik JM, Greenland P, et al: Statin use and leg functioning in patients with and without lower-extremity peripheral arterial disease. *Circulation* 2003;107:757-761.

34. *Mosby's Drug Consult.* 12th ed. St. Louis: Mosby, 2002.

35. Hiatt WR: New treatment options in intermittent claudication: the US experience. *Int J Clin Pract Suppl* 2001;119:20-27.

36. Hosomi N, Mizushige K, Ohyama H, et al: Angiotensin-converting enzyme inhibition with enalapril slows progressive intima-media thickening of the common carotid artery in patients with non-insulin-dependent diabetes mellitus. *Stroke* 2001;32:1539-1545.

37. Kodama M, Yamasaki Y, Sakamoto K, et al: Antiplatelet drugs attenuate progression of carotid intima-media thickness in subjects with type 2 diabetes. *Thromb Res* 2000;97:239-245.

38.   Shinoda-Tagawa T, Yamasaki Y, Yoshida S, et al: A phosphodiesterase inhibitor, cilostazol, prevents the onset of silent brain infarction in Japanese subjects with Type II diabetes. *Diabetologia* 2002;45:188-194.

39.   Schrier RW, Estacio RO, Esler A, et al: Effects of aggressive blood pressure control in normotensive type 2 diabetic patients on albuminuria, retinopathy, and strokes. *Kidney Int* 2002; 61:1086-1097.

40.   Kernan WN, Inzucchi SE, Viscoli CM, et al: Insulin resistance and risk for stroke. *Neurology* 2002;59:809-815.

41.   Lindholm LH, Ibsen H, Dahlof B, et al: Cardiovascular morbidity and mortality in patients with diabetes in the Losartan Intervention For Endpoint reduction in hypertension study (LIFE): a randomised trial against atenolol. *Lancet* 2002;359:1004-1010.

Chapter **7**

Hypertension and Its Treatment

The Impact of Hypertension in Diabetes

Hypertension is defined by the Joint National Committee 7 report (JNC 7)[1] as blood pressure greater than or equal to 130/80 mm Hg. It affects up to 70% of patients with type 2 diabetes[2] and is twice as prevalent in diabetics as in nondiabetics.[3] Hypertension accounts for 30% to 70% of diabetic complications[3] and worsens cardiovascular, renal, and peripheral vascular disease (PVD), stroke, and retinopathy.[4] Furthermore, hypertension accelerates diabetic cardiomyopathy, resulting in left ventricular hypertrophy[5] and, ultimately, heart failure. Serious cardiovascular events are two or three times as likely to occur in diabetic hypertensive patients as in those with either diabetes or hypertension alone.[6,7] In type 2 diabetic patients, dyslipidemia and endothelial abnormalities add to the increased cardiovascular risk from hypertension.[7] End-stage renal disease (ESRD) is five to six times more likely to develop in hypertensive patients with diabetes than in hypertensive patients without diabetes.[4] Hypertension increases diabetic mortality fourfold to fivefold because of its contribution to renal and cardiovascular disease.[7]

Treatment Rationale and Goals

Solid clinical trial data have established the effectiveness of aggressive treatment of hypertension in reducing the diabetic vascular complication rate. In the United Kingdom

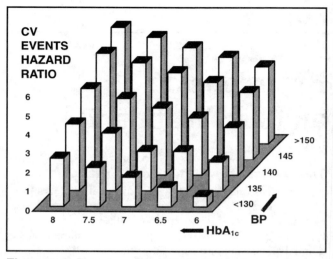

Figure 7-1: Data from the UKPD study show the strong interaction between blood glucose level expressed by Hb A_{1c} and systolic blood pressure (BP). Combinations of both abnormalities markedly amplify cardiovascular event (CV) hazard ratios. For example, when both Hb A_{1c} and blood pressure are markedly elevated, as depicted in the tallest bar in the row furthest back in the cube, the hazard ratio approaches 6. Reprinted with permission from Charles MA: *Diabetes Management. Complication Risk Assessment, Diagnosis, and Therapeutic Options.* Larchmont, NY: Mary Ann Liebert, Inc. p.33.

Prospective Diabetes Study (UKPDS), every 10 mm Hg decrease in mean systolic blood pressure reduced risk by 12% for any diabetic complication, 15% for diabetes-related death, 11% for myocardial infarction (MI), and 13% for microvascular complications, and no risk threshold was found for any end point studied.[8] A mean blood pressure of 144/82 mm Hg resulted in fewer complications, including 21% fewer MIs, 32% fewer diabetes-related deaths, and 37% less microvascular disease, compared with a mean blood pressure of 154/87 mm Hg. Tighter blood pressure control was found to reduce stroke risk by 44%, while tighter blood glucose control was not found to reduce it.[9] Figure 7-1 highlights the steep increase in cardiovascular event hazard ratios from the interaction between increasing levels of glycated hemoglobin (Hb A_{1c}) and blood pressure.

The Hypertension Optimal Treatment (HOT) trial revealed that reaching a diastolic blood pressure goal of 80 mm Hg resulted in 51% fewer cardiovascular events than reaching a goal of 90 mm Hg, supporting the importance of targeting lower blood pressures.[3,8] Elevated systolic pressure may contribute more to cardiovascular risk than elevated diastolic pressure,[10] and pressures of 120/70 mm Hg or more are linked to increased event rates and mortality in diabetic patients. Other studies also illustrated the benefits of diastolic goals of 80 mm Hg or less.[8] Retrospective analysis of studies of diabetic renal insufficiency found that long-term renal functional decline slowed when blood pressure was 130/80 mm Hg or less.[4] Therefore, the American Diabetes Association (ADA), the National Kidney Foundation Hypertension and Diabetes Executive Committees Working Group, and JNC 7 recommend a goal pressure of 130/80 mm Hg or less.[4,8] For isolated systolic hypertension, defined by the ADA as a systolic blood pressure greater than or equal to 180 mm Hg with a normal diastolic blood pressure, the initial treatment goal is to reduce systolic blood pressure to below 160 mm Hg. If the diastolic blood pressure is normal but the systolic blood pressure is between 160 and 179 mm Hg, the initial goal is to reduce systolic blood pressure by 20 mm Hg.[8]

Treatment Strategies

Antihypertensive therapy should start with lifestyle modifications, including weight loss, increased exercise, decreased salt and alcohol intake, and smoking cessation. If goal blood pressure cannot be reached with these measures after 3 months, pharmacotherapy is indicated.[3,11] Because lifestyle modifications improve responsiveness to antihypertensives, particularly in insulin-resistant patients, these modifications should continue after pharmacotherapy is begun.[12]

Lifestyle Interventions

Successful intervention requires education to help patients adopt long-term behaviors that lower blood pressure. Lifestyle interventions, such as the Dietary Approaches to Stop Hypertension (DASH) diet, reduce blood pressure without drug therapy and should be used by most, if not all, diabetic hypertensive patients.[4] Counseling to decrease fat, sodium, and alcohol intake and to increase physical activity for weight loss lowered blood pressure in the 4-year Treatment of Mild Hypertension Study. Patients who also received antihypertensives reached lower blood pressures than those who did not.[3]

Mild to moderate hypertension without nephropathy requires daily sodium restriction to 2,400 mg or less; hypertension with nephropathy requires 2,000 mg or less,[13] but individual differences in sodium sensitivity should be considered. Patients should eat a diet rich in potassium, calcium, and magnesium if they have normal renal function.[12] In controlled clinical trials in essential hypertension, decreasing sodium intake from 4,600 mg to 2,300 mg daily decreased systolic blood pressure by approximately 5 mm Hg and diastolic blood pressure by 2 to 3 mm Hg. Such restriction exerts a dose-response effect on blood pressure. Because diabetic hypertension is volume dependent, sodium restriction often enhances drug response.[8]

Weight reduction is another key factor; a 1-kg weight loss can decrease mean arterial blood pressure by 1 mm Hg. However, some appetite suppressants may increase blood pressure. Moderately intense physical activity such as 30 to 45 minutes of brisk walking almost daily can decrease blood pressure.[8] Exercise decreases blood pressure most consistently in hyperinsulinemic subjects, which is consistent with evidence linking insulin resistance to diabetic hypertension.[14]

Pharmacotherapy

Because lifestyle interventions alone often cannot enable patients to reach blood pressure goals, pharmacotherapy usually must be added. Figure 4-3 in Chapter 4, 'Goals of Therapy,' illustrates a pharmacotherapeutic paradigm for reaching blood pressure goals in diabetic patients. Treatment decisions must be based on mortality and morbidity reduction in comparative trials, as well as potency and side effects.[15] In addition, pharmacotherapy should not produce intolerable side effects or adversely affect metabolic control, lipid levels, or other conditions.[3]

Aggressive blood pressure reduction has yielded similar improvement in outcomes in many trials, regardless of the agent used (Table 7-1).[1,4] In patients with diabetes, thiazide diuretics, β-blockers, angiotensin-converting enzyme inhibitors (ACEIs), angiotensin II receptor blockers (ARBs), and calcium-channel blockers (CCBs) have reduced cardiovascular morbidity and mortality and stroke.[8]

The choice of which class of agents to use as first-line therapy depends on the degree of blood pressure lowering needed, presence of other compelling indications (Table 7-1), impact on metabolic parameters, side effect profile, cost, and other considerations. In general, the average number of antihypertensive agents needed to reach target blood pressure in patients with diabetes is 3.4;[4] therefore, a combination approach may be necessary as first-line therapy.

Angiotensin-converting enzyme inhibitors and ARBs decrease albuminuria and attenuate the progression of diabetic nephropathy.[8] Angiotensin II receptor blockers also prevent progression to ESRD in patients with type 2 diabetes and frank proteinuria.[16] Inhibition of the renin-angiotensin system has favorable effects on other compelling indications, including heart failure, MI, high coronary disease

Table 7-1: Clinical Trial and Guideline Basis for Compelling Indications for Individual Drug Classes

Compelling Indication*

Heart failure

Post-myocardial infarction

High coronary disease risk

Diabetes

Chronic kidney disease

Recurrent stroke prevention

* Compelling indications for antihypertensive drugs are based on
   benefits from outcome studies or existing clinical guidelines;
   the compelling indication is managed in parallel with the
   blood pressure.
**Conditions for which clinical trials demonstrate
   benefit of specific classes of antihypertensive drugs
   BB = β-blocker; ACEI = angiotensin-converting enzyme

Recommended Drugs

Diuretic	BB	ACEI	ARB	CCB	Aldo ANT	Clinical Trial Basis**
•	•	•	•		•	ACC/AHA Heart Failure Guideline, MERIT-HF, COPERNICUS, CIBIS, SOLVD, AIRE, TRACE, ValHEFT, RALES
	•	•			•	ACC/AHA Post-MI Guideline, BHAT, SAVE, CAPRICORN, EPHESUS
•	•	•		•		ALLHAT, HOPE, ANBP2, LIFE, CONVINCE
•	•	•	•	•		NKF-ADA Guideline, UKPDS, ALLHAT
		•	•			NKF Guideline, Captopril Trial, RENAAL, IDNT, REIN, AASK
•		•				PROGRESS

inhibitor; ARB = angiotensin II receptor blocker; CCB = calcium-channel blocker; Aldo ANT = aldosterone antagonist

National Heart, Lung, and Blood Institute: *JNC 7 Express: The Seventh Report of the Joint National Committee on Prevention, Detection, Evaluation, and Treatment of High Blood Pressure.* Rockville, MD, US Department of Health and Human Services; May 2003. NIH Publication no. 03-5233.

risk, and need for recurrent stroke prevention. Aldosterone antagonists have not been examined in large numbers of patients with diabetes but are useful in the heart failure and post-MI settings. β-Blockers are also useful in these settings, as well as in high coronary risk. Calcium-channel blockers have also proved useful in patients with high coronary risk. Angiotensin-converting enzyme inhibitors, ARBs, α-adrenoceptor antagonists, calcium-channel agonists, or low-dose diuretics have few adverse effects on glucose homeostasis, lipid profile, and renal function.

Because diabetes and hypertension require lifetime treatment, regimens should be simple to optimize long-term compliance. Dosing once or twice daily and prescribing the fewest medications is key.[3] Understanding the socioeconomic, educational, cultural, and ethnic factors affecting compliance is also important.[3] Many patients in groups at high risk for diabetes are convinced that antihypertensives cause erectile dysfunction, although incidence rates with these agents are similar to those for placebo and patients with lower blood pressure have the best sexual health.[4] This example stresses the need to regularly assess compliance and educate patients to maximize compliance.

Monotherapy

Tables 7-2 through 7-5 detail dosing and administration for the antihypertensives now used. Although the tables contain information on central α-adrenoceptor agonists, peripheral adrenergic antagonists, and direct vasodilators, these are older agents and are not examined in detail in this chapter.

Angiotensin-converting Enzyme Inhibitors

Most ACEIs belong to the dicarboxyl-containing class. In contrast, captopril (Capoten®) has a sulfhydryl moiety and fosinopril sodium (Monopril®) has a phosphorus moiety.[3,17] The ACEIs now available in the United States for treating hypertension are listed in Table 7-2 with dosing and administration details.

Indications

Angiotensin-converting enzyme inhibitors, either alone or with a thiazide diuretic, are indicated for treating hypertension, including renovascular, malignant, refractory, or accelerated types.[17] Because of their vasculoprotective and cardioprotective effects, ACEIs are especially valuable in patients who have microalbuminuria or heart failure or who have had an MI.[3] Ramipril (Altace®) is indicated for patients at least 55 years of age who have diabetes and at least one other cardiovascular risk factor, such as hypertension, microalbuminuria, or elevated total cholesterol levels or low high-density lipoprotein (HDL) cholesterol levels. Except for trandolapril (Mavik®), all the ACEIs may be added to diuretics and digitalis to treat congestive heart failure unresponsive to other measures. Ramipril and trandolapril are indicated for treating stable patients with congestive heart failure in the first days following MI. Enalapril (Vasotec®) is indicated for treating asymptomatic left ventricular dysfunction in stable patients; captopril and trandolapril are indicated for treating left ventricular dysfunction in stable post-MI patients; and lisinopril (Prinivil®, Zestril®) is indicated for treating hemodynamically stable patients within 24 hours of MI.[17]

Mechanism of Action

By blocking the conversion of angiotensin I (Ang I) to angiotensin II (Ang II), which exerts potent vasoconstrictive and hypertrophic effects, ACEIs increase large-artery compliance and decrease systemic vascular resistance.[3] Decreased Ang II levels increase plasma renin activity by removing negative feedback from renin release and decrease aldosterone secretion, which promotes loss of serum potassium, sodium, and fluid. Because of these effects, ACEIs may be less hypotensive in patients with low renin levels, such as African Americans, than in those with normal or high renin levels.[17] They may also increase bradykinin levels, thereby stimulating nitric oxide release[3] and production of prostacyclin and endothelial hyperpolarizing

Table 7-2: Angiotensin-converting Enzyme Inhibitors and Receptor Antagonists: Action, Dosing, and Effects

Drug Class/Subclass, Antihypertensive Agent, and Brand Name(s)	Mode of Action	Initial Daily Dosage; Maintenance Dosage Range
Angiotensin-converting Enzyme Inhibitors		
Benazepril (Lotensin®)	Partly inhibit conversion of angiotensin I to angiotensin II; decrease level of angiotensin II and aldosterone	10 mg q.d.; 20-40 mg/d*
Captopril (Capoten®)		25 mg b.i.d./t.i.d.; 25-50 mg b.i.d./t.i.d.
Enalapril (Vasotec®)		5 mg q.d.; 10-40 mg/d*
Fosinopril (Monopril®)		10 mg q.d.; 20-40 mg q.d.
Lisinopril (Prinivil®, Zestril®)		10 mg q.d.; 20-40 mg q.d.
Moexipril (Univasc®)		7.5 mg q.d.; 7.5-30 mg/d*
Perindopril (Aceon®)		4 mg q.d.; 4-8 mg q.d.
Quinapril (Accupril®)		10-20 mg q.d.; 20-80 mg/d*
Ramipril (Altace®)		2.5 mg q.d.; 2.5-20 mg/d*
Trandolapril (Mavik®)		1-2 mg q.d.**; 2-4 mg/d*

* = Can be given as a single dose or in 2 equal divided doses.
** = An initial dose of 1 mg is recommended for non-African-American patients, and an initial dose of 2 mg for African-American patients. Adjust dose weekly per response.

Administration and Follow-up Testing	Systolic Blood Pressure Decrease (mm Hg)	Diastolic Blood Pressure Decrease (mm Hg)	Other Effects
Moexipril should be taken 1 h before meals; serum creatinine may increase initially; measure blood pressure/ determine renal function periodically; do leukocyte count at baseline, then periodically; with captopril or hepatic dysfunction, test liver function at baseline	6-12	4-7	Provide renal and cardiovascular protection, lipid and glucose neutral (captopril may increase insulin sensitivity); cough, hyperkalemia, pancreatitis, angioedema (rare), neutropenia (rare), agranulocytosis (rare)
	—	—	
	—	—	
	8-9	6-7	
	—	—	
	4-11	3-6	
	9-15	5-6	
	5-11	3-7	
	4-6	4-6	
	7-10	4-5	

— = not listed
q.d = once daily; b.i.d. = twice daily; t.i.d. = three times daily

(continued on next page)

Table 7-2: Angiotensin-converting Enzyme Inhibitors and Receptor Antagonists: Action, Dosing, and Effects *(continued)*

Drug Class/Subclass, Antihypertensive Agent, and Brand Name(s)	Mode of Action	Initial Daily Dosage; Maintenance Dosage Range
Angiotensin II Receptor Antagonists		
Candesartan (Atacand®)	Inhibit binding of angiotensin II to angiotensin tissue receptor subtype 1; completely inhibit conversion of angiotensin I to angiotensin II	16 mg q.d.; 8-32 mg/d*
Eprosartan (Teveten®)		600 mg q.d.; 400-800 mg/d*
Irbesartan (Avapro®)		150 mg q.d.; 150-300 mg q.d.
Losartan (Cozaar®)		25-50 mg q.d.; 25-100 mg/d*
Telmisartan (Micardis®)		40 mg q.d.; 20-80 mg q.d.
Valsartan (Diovan®)		80-160 mg q.d.; 80-320 mg q.d.

* = Can be given as a single dose or in 2 equal divided doses.
ACEIs = angiotensin-converting enzyme inhibitors
ARBs = angiotensin II receptor antagonists
q.d.= once daily; b.i.d = twice daily; t.i.d = three times daily

Administration and Follow-up Testing	Systolic Blood Pressure Decrease (mm Hg)	Diastolic Blood Pressure Decrease (mm Hg)	Other Effects
Determine renal function periodically; correct volume or salt depletion before giving ARBs or supervise therapy closely to avoid hypotension in patients concomitantly treated with diuretics (such patients require a 75-mg initial dose of irbesartan and a 25-mg initial dose of losartan)	8-12 5-10 8-12 5.5-10.5 6-13 6-9	4-8 3-6 5-8 3.5-7.5 6-8 3-6	Provide renal and cardiovascular protection, glucose neutral; cough (lower incidence than with ACEIs), hyperkalemia, increased triglyceride level, angioedema (rare)

Data obtained from US Pharmacopeia[17] and Nissen.[18]

factor, accounting for some of their benefits.[19] By improving endothelial function, ACEIs improve endothelium-dependent vasodilation and may maintain endothelial antithrombotic and antiproliferative properties. In the long term, ACEIs dilate the renal vasculature, increasing its blood flow.[3] In congestive heart failure, ACEIs decrease peripheral and pulmonary vascular resistance and pulmonary capillary wedge pressure.[17]

Effectiveness

In mild to moderate hypertension, ACEIs reduced blood pressure by 4 to 12 mm Hg (systolic) and by 3 to 7 mm Hg (diastolic), depending on the dosage. Benazepril (Lotensin®) and quinapril (Accupril®) were as effective as captopril, propranolol (Inderal®), and thiazide diuretics. In contrast, lisinopril was superior to a thiazide in a mostly white population and more effective in reducing systolic blood pressure than β-blockers. In contrast, although ramipril was as effective as other ACEIs and atenolol (Tenormin®), it was significantly less effective than a thiazide.[18] Moreover, combination therapy is often required to reach blood pressure goals with ACEIs.[5]

Adverse Effects

Although generally well tolerated, ACEIs can cause cough[3] in as many as 15% of patients, more commonly women, because they elevate bradykinin levels.[10] When plasma renin activity is high, the first ACEI dose may cause hypotension, so therapy should be initiated at low doses or salt intake should be increased and diuretic therapy withdrawn. Patients with renal dysfunction or who are receiving postassium-sparing diuretics, β-blockers, or nonsteroidal antiinflammatory drugs (NSAIDs) may get hyperkalemia during ACEI therapy,[3] although it is uncommon with serum creatinine levels of 2.5 mg/dL or less. Angiotensin-converting enyzme inhibitors should be used cautiously in elderly patients with normal serum creatinine levels because the glomerular filtration rate may decline with age, and elderly patients are more likely to have increased risk from hypoaldosteronism. Angioedema is a rare, serious ACEI side effect that may be more common in African Americans.[10] Other side effects include rash, itch, fever, chest or joint pain, neutropenia, agranulocytosis, pancreatitis, headache, diarrhea, dysgeusia, fatigue, and nausea.[17]

Drug Interactions

Concomitant use of NSAIDs or potassium supplements may increase hyperkalemia risk.[10] Indomethacin (Indocin®) and other NSAIDs may decrease ACEIs' anti-hypertensive effects. Taking agents that contain potassium, consuming potassium-rich salt substitutes or low-salt milk, or receiving blood treated with potassium also elevate hy-perkalemia risk. Angiotensin-converting enzyme inhibi-tors may interact with alcohol, allopurinol (Lopurin®, Zyloprim®), antacids, bone-marrow depressants, cyclosporine (Neoral®, Sandimmune®), cytostatic agents, diuretics or hypotensives, lithium, procainamide (Procan®, Procanbid®, Pronestyl®), sympathomimetics, or systemic corticosteroids. Quinapril may interfere with absorption of tetracyclines or drugs that interact with magnesium.[17]

Contraindications and Precautions

In patients with renal artery stenosis bilaterally or when only a solitary kidney remains unilaterally, ACEIs can cause renal functional deterioration[10] and should be pre-scribed only when benefits exceed risk. Risk/benefit should also be considered for pregnant or renal transplant patients or those with impaired renal or hepatic function, angioedema, hyperkalemia, severe dietary sodium restric-tion, dialysis, or ACEI sensitivity.[17]

Angiotensin II Receptor Blockers

Angiotensin II receptor blockers have effects similar to those of ACEIs, and recent trials (the Irbesartan Dia-betic Nephropathy Trial [IDNT], Reduction of Endpoints in Non-Insulin-Dependent Diabetes Mellitus with the Angiotensin Antagonist Losartan [RENAAL] Study, Losartan Intervention for Endpoint Reduction in Hypertension [LIFE] Study, and Valsartan Heart Failure Trial [ValHEFT]) suggest that they are renoprotective and cardioprotective.[16,20-22] However, they do not have the side effects of ACEIs, particularly cough, and are often useful in patients who cannot tolerate ACEIs because of cough.[10] The six ARBs now available and approved by the US Food and Drug Administration (FDA) for use in treating hypertension are listed in Table 7-2 with details on their dosing and administration.[23]

Indications

Angiotensin II receptor blockers, either alone or with other antihypertensives, are indicated for treating hypertension.[18] The IDNT compared the ability of irbesartan (Avapro®), amlodipine (Norvasc®), or placebo to delay renal disease progression and sequelae in hypertensive type 2 diabetic patients.[16] This study showed that, compared with amlodipine, irbesartan significantly reduced the composite end point of mortality, worsened renal function indicated by doubled serum creatinine level, and new ESRD. However, only the reduction in doubling of serum creatinine level approached statistical significance independently. The RENAAL Study, which compared losartan with placebo, found significant reduction in the same primary end point studied in IDNT, as well as in two of its three components, doubling of the serum creatinine level and new ESRD, after 3.5 years.[20] However, except for a 35% reduction in the rate of heart-failure hospitalization, all-cause mortality and prespecified cardiovascular end points were not significantly reduced. Nevertheless, because ARBs have proven effects on hard end points, their use as first-line antihypertensive therapy in type 2 diabetic patients may now be appropriate.[24]

Mechanism of Action

Angiotensin II receptor blockers inhibit the binding of Ang II to Ang tissue receptor subtype 1.[10] By interrupting the renin-angiotensin system at the receptor level, ARBs offer more complete and pharmacologically desirable blockade of this system than ACEIs, which may not completely block the conversion of Ang I to Ang II because of the activation of alternative pathways. Additionally, ARBs increase activation of Ang II AT2 receptor, which has vasodilating, natriuretic, and vasculoprotective properties.[25]

Effectiveness

In placebo-controlled trials in mild to moderate hypertension, ARBs reduced blood pressure by 5 to 13 mm Hg (systolic) and by 3 to 8 mm Hg (diastolic), depending on the dosage. Although low-renin hypertensives (frequently African Americans) are less responsive to ARBs and ACEIs than high-renin hypertensives (frequently whites), this difference has not been found with valsartan (Diovan®).[18] In patients with severe diastolic hypertension, eprosartan's (Teveten®) effects were similar to those of enalapril, and telmisartan's (Micardis®) effects were similar to those of enalapril and lisinopril. In treating mild to moderate hypertension, valsartan's and hydrochlorothiazide's (Esidrix®, HydroDIURIL®, Oretic®) antihypertensive effects were similar.[23]

Adverse Effects

The ARBs are remarkably safe. Hyperkalemia, short-term initial increases in serum creatinine level, and hematologic adverse effects have been extremely rare in clinical studies.[19] However, in rare cases, losartan treatment has been associated with angioedema causing airway obstruction; some cases occurred in patients who had this side effect with other drugs, including ACEIs. Adverse effects that were reported by at least 1% of patients taking ARBs and were more frequent in them than in those taking placebo include cough, headache, depression, diarrhea, dyspepsia, dizziness, edema, fatigue, hypertriglyceridemia, insomnia, and myalgia/arthralgia.[18]

Drug Interactions

No significant drug interactions have been reported in most studies of ARBs, when given with other drugs. Because ARBs are not significantly metabolized by the cytochrome P450 system and, at therapeutic concentrations, have no effect on the enzymes of this system, interactions with drugs that inhibit or are metabolized by these enzymes are unlikely. No interaction or effect on pharmacokinetics has been reported when eprosartan or irbesartan is combined with hydrochlorothiazide or nifedipine (Adalat®, Procardia®). However, similar to other drugs that block Ang II or its effects, ARBs may increase serum potassium levels when used with potassium-sparing diuretics, potassium supplements, or salt substitutes containing potassium. Digoxin levels should be monitored when digoxin is given with telmisartan.[18]

Contraindications and Precautions

Angiotensin II receptor blockers should not be used to treat pregnant patients[10] or nursing mothers and should be used with caution in patients with hepatic or renal dysfunction or renal artery stenosis.[18]

α-Adrenoceptor Antagonists

In type 2 diabetic patients, α-blockers have a greater effect on insulin sensitivity than other antihypertensive agents, but do not reduce blood pressure as other antihypertensives do. Moreover, except for prazosin (Minipress®), tolerance to α-blockers may develop.[3,12,18]

Indications

Although initially approved only for treating hypertension, α-blockers also relieve symptoms of prostatic obstruction of the bladder outlet, and this indication has also received FDA approval.[18] Because of this as well as their metabolic benefit, α-blockers may be especially useful in treating hypertensive diabetic patients with benign prostatic hypertrophy (BPH).[3,5,18]

Mechanism of Action

By selectively blocking postsynaptic α_1-adrenoceptors, these agents indirectly produce vasodilation by relaxing vascular smooth muscle and reducing peripheral vascular resistance.[3,10] The peripheral vascular effect of the short-acting agent prazosin is confined mainly to the level of the resistance vessels, or arterioles.[18]

Effectiveness

Details on the amount of blood pressure reduction produced by α-blockers are shown in Table 7-3.[18]

Adverse Effects

α-Blockers have a greater effect on standing than on seated blood pressure and heart rate.[18] Initial doses can produce dizziness, lightheadedness, syncope, and orthostatic hypotension, especially in diabetic patients with autonomic dysfunction or when the short-acting agent prazosin is used.[3,10] Use of the long-acting agents doxazosin and terazosin minimizes risk of orthostatic hypotension.[3] Doxazosin and terazosin may cause slight weight gain. α-Blockers may decrease hematocrit, hemoglobin, and leukocyte count via hemodilution. Other adverse effects include asthenia, headache, nasal congestion, nausea, palpitations, peripheral edema, and somnolence, and doxazosin may have caused rare cases of priapism.[18]

In the Antihypertensive and Lipid-Lowering Treatment to Prevent Heart Attack Trial (ALLHAT), doxazosin was associated with a 25% higher risk of major cardiovascular events, defined as heart failure, stroke, angina, and coronary revascularizations, when compared with that for the diuretic chlorthalidone (Hygroton®, Thalitone®). This highly statistically significant finding suggested that, despite its equivalent hypotensive effect, doxazosin is inferior to chlorthalidone as first-line therapy.[15] In addition, this finding raised the question of whether doxazosin should be used as add-on therapy.[26] However, the higher cardiovascular risk found in ALLHAT was attributed to a doubling in risk of additional treatment or hospitalization for heart failure associated with doxazosin over that associated with chlorthalidone.[15] Moreover, the mean baseline systolic blood pressure in the doxazosin group was 3 mm Hg higher than in the chlorthalidone group, which, in the high-risk patients studied, could explain some of the difference in heart failure rates. Because of these limitations,

Table 7-3: Adrenoceptor Antagonists: Action, Dosing, and Effects

Drug Class/Subclass, Antihypertensive Agent, and Brand Name(s)	Mode of Action	Initial Daily Dosage; Maintenance Dosage Range
α-Adrenoceptor Antagonists (α-Blockers)		
Doxazosin (Cardura®)	Block α_1-adrenoceptors, relax vascular smooth muscle, reduce peripheral vascular resistance	1 mg q.d.; 1-16 mg q.d.
Prazosin (Minipress®)		1 mg b.i.d./t.i.d.; 1-20 mg/d*
Terazosin (Hytrin®)		1 mg q.d.; 1-20 mg q.d.
β-Adrenoceptor Antagonists (β-Blockers)		
Cardioselective Agents		
Acebutolol* (Sectral®)	Block β-1 and/or β-2 adrenoceptors on peripheral and cardiac neurons	400 mg**; 400-800 mg/d
Atenolol (Tenormin®)		25-50 mg q.d.; 50-100 mg/d
Betaxolol (Kerlone®)		10 mg q.d., 10-20 mg q.d.
Bisoprolol (Zebeta®)		5 mg q.d., 5-10 mg q.d.

* must be given in divided doses
** may be given in divided doses
— not listed

Administration and Follow-up Testing	Systolic Blood Pressure Decrease (mm Hg)	Diastolic Blood Pressure Decrease (mm Hg)	Other Effects
Initial dose should be given at bedtime; warn patient that drug may cause dizziness or fainting after the first dose is taken and increase dosage slowly to minimize risk of syncope	9-10 — 5-10	5-8 — 3.5-8	Increase insulin sensitivity, modestly improve lipid profile; orthostatic hypotension, weight gain, hemodilution, priapism (rare)
Because β-blockers may inhibit insulin release in response to hyperglycemia, more intensive diet therapy and more frequent blood glucose monitoring may be required	— — — 4.6-7.4	— — — 4.4-8.7	Reduce coronary mortality in patients with ischemic heart disease; impair glucose tolerance

(continued on next page)

Table 7-3: Adrenoceptor Antagonists: Action, Dosing, and Effects *(continued)*

Drug Class/Subclass, Antihypertensive Agent, and Brand Name(s)	Mode of Action	Initial Daily Dosage; Maintenance Dosage Range
Cardioselective Agents *(continued)*		
Carvedilol (Coreg®)	Inhibit agonistic effect of sympathetic neurotransmitters, decrease cardiac output. May diminish tonic sympathetic nerve outflow from brain and suppress renin secretion.	6.25 mg b.i.d.; 12.5 mg b.i.d.
Metoprolol		
Succinate, extended-release (Toprol XL®)		50-10 mg q.d.; 50-400 mg/d
Tartrate (Lopressor®)		100 mg*; 100-450 mg/d
Noncardioselective Agents		
Carteolol (Cartrol®)		2.5 mg q.d.; 2.5-10 mg q.d.
Labetalol (Normodyne®, Trandate®)		100 mg b.i.d.; 200-400 mg b.i.d.
Nadolol (Corgard®)		40 mg q.d.; 40-320 mg/d
Penbutolol (Levatol®)		20 mg q.d.; 20 mg q.d.
Pindolol (Visken®)		5 mg b.i.d.; 5-60 mg/d
Propranolol (Inderal®)		80 mg q.d.; 80-160 mg q.d
Timolol (Blocadren®)		10 mg b.i.d.; 20-60 mg/d

* may be given in divided doses
** data not provided
— not listed
ISA = intrinsic sympathomimetic activity

Administration and Follow-up Testing	Systolic Blood Pressure Decrease (mm Hg)	Diastolic Blood Pressure Decrease (mm Hg)	Other Effects
	7.5-9	3.5-5.5	Mask hypoglycemic symptoms (less likely with cardioselective agents), worsen lipid profile (except bisoprolol and carvedilol), agents with ISA increase heart rate, produce bronchospasm (less likely with cardioselective agents)
	—	—	
	—	—	
	—	3.1-6.7	
	—	—	
	—	—	
	5-8	3-5	
	—	—	
	—	—	
	**	**	

Data obtained from US Pharmacopeia[17] and Nissen.[18]

additional data are needed on which to base decisions on α-blocker use for diabetic hypertension,[26] particularly as add-on therapy. However, it appears prudent to reserve α-blockers for use as add-on drugs until clinical trial data can support a more prominent role for them.[15]

Drug Interactions

No significant adverse drug interactions have been reported from combining α-blockers and other commonly used agents.[18]

Contraindications and Precautions

Because the first dose of α-blockers may cause syncope, therapy should always be initiated with a 1-mg dose, and patients should be advised to avoid situations in which injury could occur during syncope. Dose should be titrated slowly, and additional antihypertensives should be added with caution. Hypotension may develop when α-blockers are combined with β-blockers. Although α-blockers have not been associated with teratogenic effects, they should be used during pregnancy only if benefits justify risks. Because some α-blockers are excreted in breast milk, they should be used cautiously in nursing mothers.[18]

β-Adrenoceptor Antagonists

In diabetic patients, long-term use of β-blockers decreases blood pressure and reduces cardiovascular morbidity and mortality.[3] Two categories exist based on the primary type of receptor to which they bind. Cardioselective agents predominantly block the β-1 receptors, which are located in cardiac tissue, whereas noncardioselective agents block β-1 and β-2 receptors, which are primarily located in noncardiac tissue. However, as dose increases, cardioselective agents begin blocking β-2 receptors as well as β-1 receptors. Additionally, betaxolol (Kerlone®), bisoprolol (Zebeta®), metoprolol (Toprol XL®, Lopressor®), penbutolol (Levatol®), pindolol (Visken®), propranolol, and timolol (Blocadren®) are more lipophilic than other β-blockers.[17]

Indications

Long-term β-blocker therapy is generally indicated after MI, and, in one study of diabetic patients, mortality 1 year after such infarction was 10% in those receiving β-blockers vs 23% in those not receiving them.[10] When diabetic patients take β-blockers for hypertension, their rate of coronary heart disease and cardiovascular events is reduced as much as or more than this event rate is reduced when nondiabetic individuals take β-blockers.[3,7] Thus, β-blockers may be the treatment of choice for hypertensive diabetic patients with coronary artery disease (CAD).[7] In large post-MI trials, the β-blockers that reduced mortality and sudden death were all lipophilic, although the importance of this property has not been definitively established.[7] β-Blocker therapy is also indicated for treating angina, certain cardiac arrhythmias, and mitral valve prolapse. Propranolol is also indicated for preventing vascular headache and migraine and treating tremors and performance anxiety.[17]

Mechanism of Action

By competing for receptor binding sites on peripheral and, especially, cardiac adrenergic neurons, β-blockers inhibit the agonistic effect of the sympathetic neurotransmitters[17,18] and thereby decrease cardiac output. Moreover, they may diminish tonic sympathetic nerve outflow from the cerebral vasomotor centers to the peripheral nervous system, thereby decreasing sympathetic stimulation and blood pressure, and may suppress renin secretion by blocking the β-adrenoceptors responsible for renal renin release.[18] However, unlike most antihypertensives, β-blockers do not reverse arteriolar hypertrophy.[2]

Effectiveness

Atenolol was as effective as captopril in reaching blood pressure goals and reducing macrovascular and microvascular complications in type 2 diabetic patients in the UKPDS, and incidence of hypoglycemic episodes did not differ between treatment groups. However, after 8 years, treatment compliance was significantly less, and additional glucose-decreasing medication was significantly more likely to be required with atenolol than with captopril.[3] Dosing and administration of β-blockers are shown in Table 7-3.

Adverse Effects

By directly inhibiting pancreatic insulin release and decreasing serum insulin levels, β-blockers can worsen glucose tolerance.[10] As a class, these agents and diuretics pose a high risk for development of new onset diabetes.[27] Additionally, some β-blockers decrease HDL cholesterol and increase triglyceride levels, although bisoprolol has no adverse effect on lipid profiles and carvedilol may even improve them. Adverse lipid effects result from blockade of β-2 receptors, which are present in noncardiac tissue. Therefore, cardioselective agents, which preferentially block the β-1 receptors present in cardiac tissue, are preferred for most patients and have been used extensively in patients with type 2 diabetes. Using low doses of β-blockers with other agents minimizes their adverse metabolic effect while exploiting their known cardioprotective effect, and lipid effects can be treated by increasing statin or fibrate doses.[7]

By interfering with the counterregulatory effects of catecholamine secretion during hypoglycemic episodes, β-blockers can mask hypoglycemic tachycardia, palpitations, nervousness, and tremor and delay normoglycemia.[7] During β-blocker therapy, hypoglycemia can increase diastolic blood pressure and reflex bradycardia via unopposed α-stimulation.[10] Cardioselective agents are less likely than nonselective ones to have these effects. However, in one study, β-blockers were not associated with increased risk of hypoglycemia. They have been well tolerated in trials, and large numbers of withdrawals related to hyperglycemic or hypoglycemic episodes have not occurred. Inability to recognize hypoglycemic symptoms is rarely a serious problem in patients with type 2 diabetes, particularly when cardioselective agents are used.[7]

Other adverse effects of β-blockers include bronchospasm, cough, decreased exercise tolerance, dizziness, fatigue, headache, insomnia, and intermittent claudication. Like α-blockers, the combined α-/β-blockers carvedilol and labetalol (Normodyne®, Trandate®) may cause postural hypotension.[18]

Drug Interactions

Combining β-blockers with CCBs, such as verapamil (Calan®, Isoptin®, Verelan®) and diltiazem (Cardizem®, Dilacor-XR®, Tiazac®), or antiarrhythmic agents, such as disopyramide (Norpace®), should be undertaken with care. When β-blockers are given with catecholamine-depleting agents, such as reserpine (Serpalan®, Serpasil®) or guanethidine (Ismelin®), excessive sympathetic suppression may result. β-Blockers should be withdrawn several days before clonidine (Catapres®) is withdrawn in patients receiving combination therapy. Combining carvedilol with insulin or sulfonylureas may increase their glucose-lowering effects and require regular blood glucose monitoring. β-Blockers should be continued perioperatively with caution, particularly when anesthesia is being induced with agents that depress myocardial function.[18]

Contraindications and Precautions

β-Blocker use is contraindicated by the presence of cardiogenic shock, overt cardiac failure, second- or third-degree atrioventricular block, and marked sinus bradycardia. Some patients with compensated heart failure may require β-blockers, but they should be used cautiously. Because abrupt cessation of β-blocker therapy may provoke or worsen angina and even precipitate MI or ventricular arrhythmia, the dose should be tapered gradually. Because they can provoke or worsen symptoms of arterial insufficiency in patients with PVD, with the possible exception of labetalol, β-blockers should be used cautiously in such patients.[17,18] β-Blocker use is relatively contraindicated by asthma, bronchospasm, and chronic airflow obstruction.[7,10] Caution should be used in adjusting the dose of some β-blockers if renal or hepatic impairment is present. In patients who have had severe anaphylactic reactions to numerous allergens, β-blocker therapy may intensify reactivity and render them unresponsive to epinephrine. β-Blockers should only be used during pregnancy if benefits justify risks and should be used cautiously in nursing mothers.[18] β-Blockers may not be effective in African-American hypertensive patients unless given with diuretics.[7]

Calcium-channel Antagonists

The second most widely used antihypertensives,[28] calcium-channel antagonists, or CCBs, are heterogeneous. Most CCBs are dihydropyridine derivatives, which do not decrease heart rate. In contrast, the nondihydropyridines do. All CCBs are potent vasodilators, although potency and effect on coronary and peripheral blood vessels vary.[3]

Indications

Except for nisoldipine (Sular®),[18] the CCBs indicated for treating hypertension are also indicated for managing nonvasospastic angina. They are also indicated for managing vasospastic or unstable angina in patients who cannot tolerate β-blockers or nitrates or whose symptoms are not relieved by them. Felodipine (Plendil®), isradipine (DynaCirc®), nicardipine (Cardene®), and nifedipine can also treat Raynaud's phenomenon, and verapamil can relieve ventricular outflow obstruction in hypertrophic cardiomyopathy and reduce the frequency and severity of vascular headaches. Verapamil and parenteral diltiazem are indicated for treating supraventricular tachyarrhythmia.[17]

Mechanism of Action

Calcium-channel blockers decrease elevated peripheral vascular resistance, an important component of diabetic hypertension,[10] by interfering with voltage-dependent calcium channels and decreasing calcium influx and tone in vascular smooth muscle cells. This process also inhibits the vasoconstrictive, hypertrophic, and hyperplastic effects of Ang II and other mitogens on these cells. Although they do not stimulate nitric oxide release or decrease endothelin production, CCBs enhance endothelium-dependent vasodilation by aiding the effects of nitric oxide in these cells and inhibiting endothelin-induced vascular contraction. Because insulin release is associated with calcium influx into pancreatic β cells, CCBs aid this process as well.[3]

Effectiveness

In mild to moderate hypertension, CCBs reduced blood pressure by 5.3 to 18 mm Hg (systolic) and by 3 to 15.4 mm Hg (diastolic) depending on the dosage. Little difference between peak and trough effects was observed, and tolerance did not develop after 1 year.[18] Calcium-channel blockers are particularly useful in reducing systolic blood pressure, which appears more important than reducing diastolic pressure in minimizing cardiovascular risk.[29] Dosing and administration of CCBs are shown in Table 7-4.

Adverse Effects

Calcium-channel blockers generally have no adverse effects on lipid profile or insulin sensitivity. Some of the most common adverse effects of CCB therapy in diabetic hypertensive patients include edema, headache, cough, and gastrointestinal tract disease,[30] particularly bleeding.[6] Calcium-channel blockers decrease esophageal contraction amplitude, and verapamil decreases gastrointestinal transit time[17] and may cause constipation.[31] Because CCBs decrease platelet aggregation, they have increased bleeding time in some. Elevations in hepatic enzyme levels and rare instances of allergic hepatitis have been reported with nifedipine. Other common adverse effects include asthenia, chest pain, dizziness, dry mouth, dyspepsia, dyspnea, fatigue, flushing, nausea, palpitation, polyuria, rash, somnolence, and tachycardia. Nondihydropyridine CCBs may cause conduction defects and worsen systolic dysfunction.[31] First-degree atrioventricular block, bradycardia, and electrocardiographic abnormalities have been reported during antihypertensive therapy with diltiazem.[18] Because CCBs may cause gingival hyperplasia, intensive concurrent plaque control is paramount.[17,31]

Table 7-4: Calcium-channel Antagonists: Action, Dosing, and Effects

Drug Class/Subclass, Antihypertensive Agent, and Brand Name(s)	Mode of Action	Initial Daily Dosage; Maintenance Dosage Range
Dihydropyridine Subclass		
Amlodipine (Norvasc®)	Decrease peripheral vascular resistance by interfering with voltage-dependent calcium channels, decreasing calcium influx, and decreasing tone in vascular smooth muscle cells. Inhibit the vasoconstrictive effects of angiotensin II on vascular smooth muscle cells.	5 mg q.d.; 5-10 mg q.d.
Felodipine (Plendil®)		5 mg q.d.; 5-10 mg q.d.
Isradipine (DynaCirc®/ DynaCirc CR®)		2.5 mg b.i.d.; 2.5-10 mg b.i.d.
Nicardipine (Cardene®)		20 mg t.i.d.; 20 mg t.i.d.
Nifedipine (Adalat®, Procardia®)		
Adalat® CC		30 mg q.d.; 30-60 mg q.d.
Adalat® PA		10-20 mg b.i.d.; 20 mg b.i.d.
Adalat® XL		30-60 mg q.d.; 60-90 mg q.d.
Procardia XL		30-60 mg q.d.; 30-60 mg q.d.
Nisoldipine, extended release (Sular®)		20 mg q.d.; 20-40 mg q.d.

— = not listed, GI = gastrointestinal

Administration and Follow-up Testing	Systolic Blood Pressure Decrease (mm Hg)	Diastolic Blood Pressure Decrease (mm Hg)	Other Effects
For elderly and those with hepatic dysfunction, 2.5 mg q.d. initial dosage is recommended for amlodipine, felodipine, and isradipine and 20 mg q.d. for nisoldipine. Blood pressure should be measured periodically; heart rate determinations are recommended during dosage titration, increase from established maintenance dosage, or addition of other antihypertensives or drugs affecting cardiac conduction.	12-13 5.3-18 — 10.3-16.3 — 6-15	6-7 4.7-10.8 — 9-15.4 — 3-10	Lipid and glucose neutral; inhibit platelet aggregation, prevent atherosclerotic lesions, improve diastolic function, reverse ventricular remodeling; edema, headache, cough, GI disease, gingival hyperplasia, allergic hepatitis (rare)

(continued on next page)

Table 7-4: Calcium-channel Antagonists: Action, Dosing, and Effects *(continued)*

Drug Class/Subclass, Antihypertensive Agent, and Brand Name(s)	Mode of Action	Initial Daily Dosage; Maintenance Dosage Range
Nondihydropyridine Subclass		
Diltiazem (Cardizem® SR, Cardizem® CD, Dilacor-XR®, Tiazac®) Cardizem® CD		180-240 mg q.d.; 240-360 mg/d
Cardizem® SR		60-120 mg b.i.d.; 60-120 mg b.i.d.
Dilacor-XR®		180-240 mg q.d.; 240-360 mg/d
Verapamil Tablets (Calan®, Isoptin®)		80-120 mg t.i.d.; 240-480 mg/d
Tablets, extended-release (Calan® SR, Isoptin® SR)		180 mg q.d.; 240-480 mg/d
Extended-release capsules (Verelan®)		240 mg q.d.; 240-480 mg/d

— = not listed, GI = gastrointestinal

Drug Interactions

Agents whose interactions with CCBs are of major clinical significance include anesthetics, aspirin, β-blockers, carbamazepine (Tegretol®, Carbatrol®), cimetidine (Tagamet®), cyclosporine, digitalis glycosides, disopyramide or flecainide (Tambocor™), hypokalemia-producing medications, procainamide, quinidine

Administration and Follow-up Testing	Systolic Blood Pressure Decrease (mm Hg)	Diastolic Blood Pressure Decrease (mm Hg)	Other Effects
Same as for dihydropyridines but ECG readings are also recommended	—	4.5-10.5	Same as for dihydropyridines but may cause conduction defects
	—	3.8-10	

Data obtained from US Pharmacopeia[17] and Nissen.[18]

(Quinidex®, Quinaglute®) or other medications that prolong the Q-T interval, theophylline (Uniphyl®), and valproate (Depacon®).[17,18]

Contraindications and Precautions

Use of sublingual nifedipine capsules in hypertensive crisis has been associated with severe hypotension, acute MI, stroke, and death and is therefore contraindicated.[17] Rarely, acute hypotension has been reported as a result of CCB therapy, particularly when severe aortic stenosis is present, and may cause dizziness, syncope, or reflex tachycardia and precipitate angina pectoris or MI, particularly in patients with severe obstructive CAD. Calcium-channel blockers should be used cautiously in patients with severe heart failure, compromised ventricular function, or hepatic or renal impairment. Diltiazem use is contraindicated by sick sinus syndrome, second- or third-degree atrioventricular block, hypotension, acute MI, and pulmonary congestion. In rare cases, erythema multiforme and exfoliative dermatitis have been reported with diltiazem, and, if they persist, it should be discontinued. Because verapamil decreases neuromuscular transmission in patients with Duchenne's muscular dystrophy, a decrease in dosage may be necessary. Calcium-channel blockers should be used during pregnancy only if benefits justify risks and should be discontinued during nursing.[18]

Diuretics

Although some diuretics can worsen hyperglycemia, diuretics are not contraindicated when diabetes is reasonably well controlled, and, because diabetic hypertension is volume-dependent, diuretics are frequently integral to its treatment.[10] Four types of diuretics exist: thiazide, thiazide-like, loop, and potassium-sparing. Table 7-5 lists the available diuretics by type with details on their dosage and administration.

Indications

Except for metolazone (Zaroxolyn®, Mykrox®), diuretics are indicated for treating edema as well as hypertension. Unlike thiazide and thiazide-like diuretics, loop diuretics are not considered primary agents for treating essential hypertension, but they can be combined with other agents to treat renal hypertension. Like loop diuretics, potassium-sparing diuretics are indicated for adjunctive treatment of hypertension, especially when potassium-sparing is desired. Thiazide and thiazide-like diuretics are also indicated for treating diabetes insipidus and for preventing calcium-containing kidney stones, and loop and potassium-sparing diuretics, for treating and preventing hypercalcemia. Because it is a competitive inhibitor of aldosterone, spironolactone (Aldactone®) is indicated for treating primary hyperaldosteronism. It may also have an antiandrogenic effect and is indicated for treating female hirsutism as well as polycystic ovary syndrome, an insulin-resistant condition. It may also be used adjunctively to reduce morbidity and mortality in severe congestive heart failure.[17] Because ethacrynic acid (Edecrin®) is the only nonsulfonamide diuretic, it may be useful for patients who are allergic to sulfa drugs.[31]

Mechanisms of Action

Diuretics decrease blood pressure initially by reducing plasma and extracellular fluid volume. They decrease cardiac output, which eventually normalizes. Thiazides exert a direct effect on peripheral arterioles, thereby decreasing peripheral resistance,[17] and interfere with the renal tubular mechanism of electrolyte reabsorption, increasing excretion of sodium and chloride in equivalent amounts by blocking sodium reabsorption and causing secondary loss of potassium, bicarbonate, and water. Their continued use may cause sodium depletion, which helps reduce blood pressure but may cause excessive potassium, magnesium, chloride, and hydrogen loss. Calcium and uric acid excretion and glomerular filtration rate may decrease, and iodide excretion may increase. Although their long-term use in high doses can cause mild alkalosis from hypokalemia and hypochloremia, metabolic toxicity from electrolyte imbalance can be avoided by using low doses. Thiazides also increase plasma renin activity and aldosterone secretion.[18,32] Loop diuretics act on the ascending limb of the loop of Henle and the proximal and, except for bumetanide (Bumex®), distal tubule to inhibit chloride more than sodium reabsorption and increase water and electrolyte excretion several times more than thiazides.

Table 7-5: Older Antihypertensive Agents: Action, Dosing, and Effects

Drug Class/Subclass, Antihypertensive Agent, and Brand Name(s)	Mode of Action	Initial Daily Dosage; Maintenance Dosage Range
Central α-Adrenoceptor Agonists		
Clonidine (Catapres®)	Stimulate α-adrenoceptors in brain stem, reduce sympathetic outflow from central nervous system, decrease peripheral and renal vascular resistance, heart rate, and blood pressure	0.1 mg b.i.d.; 0.2-0.6 mg/d
Guanabenz (Wytensin®)		4 mg b.i.d.; 8-64 mg/d
Guanfacine (Tenex®)		1 mg q.d.; 1-3 mg q.d.
Methyldopa (Aldomet®)		250 mg b.i.d./t.i.d; 500 mg-2 g/d in 2-4 doses
Diuretics		
Thiazide	Reduce plasma and extracellular fluid volume	
Bendroflumethiazide (Naturetin®)		2.5-20 mg/d; 2.5-20 mg/d*
Chlorothiazide (Diuril®)		250 mg-1 g/d; 500 mg-1g/d*

* Can be given as a single dose or in 2 equal divided doses.

Administration and Follow-up Testing	**Other Effects**
Transdermal clonidine patches are also available; change weekly. Initial effects take 2-3 days. For methyldopa, obtain initial and periodic blood count, Coombs' test, and liver function test results.	Guanabenz promotes minor weight loss and lipid profile improvement; constipation, dizziness, sedation (methyldopa can cause hepatic and autoimmune disease and hemolytic anemia)
Periodically measure serum electrolyte levels.	Reduce cardiovascular morbidity and mortality

(continued on next page)

Table 7-5: Older Antihypertensive Agents: Action, Dosing, and Effects *(continued)*

Drug Class/Subclass, Antihypertensive Agent, and Brand Name(s)	Mode of Action	Initial Daily Dosage; Maintenance Dosage Range
Thiazide *(continued)*		
Hydrochlorothiazide Tablets (Esidrix, HydroDIURIL®, Oretic®) Capsules (Microzide®)	Directly dilate peripheral arterioles and decrease peripheral resistance, interfere with renal tubular electrolyte reabsorption, increase sodium and chloride excretion, block sodium reabsorption, thereby causing loss of potassium, bicarbonate, and water. Continued use may cause sodium depletion, aiding blood pressure reduction.	25-100 mg/d; 25-100 mg/d* 12.5 mg q.d.; 12.5-50 mg/d
Hydroflumethiazide (Diucardin®, Saluron®)		50-100 mg/d; 50-100 mg/d*
Methyclothiazide (Aquatensen®, Enduron®)		2.5-5 mg q.d.; 2.5-5 mg q.d.
Polythiazide (Renese®)		2-4 mg q.d.; 2-4 mg q.d.
Trichlormethiazide (Naqua®)		2-4 mg q.d.; 2-4 mg q.d.
Thiazide-like		
Chlorthalidone (Hygroton®, Thalitone®)		25 mg q.d.; 25-100 mg q.d.
Indapamide (Lozol®)		1.25 mg q.d.; 1.25-5 q.d.
Metolazone Zaroxolyn®		2.5-5 mg q.d.; 2.5-5 mg q.d.
Mykrox® (rapidly available formulation)		0.5 mg q.d.; 1 mg q.d.
Quinethazone (Hydromox®)		25/50 mg/d; 50-200 mg/d*

* Can be given as a single dose or in 2 equal divided doses.

Administration and Follow-up Testing

For indapamide, periodically measure uric acid levels as well as serum electrolyte levels.

Other Effects

Electrolyte imbalance, hypovolemia, may increase insulin resistance, dyslipidemia, and uric acid levels; may in rare cases cause blood dyscrasias, liver damage, pancreatitis, and photosensitivity

(continued on next page)

Table 7-5: Older Antihypertensive Agents: Action, Dosing, and Effects *(continued)*

Drug Class/Subclass, Antihypertensive Agent, and Brand Name(s)	Mode of Action	Initial Daily Dosage; Maintenance Dosage Range
Loop Bumetanide (Bumex®)	Inhibit chloride reabsorption more than	0.5 mg-2 mg q.d.; 0.5-10 mg/d**
Ethacrynic acid (Edecrin®)	sodium re-absorption and	50-100 mg/d; 50-400 mg/d*
Furosemide (Lasix®)	increase water and electrolyte	40 mg b.i.d.; 40-600 mg/d
Torsemide (Demadex®)	excretion	5 mg q.d.; 5-10 mg q.d.
Potassium-sparing Amiloride (Midamor®)	Inhibit exchange of sodium for potassium,	5-10 mg q.d.; 5-20 mg/d
Spironolactone (Aldactone®)	sodium reabsorption;	50-100 mg q.d.; 50-200 mg/d†
Triamterene (Dyrenium®)	increase sodium and water excretion while sparing potassium	100 mg b.i.d.; 200-300 mg/d

* May be given as a single dose or in 2 equal divided doses.
** May be given in 2 or 3 daily doses or on alternate days or by incorporating 1- to 2-day medication-free periods in between 3- to 4-day dosing periods.
† May be given as a single daily dose or in 2-4 divided doses.

Administration and Follow-up Testing

Periodically measure serum electrolyte levels. Use potassium supplements or potassium-sparing agents with ethacrynic acid.

Take amiloride with or after meals. Periodically measure serum electrolyte levels.

Other Effects

Same as thiazides plus risk of hyperkalemia; spironolactone may cause gynecomastia and breast cancer

Same as thiazides plus ototoxicity

(continued on next page)

Table 7-5: Older Antihypertensive Agents: Action, Dosing, and Effects *(continued)*

Drug Class/Subclass, Antihypertensive Agent, and Brand Name(s)	Mode of Action	Initial Daily Dosage; Maintenance Dosage Range
Peripheral Adrenergic Antagonists		
Reserpine	Deplete stores and/or inhibit release of catecholamines, depress sympathetic function, relax vascular smooth muscle, decrease heart rate and arterial blood pressure	0.5 mg/d; 0.1-0.25 mg/d
Guanadrel (Hylorel®)		10 mg/d; 20-75 mg/d‡
Guanethidine (Ismelin®)		10 mg/d; 25-50 mg/d
Vasodilators, Direct		
Hydralazine (Apresoline®)	Decrease peripheral resistance through direct vasodilation	40 mg/d; 40-300 mg/d§
Minoxidil (Loniten®)		5 mg q.d.; 10-40 mg/d†

† May be given as a single daily dose or in 2-4 divided doses.

‡ Should be given in divided doses.

§ Initial dosage should be used for the first 2-4 days and divided into 4 daily doses, and daily dosage for the rest of the first week should be 100 mg divided into 4 daily doses. Daily dosage should

Administration and Follow-up Testing	Other Effects
For guanethidine, increase dosage gradually every 5-7 days and only if standing blood pressure has not decreased from previous levels.	Orthostatic hypotension, worsened peptic ulcer/colitis, biliary colic, depression, nasal congestion, weight gain, sedation, impotence
For minoxidil, if supine diastolic pressure was reduced <30 mm Hg, dose q.d.; if it was reduced >30 mm Hg, give two divided doses daily.	Increase renal blood flow; tachycardia, chest pain, edema, tamponade, lupus-like syndrome, peripheral neuritis

be 200 mg divided into 4 daily doses in the subsequent weeks. Adjust maintenance dosage to lowest effective level.

— = not listed

Data obtained from U.S. Pharmacopeia,[17] Nissen,[18] and Noueihed.[32]

With long-term use, chloride excretion decreases and potassium and hydrogen excretion may increase. Except when diuresis is rapid and plasma volume is severely reduced, loop diuretics produce more favorable sodium/potassium excretion ratios than thiazides and, unlike thiazides, do not affect glomerular filtration or renal blood flow, so they are effective in patients with renal insufficiency.[32] In the distal convoluted tubule, spironolactone competitively binds with receptors at the aldosterone-dependent sodium-potassium exchange site to inhibit the exchange of sodium for potassium, increasing the amount of sodium and water for excretion, while sparing potassium. Other potassium-sparing diuretics act at this site as well as the cortical collecting tubule and collecting duct to inhibit sodium reabsorption, decrease the tubular lumen's negative potential, and, thus, reduce potassium and hydrogen secretion and excretion. Their weak natriuretic, diuretic, and hypotensive effects are partially additive to those of thiazides, and they decrease magnesium excretion when given with them.[18]

Effectiveness and Clinical Benefits

Diuretics not only lower blood pressure effectively but also reduce cardiovascular morbidity and mortality when used as monotherapy or in combination therapy,[3] and their ability to provide these benefits in diabetic patients with systolic hypertension is proven.[5] In a large cohort of elderly diabetic patients with isolated systolic hypertension studied for 5 years by the Systolic Hypertension in the Elderly Program (SHEP), low-dose chlorthalidone-based treatment lowered blood pressure, prevented major cardiovascular events, and produced few adverse effects relative to placebo treatment.[3,33] Although the relative treatment benefit in patients with diabetes was similar to that in individuals without diabetes, the absolute benefit in terms of number of patients needed to treat to prevent one cardiovascular complication was lower in diabetic patients than in nondiabetic individuals. These results also refuted the notion that diuretics should be avoided in diabetic patients because they increase blood glucose levels.[33] More recently, ALLHAT found chlorthalidone to be superior to amlodipine and lisinopril in reducing systolic blood pressure and in preventing heart failure and superior to lisinopril in preventing stroke. As a result, the ALLHAT investigators recommended that thiazides be used as initial antihypertensive therapy in patients with hypertension and at least one other CAD risk factor.[34]

Adverse Effects

Diuretics may cause hypovolemia and electrolyte imbalance.[18] Although diuretics are recommended for hypertensive diabetic patients, no consensus exists regarding their use in clinical practice. Many do not prescribe thiazides because they may alter carbohydrate metabolism, increase insulin resistance, promote hyperinsulinemia and dyslipidemia, and cause electrolyte imbalance[3] by decreasing potassium, sodium, and magnesium and increasing calcium levels. Although the loop diuretics bumetanide and furosemide (Lasix®) do not induce hypercalcemia, their duration of action is short.[31] Thiazide diuretics have been the diuretics most closely associated with promoting diabetes, and thiazide-like diuretics and the loop diuretic furosemide also have this effect. One exception is indapamide (Lozol®), which, in low doses, can reduce blood pressure without worsening glucose control or lipid profile.[10] Although some reports indicated that long-term diuretic therapy can worsen glucose tolerance, others showed no increased incidence of diabetes compared with that associated with other agents.[10] Low-dose thiazide therapy is not generally associated with an adverse metabolic effect, which may respond to diet therapy if it does occur.[3] Because this effect is mediated by impaired insulin release induced by hypokalemia, it can be avoided by maintaining normokalemia with potassium supplementation, which can also control blood pressure.

High-dose diuretics should be avoided because of risk of hypokalemia, hypomagnesemia, ventricular arrhythmia, and sudden death in susceptible patients.[10] Although judicious use of thiazides can reduce risk of stroke and congestive heart failure, high doses have been associated with increased mortality from cardiovascular disease. However, smaller doses (eg, 12.5 mg hydrochlorothiazide or less daily) have the same hypotensive effects but no clinically significant adverse effects.[5] Potassium-sparing diuretics pose a risk of hyperkalemia that is greater in diabetic patients than in nondiabetic individuals.[3] Spironolactone may cause gynecomastia[31] and should be avoided in patients with breast enlargement or menstrual abnormalities. Breast carcinoma has been reported in men and women during spironolactone therapy.[17] Although, in short-term trials, most diuretics increased cholesterol and triglyceride levels, in most longer-term trials, these levels returned to normal.[10] Diuretics can also increase uric acid levels and, in rare cases, cause blood dyscrasias, liver damage, photosensitivity, pancreatitis, and hyponatremia. Loop diuretics can be ototoxic.[32] Other adverse effects include abdominal pain, anorexia, confusion, constipation, diarrhea, dysphagia, fatigue, flatulence, headache, irritability, muscle cramps, nausea, orthostatic hypotension, skin rash, vomiting, and weakness.[17,18]

Drug Interactions

Patients sensitive to sulfonamides may be sensitive to most diuretics. Combining diuretics with lithium should be avoided because they reduce its clearance and increase toxicity risk. Thiazides may increase risk of digitalis toxicity from hypomagnesemia or hypokalemia, and their use with amiodarone (Cordarone®, Pacerone®) may increase risk of arrhythmias associated with hypokalemia. Combining thiazides with other agents that cause hypokalemia requires careful monitoring of serum potassium level and cardiac function and, possibly, potassium supplementation. Combining thiazides with agents that contain calcium may cause hypercalcemia. Thiazide therapy may require adjusting anticoagulant or antidiabetic dosages. Combining thiazides with other antihypertensives may potentiate their effects to excess, and sympathomimetics may antagonize thiazides' hypotensive effect. Use of NSAIDs with thiazides may increase plasma renin activity or risk of renal failure.[17] Using two loop diuretics or combining them with aminoglycosides or cephalosporins increases risk of ototoxicity and should be avoided. Use of ethacrynic acid with warfarin (Coumadin®) may require reduction in warfarin dose.[32] Combining torsemide (Demadex®) with salicylates may produce salicylate toxicity. In some patients, NSAIDs, particularly indomethacin (Indocin® IV), may reduce the hypotensive effects of diuretics. Severe hyperkalemia may result when potassium-sparing diuretics are given with NSAIDs, ACEIs, or potassium supplements.[18] Spironolactone may increase digoxin (Digitek®, Lanoxicaps®, Lanoxin®) half-life, and triamterene (Dyrenium®) may antagonize allopurinol, colchicine, probenecid (Benemid®, Probalan®), or sulfinpyrazone (Anturane®),[17] whereas probenecid may antagonize bumetanide.[18]

Contraindications and Precautions

Patients treated with diuretics should be carefully observed for evidence of fluid or electrolyte imbalance.[18] In patients with advanced renal insufficiency and serum creatinine level greater than 2 to 3 mg/dL, thiazides are ineffective, and loop diuretics are usually required.[10,35] Use of thiazides may worsen lupus in patients with a history of this disease,[17] and risk vs benefit should be carefully considered in patients with hyperuricemia, a history of gout, or pancreatitis. Loop diuretics may cause hyperuricemia and, in dehydrated patients with renal insufficiency, reversible elevations in blood urea nitrogen (BUN) and creatinine level.[17] In patients with cirrhosis, loop diuresis should be initiated in the hospital.[17] Because potassium-sparing diuretics may cause or worsen hyperkalemia, especially in diabetic patients, their use is contraindicated by anuria, impaired renal function, or hyperkalemia.[18] They may elevate BUN levels when combined with other diuretics and should be avoided in patients with hepatic impairment, who are more sensitive to electrolyte changes. Hyperuricemia, gout, or a history of nephrolithiasis contraindicates triamterene use. Use of diuretics should be avoided in pregnant patients unless benefits justify risks.[17] Diuretics do not prevent toxemia of pregnancy and have not been proven useful in treating it.[18] Thiazides should be avoided during the first month of nursing because they may suppress lactation.[17]

Combination Therapy

Because hypertension is a multifactorial disease, interrupting a single contributory physiologic pathway is frequently insufficient to reach target blood pressure. Combining agents from different drug classes that affect different physiologic pathways may be required for adequate control.[36] Furthermore, adding a second antihypertensive agent is recommended if target blood pressure cannot be achieved with a single agent,[37] and many, if not most, type 2 diabetic patients require combination therapy. For example, more than 65% of micro- or macroalbuminuric diabetic hypertensive patients studied in a review of clinical trials needed at least two antihypertensive agents to attain the current recommended target of 130/85 mm Hg.[4,38] In the UKPDS, almost one third of patients (29%) required at least three antihypertensive agents to achieve an average blood pressure of 144/82 mm Hg, which, by current standards, would be considered high.[37] In HOT, 73% of patients required about 2.7 different antihypertensive agents to reach a diastolic blood pressure of less than 80 mm Hg.[4] Diabetic patients with renal insufficiency often require moderate to high doses of three different antihypertensives to reach lower blood pressure targets.[38] Thus, for most diabetic patients, reaching goals with monotherapy is challenging, particularly because fear of increased side effects and patient resistance make many clinicians reluctant to titrate the dose or change agents. Nevertheless, the most important factor in decreasing their high incidence of CAD may be aggressive early hypertension control,[36] and one of the most important factors in slowing renal disease progression in patients with type 2 diabetes is the level of arterial pressure reduction, particularly systolic.[37]

Using low-dose combination antihypertensive therapy either as first-line treatment or early in the disease course can meet many of these challenges, and it has been recommended as an alternative to standard first-line monotherapy in reducing hypertension. Low-dose combinations are more effective than monotherapy because of the additive and sometimes even synergistic hypotensive effects of their complementary agents. Because they typically incorporate long-acting components, they can be given once daily in a single tablet or capsule to conveniently provide 24-hour effects and control surges during the crucial early morning hours when cardiovascular risk is highest. Their response rates, which range from 75% to 90%, are considerably higher than the 30% to 60% for monotherapy. Although some type 2 diabetic patients have severe hypertension that requires conventional fixed-dose combination therapy, in which the highest recommended doses of each agent are combined in one tablet for convenience, most patients with type 2 diabetes have mild hypertension and, therefore, do not. In contrast with conventional fixed-dose agents, low-dose combinations cause fewer dose-dependent side effects, including metabolic ones, than monotherapy. The benefits of low-dose combinations, as well as their frequently lower cost, may enhance patient compliance, the most important factor in adequately controlling blood pressure.[36] Table 7-6 lists the low-dose combinations now available for treating hypertension.

Indications

Combination therapy may be particularly valuable in reaching the even lower target blood pressures recommended for type 2 diabetic patients with comorbidities than those generally recommended for diabetic patients. In patients with CAD, the recommended blood pressure target is 120/80 mm Hg, and, in those with diabetic neph-

Table 7-6: Low-dose Combination Antihypertensive Agents

Drug Class/Brand Name	Available Low Doses (mg)
β-*Blocker/Diuretic*	
Bisoprolol/hydrochlorothiazide (Ziac®)	2.5/6.25; 5/6.25; 10/12.5
Metoprolol tartrate/hydrochlorothiazide (Lopressor HCT®)	50/25; 100/25
Propranolol/hydrochlorothiazide (Inderide®)	40/25; 80/25
Timolol/hydrochlorothiazide (Timolide®)	10/25
ACEI/Diuretic	
Benazepril/hydrochlorothiazide (Lotensin HCT®)	5/6.25; 10/12.5; 20/12.5; 20/25
Captopril/hydrochlorothiazide (Capozide)	25/15; 25/25; 50/15; 50/25
Enalapril/hydrochlorothiazide (Vaseretic®)	5/12.5; 10/25
Fosinopril/hydrochlorothiazide (Monopril HCT®)	10/12.5; 20/12.5
Lisinopril/hydrochlorothiazide (Prinzide®, Zestoretic®)	10/12.5; 20/12.5; 20/25
Moexipril/hydrochlorothiazide (Uniretic™)	7.5/12.5; 15/25
Quinapril/hydrochlorothiazide (Accuretic®)	10/12.5; 20/12.5; 20/25

ACEI = angiotensin-converting enzyme inhibitor
ARB = angiotensin II receptor blocker
CCB = calcium-channel blocker

Drug Class/Brand Name	Available Low Doses (mg)
ARB/*Diuretic*	
Irbesartan/hydrochlorothiazide (Avalide®)	150/12.5
Losartan/hydrochlorothiazide (Hyzaar®)	50/12.5; 100/25
Telmisartan/hydrochlorothiazide (Micardis HCT®)	40/12.5; 80/12.5
Valsartan/hydrochlorothiazide (Diovan HCT®)	80/12.5; 160/12.5; 160/25
CCB/*ACEI*	
Amlodipine/benazepril (Lotrel®)	2.5/10; 5/10; 5/20
Diltiazem/enalapril (Teczem®)	180/5
Felodipine/enalapril (Lexxel®)	5/2.5; 5/5
Verapamil (extended release)/ trandolapril (Tarka®)	180/1; 180/2; 180/4; 240/1; 240/2; 240/4

Data obtained from US Pharmacopeia,[17] Nissen,[18] and Neutel.[36]

ropathy, the rate of decline in renal function appears to be a continuous function of arterial pressure down to levels of 125 to 130 mm Hg (systolic) and 70 to 75 mm Hg (diastolic).[37] Reducing blood pressure to 110/75 mm Hg is associated with significant renal protection in type 2 diabetic patients, regardless of agent used.[36]

Reducing Adverse Effects

Except for ACEI-induced cough, most adverse effects of antihypertensive treatment, such as the hypokalemia and hyperglycemia associated with thiazides and the decreases in HDL cholesterol induced by some β-blockers, are dose-dependent. However, when β-blockers and diuretics are combined in low doses, they may have slightly beneficial effects on glucose and lipid levels. In other cases as well, although high-dose monotherapy is frequently associated with more side effects than low-dose combination therapy, in some cases, the side-effect profile of the combination may be more favorable than that for either drug used as monotherapy at the same dose. For example, when an ACEI is combined with a dihydropyridine CCB, ACEI-induced venodilation counteracts and mitigates the unopposed arterial vasodilation produced by the dihydropyridine, reducing capillary perfusion pressure and risk of capillary leak syndrome and peripheral edema. Diuretics are useful in combination therapy because they can reduce the compensatory fluid retention often associated with vasodilators. Ziac® and Capozide®, the two low-dose combination agents approved by the FDA for use as first-line agents in initial therapy, incorporate hydrochlorothiazide.[36]

References

1. Chobanian AV, Bakris GL, Black HR, et al: The Seventh Report of the Joint National Committee on Prevention, Detection, Evaluation, and Treatment of High Blood Pressure: The JNC 7 Report. *JAMA* 2003;289:2560-2571.

2. Julius S, Majahalme S, Palatini P: Antihypertensive treatment of patients with diabetes and hypertension. *Am J Hypertens* 2001; 14:310S-316S.

3.   Garber AJ: Treatment of hypertension in patients with diabetes mellitus. In: *Current Review of Diabetes*. Taylor SI, ed. Philadelphia, Current Medicine, Inc, 1999, pp 105-113.

4.   Bakris GL, Williams M, Dworkin L, et al: Preserving renal function in adults with hypertension and diabetes: a consensus approach. *Am J Kidney Dis* 2000;36:646-661.

5.   Fineberg SE: The treatment of hypertension and dyslipidemia in diabetes mellitus. *Prim Care* 1999;26:951-964.

6.   Kaplan RC, Heckbert SR, Koepsell TD, et al: Use of calcium channel blockers and risk of hospitalized gastrointestinal tract bleeding. *Arch Intern Med* 2000;160:1849-1855.

7.   Dunne F, Kendall MJ, Martin U: β-blockers in the management of hypertension in patients with type 2 diabetes mellitus: is there a role? *Drugs* 2001;61:429-435.

8.   American Diabetes Association. Treatment of hypertension in adults with diabetes. *Diabetes Care* 2003;26(suppl 1):S80-S82.

9.   Laakso M: Benefits of strict glucose and blood pressure control in type 2 diabetes: lessons from the UK Prospective Diabetes Study. *Circulation* 1999;99:461-462.

10.   Hall WD: Hypertension in the patients with diabetes. In: Davidson JK, ed: *Clinical Diabetes Mellitus: a Problem-Oriented Approach*. New York, Thieme Medical Publishers, 2000, pp 663-674.

11.   Sowers JR: Diabetes and hypertension. In: Johnstone MT, Veves A, eds: *Contemporary Cardiology: Diabetes and Cardiovascular Disease*. Totowa (NJ), Humana Press, 2001, pp 123-129.

12.   Landsberg L: Insulin resistance and hypertension. *Clin Exp Hypertens* 1999;21:885-894.

13.   American Diabetes Association. Position statement: Diabetes mellitus and exercise. *Diabetes Care* 2001;24(suppl 1). Available at http://www.diabetes.org/clinicalrecommentations/Supplement101/S51.htm.

14.   American Diabetes Association: Position statement: Nutrition recommendations and principles for people with diabetes mellitus. *Diabetes Care* 2001;24(suppl 1). Available at http://www.diabetes.org/clinicalrecommentations/Supplement101/S44.htm.

15.   Furberg CD, Psaty BM, Pahor M, et al: Clinical implications of recent findings from the Antihypertensive and Lipid-Lowering Treatment to Prevent Heart Attack Trial (ALLHAT) and other studies of hypertension. *Ann Intern Med* 2001;135:1074-1078.

16. Lewis EJ, Hunsicker LG, Clarke WR, et al: Renoprotective effect of the angiotensin-receptor antagonist irbesartan in patients with nephropathy due to type 2 diabetes. *N Engl J Med* 2001;345: 851-860.

17. US Pharmacopeial Convention, Inc: US Pharmacopeia Dispensing Information, Volume II-Drug Information for the Health Care Professional. Greenwood Village, CO, MICROMEDIX Thomson Healthcare, 2002.

18. Nissen D, ed: 2002 *Mosby's Drug Consult.* St. Louis (MO), Mosby, 2002.

19. Deedwania PC: Hypertension and diabetes: new therapeutic options. *Arch Intern Med* 2000;160:1585-1594.

20. Brenner BM, Cooper ME, de Zeeuw D, et al: Effects of losartan on renal and cardiovascular outcomes in patients with type 2 diabetes and nephropathy. *N Engl J Med* 2001;345:861-869.

21. Dahlof B, Devereux RB, Kjeldsen SE, et al: Cardiovascular morbidity and mortality in the Losartan Intervention For Endpoint reduction in hypertension study (LIFE): a randomised trial against atenolol. *Lancet* 2002;359:995-1003.

22. Cohn JN, Tognoni G: A randomized trial of the angiotensin-receptor blocker valsartan in chronic heart failure. *N Engl J Med* 2001;345:1667-1675.

23. Manzo BA, Matalka MS: Hypertension management: future therapeutic options (Web page). California Society of Health-System Pharmacists Web site. Available at http://www.continuingeducation.com/pharmacy/hyper-management. Posted April 1, 2001; accessed August 3, 2002.

24. Coats AJ: Angiotensin receptor blockers–finally the evidence is coming in: IDNT and RENAAL. *Int J Cardiol* 2001;79:99-102.

25. Siragy HM, Carey RM: Angiotensin type 2 receptors: potential importance in the regulation of blood pressure. *Curr Opin Nephrol Hypertens* 2001;10:99-103.

26. Poulter N, Williams B: Doxazosin for the management of hypertension: implications of the findings of the ALLHAT trial. *Am J Hypertens* 2001;14:1170-1171.

27. Cressman MD, Vidt DG, Mohler H, et al: Glucose tolerance during chronic propranolol treatment. *J Clin Hypertens* 1985;1:138-144.

28. Moser M: Is it time for a new approach to the initial treatment of hypertension? *Arch Intern Med* 2001;161:1140-1144.

29.   Bakris GL: New concepts in hypertension therapy and cardio-vascular disease: the role of calcium channel blockers (Web presentation). Medscape.com Web page. School of Medicine, Medical College of Virginia, Virginia Commonwealth University, 2002. www.medscape.com/viewprogram/1001_pnt. Posted March 22, 2002; accessed August 3, 2002.

30.   Grossman E, Messerli FH, Goldbourt U: High blood pressure and diabetes mellitus: are all antihypertensive drugs created equal? *Arch Intern Med* 2000;160:2447-2452.

31.   The sixth report of the Joint National Committee on prevention, detection, evaluation and treatment of high blood pressure. *Arch Intern Med* 1997;157:2413-2446.

32.   Noueihed LA, ed: *PDR Generics*. Montvale, NJ, Medical Economics Co, 1998.

33.   Furberg CD: Hypertension and diabetes: current issues. *Am Heart J* 1999;138:S400-S405.

34.   Major outcomes in high-risk hypertensive patients randomized to angiotensin-converting enzyme inhibitor or calcium-channel blocker vs diuretic: The Antihypertensive and Lipid-Lowering Treatment to Prevent Heart Attack Trial (ALLHAT). *JAMA* 2002;288:2981-2997.

35.   Bakris GL: A practical approach to achieving recommended blood pressure goals in diabetic patients. *Arch Intern Med* 2001; 161:2661-2667.

36.   Neutel JM: The use of combination drug therapy in the treatment of hypertension. *Prog Cardiovasc Nurs* 2002;17:81-88.

37.   Sheinfeld GR, Bakris GL: Benefits of combination angiotensin-converting enzyme inhibitor and calcium antagonist therapy for diabetic patients. *Am J Hypertens* 1999;12:80S-85S.

38.   Odama UO, Bakris GL: Combination therapy for hypertension and renal disease in diabetes. Chapter 42. In Mogensen CE, ed: *The Kidney and Hypertension in Diabetes Mellitus*. 5th ed. Boston: Kluwer Academic Publishers, 2000, pp 559-573.

Chapter 8

Dyslipidemia: Reaching New Targets

Diabetic Dyslipidemia Defined

Elevated levels of triglyceride, decreased levels of high-density lipoprotein (HDL) cholesterol, and a preponderance of small, dense, atherogenic low-density lipoprotein (LDL) particles are the chief lipid abnormalities in type 2 diabetic dyslipidemia. These lipid abnormalities persist to some extent even when blood glucose levels approach normal.[1] They constitute the most common pattern of dyslipidemia in patients with type 2 diabetes[2] and generally precede the onset of diabetes.[1] As many as 95% of patients with type 2 diabetes have triglyceride levels below 400 mg/dL, and the median triglyceride level of this group is less than 200 mg/dL.[2] However, poor glycemic control can be expected to worsen hypertriglyceridemia in patients whose triglyceride levels are already elevated.

Diabetic nephropathy is associated with increased levels of triglycerides, even during the early stages of microalbuminuria, while HDL cholesterol levels may fall and LDL cholesterol and lipoprotein(a) [Lp(a)] levels may rise.[1] Lp(a) is an LDL globule enveloped by the adhesive molecule apoprotein(a), which attaches lipoprotein to vessel walls, thereby promoting atherogenesis. An elevated Lp(a) level has been shown to pose 10 times the coronary heart disease (CHD) risk of an elevated LDL cholesterol level.[3] Such proatherogenic changes probably contribute to the increased risk for CHD posed by diabetic nephropathy.[1]

In general, LDL cholesterol levels in patients with type 2 diabetes are not significantly different from those in nondiabetic individuals, and the prevalence of hypercholesterolemia is the same in both groups. However, the relative risk of CHD is substantially elevated at each cholesterol level in patients with type 2 diabetes, possibly because these patients have more atherogenic, small, dense LDL particles and a lack of the more cardioprotective HDL_2 subfraction.[2]

Patients with type 2 diabetes can have lipid abnormalities other than hypertriglyceridemia or low HDL cholesterol levels, including hyperchylomicronemia and elevated levels of very low density lipoprotein (VLDL).[4] Chylomicrons contain a truncated form of apolipoprotein B, called apoB48, which is only 48% of the length of the complete molecule, lacks the protein that interacts with the LDL receptor, and has been implicated in atherogenesis in many animal models.[5] Patients with type 2 diabetes also often have elevated levels of small, dense VLDL particles and intermediate-density lipoprotein, which have both been associated with increased atherogenesis.[4] As in nondiabetic individuals, lipid levels in patients with type 2 diabetes may be affected by genetically determined lipoprotein disorders, such as familial combined hyperlipidemia and familial hypertriglyceridemia.[6]

Treatment Rationale

Patients with type 2 diabetes have a CHD risk two to four times that of nondiabetic individuals. As many as 80% of adult diabetic patients die of diseases associated with atherosclerosis, including CHD, cerebrovascular disease, and peripheral vascular disease.[6] As a result, controlling risk factors associated with atherosclerosis in these patients is paramount. However, hyperglycemia is only modestly related to the development of macrovascular disease in patients with type 2 diabetes, and cardiovascular risk factors increase even before the onset of type 2 diabetes. These findings indicate that aggressive diabetes screening and improvements in glycemic control alone cannot eliminate excess cardiovascular risk in patients with type 2 diabetes. Instead, a multifactorial approach to cardiovascular disease prevention is required.[2]

The Multiple Risk Factor Intervention Trial (MRFIT) showed that elevated total cholesterol levels are associated with an increased incidence of coronary artery disease (CAD) in patients with diabetes.[7] This finding indicates that reducing the total cholesterol level is one logical means of reducing cardiovascular disease in these patients; however, an elevated LDL cholesterol level is considered the most important CHD risk indicator and is the primary target for intervention in treatment guidelines for dyslipidemia.[6] LDL cholesterol reduction has become the focus of dyslipidemia treatment efforts for several reasons. Experimental animal research, laboratory investigations, epidemiologic studies, and evaluations of genetic hypercholesterolemia have all indicated that elevated LDL cholesterol is a major cause of CHD, and clinical trials have established that LDL-lowering therapy reduces CHD risk.[8] However, both decreased HDL and elevated LDL levels predicted CHD in the United Kingdom Prospective Diabetes Study (UKPDS).[2] Taken together, the results of these studies suggest that increasing HDL cholesterol levels while reducing LDL and total cholesterol levels may be a better means of reducing cardiovascular disease risk than simply reducing total cholesterol.

Much of the elevation in cardiovascular disease risk attributable to type 2 diabetes may stem from hypertriglyceridemia. For example, epidemiologic surveys have shown a consistent univariate relationship between hypertriglyceridemia and cardiovascular risk. In the Copenhagen Male Study,[9] the cumulative incidence rate attributable to triglycerides was 4.6%, or a 1.5 risk ratio, for the lowest tertile of triglyceride levels, and 11.5%, or a 2.2 risk ratio, for the highest tertile. Even when risk was stratified by increasing HDL cholesterol, a clear risk gradient was seen from the lowest to the highest tertile. These findings suggest that, as triglyceride levels increase, HDL-cholesterol-related cardioprotection is lost. Further support for the role of elevated triglyceride levels in elevating the risk of cardiovascular disease has been provided by the Paris Prospective Study,[10] the Prospective Cardiovascular Mortality Munster Study (PRO-CAM),[11] and a meta-analysis of 17 other population-based prospective studies.[12] Results of these studies indicate that elevated triglyceride levels should be targeted for reduction if they remain elevated after good glycemic control has been achieved.[4] However, in a Finnish study that showed that increased triglyceride levels and decreased HDL cholesterol levels predicted CHD in patients with type 2 diabetes, neither total nor VLDL triglyceride predicted CHD after adjustment for the influence of HDL cholesterol level.[2] In fact, low HDL level appears to be the most consistent predictor of CHD in observational studies of patients with type 2 diabetes; elevated triglyceride is the next most consistent predictor, followed by elevated total cholesterol.[2] Overall, these studies indicate that therapies targeted at increasing HDL cholesterol levels while decreasing LDL cholesterol and triglyceride levels may be the best means of reducing the incidence of cardiovascular disease and its related mortality in patients with type 2 diabetes.

Treatment Goals

The National Cholesterol Education Program (NCEP) Adult Treatment Panel III (ATP III) defined optimal plasma lipid levels for adults with diabetes to be less than 200 mg/dL of total cholesterol, less than 100 mg/dL of LDL cholesterol, more than 45 mg/dL of HDL cholesterol, and less than 200 mg/dL triglyceride. Because patients with type 2 diabetes not only have a risk of CHD events about three times that of nondiabetic individuals, but also have an increased risk of mortality from a first myocardial infarction, these recommended lipid levels are the same as those for nondiabetic patients with cardiovascular disease. However, because nondiabetic women generally tend to have higher levels of HDL cholesterol than men, an HDL cholesterol level even higher than that generally recommended for all patients with type 2 diabetes (55 mg/dL) may be desirable for women with type 2 diabetes. Reducing the LDL cholesterol level is the first treatment priority,[2] and lowering triglyceride levels is the second, followed by increasing the HDL cholesterol level, and then by addressing combined hyperlipidemia.

Diet Therapy

According to the NCEP's ATP III recommendations for CHD risk reduction in patients with elevated LDL cholesterol levels, total fat consumption may range from 25% to 35% of total calories if consumption of saturated fats and transunsaturated fatty acids is kept low. This level of mostly unsaturated fat intake can help to counteract the increased triglyceride levels and decreased HDL cholesterol levels characteristic of diabetic dyslipidemia. Patients with elevated LDL cholesterol levels should reduce cholesterol consumption to less than 200 mg/d and saturated fat consumption to less than 7% of total calories. All other fat consumed should be unsaturated: as many as 20% of total calories should come from monounsaturated fat, and as many as 10% should come from polyunsaturated fats.[8] Maximal diet therapy typically reduces LDL cholesterol by 15 to 25 mg/dL.[2] Moderate physical activity should also be incorporated into the treatment plan and LDL response checked after 6 weeks. If at that time the LDL goal has not been reached, other LDL-lowering dietary elements, such as soluble fiber or plant stanols or sterols, can be incorporated into the treatment plan.[8] Large amounts of soluble fiber have been shown to exert a beneficial effect on serum lipids.[13] In addition, 1.5 to 2 g/d of sitosterol and stanol esters, used instead of regular margarine, can reduce LDL cholesterol levels 10% to 15% more than a low-fat, low-cholesterol diet can.[14-16] Because these esters inhibit cholesterol absorption from the intestinal lumen and reduce the absorption of dietary cholesterol and the secretion of cholesterol in bile, they complement dietary therapy.[17]

Weight reduction should also be pursued, particularly in overweight or obese and sedentary patients.[8] Weight loss can be aided by restricting total fat consumption to an even smaller percentage of total calories than that recommended for type 2 diabetes patients at a normal body weight.[13] In terms of treating diabetic dyslipidemia, reduction in excess weight exerts its greatest effect on triglyceride levels, increases HDL cholesterol levels slightly, and modestly decreases total and LDL cholesterol levels.[18] However, LDL levels often rise transiently as triglycerides fall, due to the increased synthesis of the buoyant, 'fluffy' LDL subtype and a corresponding decrease in formation of small, dense, atherogenic LDL particles. Because weight loss improves the lipid profile in the long term, overweight diabetic patients should be prescribed diet therapy as first-line treatment for dyslipidemia.[2] Orlistat (Xenical®), a potent and specific inhibitor of pancreatic lipase that blocks the hydrolysis of dietary fat into absorbable free fatty acids and monoglycerides, can also be used to reduce body weight and improve lipid profiles in obese patients with type 2 diabetes. In one study, such treatment of these patients was associated with significant reduction in total and LDL cholesterol levels and triglyceride levels when compared with reductions obtained from placebo and diet.[18] Beneficial effects from orlistat are proportional to fat intake. Less weight loss is seen in patients on a low-fat diet. Diarrhea resulting from the use of orlistat may be minimized by concurrent administration of fiber supplements.

Although patients with elevated triglyceride and VLDL levels may be advised to increase monounsaturated fat as a proportion of total fat intake while moderating carbohydrate intake, obese patients should be aware that increased total fat intake may perpetuate or worsen obesity. Patients with triglyceride levels of 1,000 mg/dL or higher require immediate restriction of total fat consumption to less than 10% of total calories as well as pharmacologic treatment to reduce risk of pancreatitis.[13] Transunsaturated fatty acids (TFAs) should be avoided as much as possible because they raise total and LDL cholesterol, may lower HDL cholesterol, and may worsen glycemic control in patients with type 2 diabetes. Replacement of butter by low-TFA or TFA-free soft margarines favorably affects blood lipoprotein profiles.[19]

Patients with diabetes should consume foods containing ω-3 polyunsaturated fats and their precursors, including flax seed, flax oil, and fresh salmon, tuna, trout, and sardines. Fish-oil supplements are not recommended because of rancidity and their association with increased LDL cholesterol levels,[20] as well as their possible adverse effect on clotting time.[4] Moreover, at dosages of more than 2 to 4 g daily, fish-oil capsules may worsen glycemic control.[21] Although no clinical trials in patients with diabetes have shown reduced CHD incidence from ω-3 fatty acids, there is epidemiologic evidence that increased consumption of fish is associated with lower CHD risk.[22] The ω-3 fatty acids may exert this effect by lowering triglycerides; they have minimal effects on HDL and LDL cholesterol levels.[22] As a result, they are especially useful for patients with severe hypertriglyceridemia.[1]

Exercise

Poor aerobic fitness is associated with many cardiovascular risk factors, and most patients with type 2 diabetes have a low level of fitness compared with control patients, even when their ambient activity levels are matched. Improvement in cardiovascular risk factors has been associated with decreased plasma insulin levels. Also, many of the beneficial effects of exercise on cardiovascular risk are likely to result not only from reduced weight and an improved lipid profile,[18] but also from a reduction in the amount of intra-abdominal fat and from improved insulin sensitivity. Decreased intra-abdominal fat mass and increased insulin sensitivity are associated with decreased triglyceride levels and increased HDL cholesterol levels, which can be especially important in managing diabetic dyslipidemia.[1] In addition, although its effects on LDL cholesterol levels have not been consistently documented, regular exercise has been consistently shown to reduce levels of atherogenic triglyceride-rich VLDL.[23] General recommendations and precautions for using exercise to treat type 2 diabetes, including optimal weekly activity levels for normal-weight patients and obese patients who require weight reduction, are provided in Chapter 5.

Pharmacotherapy

Glucose-Control Agents

Any treatment that enhances glycemic control improves overall diabetic dyslipidemia, especially hypertriglyceridemia.[1] Optimal control can reduce LDL cholesterol levels by 10% to 15%.[6] As a result, sulfonylurea, metformin (Glucophage®), acarbose (Precose®), thiazolidinedione (TZD), and insulin therapies have all been reported to improve the lipid profile.[1] In general, although treatment with glucose-lowering agents reduces triglyceride levels in patients with type 2 diabetes, it does not change or only modestly increases HDL cholesterol levels.[2] However, treatment with antidiabetic agents may change the composition of LDL and HDL, thereby making them less atherogenic and more vasculoprotective, respectively.

Sulfonylurea therapy can modestly decrease triglyceride levels,[24] and most studies have shown that it has neutral or slightly beneficial effects on plasma lipid levels.[24,25] These effects probably result from direct enhancement of VLDL metabolism, coupled with the indirect effects of a reduction in blood glucose on lipid levels. Meglitinides have no significant effects on plasma lipid levels despite their marked ability to decrease postprandial plasma glucose levels.[26] Metformin reduces both fasting and postprandial triglyceride concentrations,[18] and reductions in triglyceride and LDL cholesterol of 10% to 15% are sometimes, but not consistently, reported from metformin

227

Table 8-1: Effects of Glucose-control Agents on Plasma Lipid Levels in Patients With Type 2 Diabetes

Therapy	Effect on LDL-C
Sulfonylureas	None or decreases
Meglitinides	None
Metformin (Glucophage®)	Decreases
Thiazolidinediones	
-Pioglitazone (Actos®)	Increases
-Rosiglitazone (Avandia®)	Increases
Acarbose (Precose®)	None
Insulin	
-Intensive therapy	None
-Standard therapy	Decreases

HDL-C = high-density lipoprotein cholesterol

therapy. The degree of decrease in triglyceride is related to the fasting level and is to some extent independent of alteration in plasma glucose level.[26] In addition, metformin slightly decreases total cholesterol levels[18] and decreases the plasma level and oxidation of free fatty acids.[26] Metformin was shown to decrease Lp(a) levels by an average of 11% in a retrospective study of patients with type 2 diabetes who were receiving stable doses of lipid-lowering medication, although Lp(a) level rose in some patients.[27] More impressively, in a study of women with polycystic ovary disease, a condition associated with insulin

Effect on HDL-C	Effect on Triglyceride Level
None or increases	Decreases
None	None
None	Decreases
Increases	Decreases
Increases	None
None	Decreases
None	Decreases
Increases	None

LDL-C = low-density lipoprotein cholesterol

resistance and the development of type 2 diabetes, metformin therapy reduced Lp(a) levels by 42%.[27] Some of metformin's beneficial effects on plasma lipid levels may result from its ability to induce significant weight loss in patients with android obesity.[26] However, metformin has no effect on HDL cholesterol levels.[18]

When combined with metformin, rosiglitazone (Avandia®) treatment was shown to increase body weight and total and LDL cholesterol levels in a randomized trial in patients with type 2 diabetes, but the ratio of total cholesterol to HDL cholesterol did not change significantly. In patients whose rosiglitazone dose was 8 mg daily and whose baseline triglyceride level was greater than 200 mg/dL, the triglyceride level decreased significantly. However, no significant changes in triglyceride levels were found in patients with baseline triglyceride levels lower than 200 mg/dL.[6] TZD monotherapy increases HDL and LDL cholesterol levels, but the long-term effect of such changes on cardiovascular risk is not established.[2] Pioglitazone (Actos®) increases HDL levels by 12% to 19% and decreases triglyceride levels by about 9%. Although rosiglitazone decreases free fatty acid levels by as much as 22%, it does not significantly decrease triglyceride levels, but it does increase HDL levels by as much as 19%.[28] However, rosiglitazone can increase LDL as much as HDL, leaving the ratio between the two unchanged.[29] Pioglitazone may also increase LDL, although less than rosiglitazone does.[30] However, this increase is predominantly in the buoyant, less atherogenic LDL fraction.[31]

Acarbose treatment has been associated with a modest decrease in plasma triglyceride levels and stable LDL and HDL cholesterol levels in some studies.[26] α-Glucosidase inhibitor therapy may also promote weight loss, which can improve the lipid profile.

Like TZD monotherapy, insulin therapy tends to increase HDL cholesterol levels in patients with type 2 diabetes.[18] However, in the Veterans Affairs Cooperative Study in Type 2 Diabetes, intensive stepped insulin therapy resulted in significant reduction in triglyceride levels from baseline levels after 2 years of treatment but did not significantly increase HDL or decrease LDL cholesterol levels. In contrast, standard insulin therapy resulted in significant increases in HDL cholesterol levels and significant reductions in LDL cholesterol levels but did not significantly reduce triglyceride levels.[6] Table 8-1 summarizes the effects of the various glucose-control agents on plasma lipid levels in patients with type 2 diabetes.

Although interventions aimed at improving glycemic control usually decrease triglyceride levels, they may not be able to decrease them enough to reach target goals in patients with moderate to severe hypertriglyceridemia. Achieving optimal glycemic control with the aid of glucose-lowering agents can only be expected to increase HDL and decrease LDL cholesterol levels modestly, although TZDs have a large positive effect on HDL levels. Because of these limitations, lipid-lowering agents are required for many patients with type 2 diabetes.

Lipid-lowering Agent Monotherapy
HMG-CoA reductase inhibitors

The 3-hydroxy-3-methylglutaryl coenzyme A (HMG-CoA) reductase inhibitors, commonly known as statins, are the most effective agents for lowering LDL cholesterol in patients with type 2 diabetes.[1] In addition, statins can beneficially alter LDL subfraction profiles and significantly reduce triglyceride levels.[18] The first statin to receive US Food and Drug Administration (FDA) approval, lovastatin (Mevacor®), was approved in 1987. Since then, statins have become the most widely used drugs for treating hypercholesterolemia in adults. The five statins now approved for use in the United States, in order of their LDL-cholesterol-lowering potency per milligram from greatest to least, are atorvastatin (Lipitor®), simvastatin (Zocor®), lovastatin, pravastatin (Pravachol®), and fluvastatin (Lescol®).[1] The fermentation-derived statins, simvastatin, lovastatin, and pravastatin, are similar in structure. Atorvastatin and fluvastatin are synthetic statins with distinct structures that differ from each other and from that of the fermentation-derived statins. Except for atorvastatin, whose elimination half-life ranges from 12 to 16 hours, the statins have elimination half-lives of about 0.5 to 3 hours. Because of this short half-life, and because cholesterol biosynthesis is enhanced at night, they are generally more effective when taken in the evening. Choice of statin in patients previously untreated with these agents depends on the degree of hypercholesterolemia and percentage reduction in the LDL cholesterol level required to reach target goals. Other factors that should be considered in the selection of a statin are use of other medications that may cause drug interactions and the amount of clinical experience with each agent. Therapy should not be changed unless patients experience side effects or do not reach their treatment goals. Changes based on formulary decisions have caused thrombotic stroke and hepatitis and are therefore not recommended.[17]

Indications. Statin therapy should be considered for patients who are at increased risk for atherosclerosis-related events because of their cholesterol level and/or the additional cardiovascular risk posed by type 2 diabetes. In general, the NCEP ATP III recommends that medical nutritional therapy (MNT), or diet therapy initiated and supervised by qualified nutritionists or dietitians, should be tried before statin treatment is begun. However, it further recommends that diabetic patients with CHD and an LDL cholesterol level of 100 to 130 mg/dL despite adequate glycemic control and a 6-week trial of MNT should be treated with pharmacologic agents. When diabetic patients with CHD have an LDL cholesterol of 130 mg/dL or more, MNT and pharmacologic therapy should be initiated simultaneously. For diabetic patients without CHD but with an LDL cholesterol level of 130 mg/dL or more after a trial of MNT, pharmacologic therapy should be initiated with the goal of an LDL cholesterol level of 100 mg/dL or less. Diabetic patients without CHD whose LDL cholesterol level ranges between 100 and 130 mg/dL may be treated with either more aggressive MNT or a statin.[2] However, patients should continue their dietary efforts to reduce cholesterol levels during statin treatment to enhance the drug's effects and minimize the required dose. In addition to its use for decreasing LDL cholesterol levels, simvastatin was recently approved by the FDA for elevating HDL cholesterol levels because of its demonstrated ability to increase this important marker of cardiovascular health.[6] However, pravastatin is the only agent of its class that has received FDA approval for use in reducing the risk of stroke and cardiac events.[6]

Mechanism of action. Statins act in the liver to inhibit HMG-CoA reductase, the rate-limiting enzyme in cholesterol synthesis. This inhibition increases the expression of high-affinity LDL receptors in the liver, thereby reducing synthesis of LDL and VLDL and promoting LDL-receptor-mediated clearance of LDL and VLDL remnants.[17,18] The up-regulation of the LDL receptor, reduction in VLDL synthesis, and enhancement of catabolism of remnant proteins account for the statins' ability to reduce triglyceride levels in patients with moderate hypertriglyceridemia. However, statins do not have a significant effect on plasma Lp(a) levels.[17]

Effectiveness. Statins typically reduce total cholesterol levels by 10% to 15%, reduce LDL cholesterol levels by 10% to 20%, and increase HDL cholesterol levels by 5% to 10%.[6] In patients with initially low levels of HDL cholesterol, statins may increase HDL cholesterol levels even more.[1] In clinical studies, statins reduced LDL cholesterol levels in patients with and without diabetes to the same degree, and they have been shown to reduce long-term CHD-related morbidity and mortality.[1] However, although atorvastatin can reduce LDL cholesterol levels by as much as 61% in patients with primary hypercholesterolemia,[6] high-dose atorvastatin (80 mg/d) has been shown to slightly decrease HDL cholesterol levels. Pravastatin therapy has shown the earliest onset of benefit with respect to the CHD event rate (within 6 months) and significant reduction in this rate was demonstrable after less than 1 year of therapy.[6] Statin dose may need to be titrated in response to the level of LDL cholesterol reduction obtained with initial therapy and adjusted after 4 to 6 weeks.[1]

The ability of statins to reduce plasma triglyceride levels depends on the patient's baseline triglyceride level and the statin's effectiveness in reducing the LDL cholesterol level. For example, in patients with triglyceride levels of 250 to 400 mg/dL, simvastatin reduced triglyceride concentrations by 24% to 40% and pravastatin reduced them

Table 8-2: Lipid-lowering Agents for Type 2 Diabetic Dyslipidemia: Action, Dosing, and Effects

Drug Class, Lipid-lowering Agent, and Brand Name(s)	Mode of Action	Half Life/ Duration of Action
HMG-CoA Reductase Inhibitors (Statins)	Inhibit action of rate-limiting enzyme in cholesterol synthesis	
Atorvastatin (Lipitor®)		12-16 h/—
Simvastatin (Zocor®)		2-3 h/—
Pravastatin (Pravachol®)		1.3-2.7 h/—
Lovastatin (Mevacor®)		2-3 h/4-6 wk
Fluvastatin (Lescol®)		0.5-3.1 h/—
Fibric Acid Derivatives (Fibrates)	Activate PPAR-α; decrease apoprotein	
Fenofibrate, micronized (Tricor®)	CIII, hepatic triglyceride, VLDL	20 h/—
Gemfibrozil (Lopid®, Apo-Gemfibrozil®, Gen-Fibro®, Nu-Gemfibrozil®)	particle synthesis; augment lipoprotein lipase expression	1.3-1.5 h/—
Clofibrate (Atromid-S®, Abitrate®)		6-25 h/3 wk
Bile Acid Sequestrants (Resins)	Block resorption of bile acids; increase	
Cholestyramine (Questran®, Questran Light®)	bile acid synthesis from cholesterol, hepatic cholesterol	—/2-4 wk
Colestipol hydrochloride (Colestid®)	synthesis, LDL receptor expression, LDL clearance	—/1 mo
Colesevelam hydro- chloride (WelChol®)		—/—

Starting Dosage; Daily Dosage Range	Administration and Follow-up Testing
	Bedtime administration optimal; AST, ALT, and CK levels should be monitored every 6-8 wk initially, then every 6 mo
10 mg q.d.; 10-80 mg q.d.	
20 mg q.d.; 5-80 mg q.d.	
10-40 mg q.d.; 10-40 mg q.d.	
20 mg q.d.; 20-80 mg q.d.	
20 mg q.d.; 20-40 mg q.d.	
	Take gemfibrozil before meals; AST, ALT, and CK levels and renal function should be monitored every 6-8 wk initially, then every 6 mo
67 mg q.d.; 67-200 mg/d	
600 mg b.i.d.; —	
750 mg-1 g b.i.d.; 1.5-2 g/d	
	Therapy should be initiated at low doses and divided dose(s) taken before meals to reduce adverse effects; other agents should be taken either 1 h before or 3 to 4 h after
4-8 g q.d./b.i.d.; 4-24 g/d	
2 g q.d. or b.i.d.; 2-16 g/d	
5 g b.i.d.; 5-30 g/d	
1,875 mg b.i.d. or 3,750 mg q.d.; 3,750-4,375 mg/d	

(continued on next page)

Table 8-2: Lipid-lowering Agents for Type 2 Diabetic Dyslipidemia: Action, Dosing, and Effects *(continued)*

Drug Class, Lipid-lowering Agent, and Brand Name(s)	Mode of Action	Half Life/ Duration of Action
Nicotinic Acid (Niacin) Crystalline (Niacor®, Nicocap®, Nicolar®)	Reduces lipolysis; inhibits synthesis and secretion of apolipoprotein B-containing lipoproteins; reduces Lp(a) synthesis; increases levels of HDL particles	45 min/—
Extended-release (Endur-Acin®, Slo-Niacin®, Nia-Bid®, Niac®, Niacels®, Niaspan ER®, Nico-400®, Nicobid® Tempules)		—/—
Selective Cholesterol Absorption Inhibitor Ezetimibe (Zetia®)	Inhibits cholesterol absorption by small intestine	22 h/—

by 25% to 30%, depending on the dose.[17] If triglyceride reduction is an important concern, atorvastatin and high-dose simvastatin are able to reduce triglyceride levels more than other statins, although fibrates and nicotinic acid are better at reducing elevated VLDL cholesterol levels.[6] Pravastatin in particular has been shown to attenuate the postprandial increase in triglyceride-rich VLDL.[18]

Starting Dosage; Daily Dosage Range	Administration and Follow-up Testing
	Take crystalline with meals, ER in evening; take aspirin or an NSAID 30 min before to minimize flushing and paresthesias; monitor Hb A_{1c}, uric acid, and AST and ALT levels every 6-8 wk, then every 6 mo; measure baseline level of homocysteine and re-check every 4-5 mo after dose stabilizes
1 g t.i.d.; 100 mg-6 g/d 1 g t.i.d.; 500 mg q.d. or b.i.d.-2g t.i.d.	
10 mg q.d.; 10 mg q.d.	Can be taken with or without food or with a statin; should be taken ≥ 2 h before or ≥ 4 h after a resin

(continued on next page)

Because response to statins varies considerably among patients, therapy should be initiated at the recommended starting dose. Individual variation in response depends on compliance with diet and medication therapy, gender, hormone status, and body weight. Other factors influencing treatment response include differences in drug metabolism, degree of compensatory increase in hepatic HMG-CoA re-

Table 8-2: Lipid-lowering Agents for Type 2 Diabetic Dyslipidemia: Action, Dosing, and Effects (continued)

Drug Class, Lipid-lowering Agent, and Brand Name(s)	Side Effects	Mean % LDL-C Decrease
HMG-CoA Reductase Inhibitors (Statins)	Nausea, diarrhea, fatigue, headache, rash, elevated AST/ALT	20-40
Atorvastatin	levels, insomnia	36
Simvastatin	myopathy,	14-40
Pravastatin	rhabdomyolysis	21-32
Lovastatin		28
Fluvastatin		24-32
Fibric Acid Derivatives (Fibrates)	Nausea, dyspepsia, diarrhea, abdominal	
Fenofibrate, micronized	pain, headache, rash, pruritus, increased risk	5
Gemfibrozil	of gallstones, elevated hepatic enzyme levels, myopathy	0-5
Clofibrate		—

ductase level, and the presence or absence of LDL-receptor mutations common in patients with familial hypercholesterolemia or of the apolipoprotein E4 genotype, which impairs response to therapy. Statins effectively treat hypercholesterolemia of all known genetic causes, and high-dose simvastatin and atorvastatin (80 mg/d) reduce LDL cholesterol levels by 30% in patients with homozygous familial hypercholesterolemia.[17] Details on dosing and administra-

Mean % HDL-C Increase	Mean TG Decrease	Main Clinical Utility
5-10	10-20	Decrease LDL-C, triglyceride levels; treat combined hyperlipidemia (at high doses or with fibrates or niacin)
4-8	21-26	
7-10	11	
5-6	10-14	
14	—	
15	5	
		Decrease triglyceride level; increase HDL-C; decrease LDL-C (fenofibrate); treat combined hyperlipidemia (with a statin or a resin)
8	30	
5-6	22-31	
—	—	

(continued on next page)

tion of statins, as well as the amount of lipid-level reduction reported from their use in patients with type 2 diabetes, are presented in Table 8-2. The results of clinical trials of statin therapy in terms of CHD event reduction in patients with diabetes are summarized in Table 8-3.

Adverse effects. All of the available statins are well tolerated,[17] and reported rates of compliance with statin therapy are higher than those for other classes of agents that reduce

Table 8-2: Lipid-lowering Agents for Type 2 Diabetic Dyslipidemia: Action, Dosing, and Effects (continued)

Drug Class, Lipid-lowering Agent, and Brand Name(s)	Side Effects	Mean % LDL-C Decrease
Bile Acid Sequestrants (Resins) Cholestyramine	Bad taste, constipation, hemorrhoid irritation, bloating, nausea, dyspepsia, reflux esophagitis	15-20
Colestipol hydrochloride Colesevelam hydrochloride		
Nicotinic Acid (Niacin) Crystalline Extended-release	Flushing, paresthesias, abdominal discomfort, gastric irritation, pruritus, dry skin, nausea, hepatitis, blurred vision (rare)	21
Selective Cholesterol Asorption Inhibitor Ezetimibe	Chest pain, joint pain, headache, dizziness, diarrhea, pharyngitis, sinusitis	16-19

— = not provided; AST/ALT = serum transaminases; CK = creatine kinase; ER = extended-release; Hb A_{1c} = glycosylated hemoglobin; HDL-C = high-density lipoprotein cholesterol level; LDL-C = low-density lipoprotein cholesterol level; NSAID = nonsteroidal anti-inflammatory drug;

Mean % HDL-C Increase	Mean TG Decrease	Main Clinical Utility
3-8	Mild increase	Decrease LDL-C; treat combined hyperlipidemia (with a fibrate)
32	28	Increase HDL-C; decrease LDL-C, triglyceride levels; treat combined hyperlipidemia (with a statin)
1-4	6-8	Decrease LDL-C, triglyceride levels; treat combined hyperlipidemia (with a statin)

TG = triglyceride level; VLDL = very-low-density lipoprotein cholesterol. Percentage figures given for resins and nicotinic acid are general figures for the drug class and for the combined nondiabetic and diabetic populations. Data were obtained from references 1, 4, 6, 17, 18, 32, 33, 34, 35, and 36.

Table 8-3: Coronary Heart Disease Event Reduction in Patients With Type 2 Diabetes in Selected Studies of Lipid-lowering Agents

Study Name	Study Type	Number of Patients With Type 2 Diabetes
Helsinki Heart Study	Primary prevention, subgroup analysis	59
Scandinavian Simvastatin Survival Study (4S)	Secondary prevention, subgroup analysis	105
Air Force/Texas Coronary Atherosclerosis Prevention Study (AFCAPS/ TexCAPS)	Primary prevention, subgroup analysis	84
Cholesterol and Recurrent Events (CARE) Study	Secondary prevention, subgroup analysis	282

HDL-C = high-density lipoprotein cholesterol
LDL-C = low-density lipoprotein cholesterol
* = P value not significant

Lipid-lowering Agent and Dosage Used	Changes in LDL-C, HDL-C, and Triglyceride Levels	% Coronary Heart Disease Event Rate Reduction (Significance Level)
Gemfibrozil, 600 mg b.i.d.	5% reduction; 5% increase; 22% reduction	68 ($P = 0.19$*)
Simvastatin, 20-40 mg/d	36% reduction; 7% increase; 11% reduction	55 ($P = 0.0002$)
Lovastatin, 20-40 mg/d	25% reduction; 6% increase; 15% reduction**	33 ($P < 0.006$)*
Pravastatin, 40 mg/d	28% reduction; 5% increase; 14% reduction**	25 ($P = 0.05$)

** = Percentage changes reported are for the total treated cohort, including both diabetic and nondiabetic patients.

Table was adapted from reference 1 with additional data from references 11, 37, 38, 39, and 40.

(continued on next page)

Table 8-3: Coronary Heart Disease Event Reduction in Patients With Type 2 Diabetes in Selected Studies of Lipid-lowering Agents

(continued)

Study Name	Study Type	Number of Patients With Type 2 Diabetes
Diabetes Atherosclerosis Intervention Study (DAIS)	Primary and secondary prevention, diabetic patients only	418
Veterans Affairs Cooperative Studies Program HDL-C Intervention Trial (VA-HIT)	Secondary prevention, subgroup analysis	309
Long-term Intervention with Pravastatin in Ischaemic Disease (LIPID) Study	Secondary prevention, subgroup analysis	396

HDL-C = high-density lipoprotein cholesterol
LDL-C = low-density lipoprotein cholesterol
* = P value not significant

Lipid-lowering Agent and Dosage Used	Changes in LDL-C, HDL-C, and Triglyceride Levels	% Coronary Heart Disease Event Rate Reduction (Significance Level)
Fenofibrate, micronized, 200 mg/d	7% reduction; 8% increase; 29% reduction	24 (*P* not available; study was not powered to examine clinical end points)*
Gemfibrozil, 600 mg b.i.d.	No change; 6% increase; 31% reduction**	24 (*P* = 0.05)
Pravastatin, 40 mg/d	25% reduction; 5% increase 11% reduction	19 (*P* < 0.001)*

** = Percentage changes reported are for the total treated cohort, including both diabetic and nondiabetic patients.

Table was adapted from reference 1
with additional data from references 18, 37, 38, 39, and 40.

lipid levels.[6] Significant side effects, which include nausea, fatigue, headache, change in bowel function, rashes, insomnia, and myalgia, are fairly uncommon.[17] The most commonly reported adverse effect of statins is minor gastrointestinal disturbance. In clinical trials, discontinuation of therapy owing to adverse effects was unusual.[1] Less common but more serious side effects include proximal myopathy, rhabdomyolysis, and elevated liver enzyme levels, which appear to be dose dependent.[17] Transient asymptomatic increases in hepatic transaminase levels have been reported in about 1% of patients receiving statin therapy.[6] Because of the possibility of these serious adverse effects, monitoring of creatine kinase levels is recommended; an increase above five times the upper limit of normal indicates that the dose must be reduced or treatment halted.[1] Liver function must also be assessed every 6 to 8 weeks in the first 6 months of treatment and less frequently thereafter, once the statin dose stabilizes.[17] An increase of aspartate aminotransferase (AST) or alanine aminotransferase (ALT) above three times the upper limit of normal indicates that the dose must be reduced or treatment halted. However, in patients with hypertriglyceridemia, abnormal liver function tests may result from fatty infiltration and may actually improve after treatment.[1]

Drug interactions. Atorvastatin, simvastatin, and lovastatin are primarily metabolized by the cytochrome P450 3A4 isoenzyme. Fluvastatin is primarily metabolized by the 2C9 isoenzyme. Pravastatin is metabolized by multiple isoenzymes. As a result, the safety and efficacy of any statin may be affected when it is given with other drugs that use these enzymes for their metabolism. Particularly in patients with underlying muscle disorders, proximal myopathy and rhabdomyolysis are more common when statins are combined with fibrates, nicotinic acid, or cyclosporine,[17] which impairs statin metabolism. Treatment with azole antifungal agents, erythromycin, clarithromycin, human immunodeficiency virus (HIV) protease inhibitors, nefazodone, or verapamil can increase the risk of myopathy in patients receiving statin therapy, as can consuming large amounts of grapefruit juice. Patients taking some statins and coumarin anticoagulants have experienced bleeding and increased clotting times. As a result, patients taking these medications should have their blood coagulation profile measured before statin therapy is initiated and should be monitored regularly thereafter.[41] Statins do not impair glycemic control in patients with diabetes,[1] and, in one study, simvastatin enhanced the action of insulin by strongly inhibiting hepatic glucose output and stimulating the rate of glucose disappearance and metabolic clearance.[18]

Contraindications and precautions. Statin therapy is contraindicated in pregnant patients and in patients with cholestasis and should be used with caution in patients with liver dysfunction. Statin therapy should be avoided or discontinued if a pregnancy is planned and should be stopped when pregnancy is discovered and not resumed until nursing is completed. Pediatric use of statins is not recommended.[17]

Fibrates

The fibric acid derivatives, or fibrates, are similar in structure to clofibrate (Atromid-S®), the first drug in this class to be approved. Clofibrate was used in the first trial of lipid-lowering therapy for the primary prevention of CHD, which was conducted by the World Health Organization (WHO). Clofibrate, gemfibrozil (Lopid®), and micronized fenofibrate (Tricor®) are the three drugs in this class that are now approved for prescription use in the United States. As a class, fibrates are most effective in reducing plasma concentrations of triglyceride-rich lipoproteins such as VLDL and chylomicrons. However, they differ in their effectiveness in reducing LDL cholesterol concentrations and do not reduce Lp(a) levels.[17] They generally decrease triglyceride levels and increase HDL cholesterol levels more than statins.[6] Fenofibrate reduces triglyceride and LDL cholesterol levels and increases HDL cholesterol levels slightly more than gemfibrozil does.

Indications. Fibrates are the agents of choice for diabetic patients whose primary lipid abnormality is hypertriglyceridemia.[6] However, although gemfibrozil and clofibrate are indicated for the treatment of hypertriglyceridemia, they are not recommended as LDL-cholesterol reducing agents. Micronized fenofibrate is indicated for the treatment of hypertriglyceridemia and is moderately effective in reducing LDL cholesterol levels in patients with primary hypercholesterolemia or combined hyperlipidemia.[17] Although fenofibrate cannot be considered the first choice for treating primary hypercholesterolemia, it can be used for patients with combined hyperlipidemia or in combination drug therapy.

Mechanism of action. Fibrates affect lipoprotein metabolism by activating peroxisome proliferator activator receptor-α (PPAR-α), a member of the nuclear hormone receptor family. Through their effects on the PPAR-α signaling pathway, which influences a number of cellular metabolic processes, including those involved in lipoprotein metabolism, fibrates decrease apoprotein C-III synthesis, decrease hepatic synthesis of triglyceride and VLDL particles, and increase the expression of lipoprotein lipase.[17] The main result is a reduction in triglyceride levels, but HDL cholesterol levels often reciprocally increase between 5% and 15%, or more when baseline triglyceride levels are high.[1] Because apolipoprotein A-I and A-II are important structural elements of HDL cholesterol, increased transcription of the genes that encode these proteins by PPAR-α activation may be one mechanism by which fibrate therapy increases HDL cholesterol levels.[42]

Fibrates have different effects on LDL cholesterol levels, depending on the baseline triglyceride level. When the baseline triglyceride level is normal or slightly elevated, the LDL cholesterol level decreases with fibrate therapy, but when the baseline triglyceride level is high, the LDL level may increase because of enhanced VLDL metabolism.[1]

Effectiveness. Treatment with fenofibrate is most effective at reducing triglyceride concentrations. Fenofibrate also shifts the distribution of LDL particles in favor of the larger, possibly less atherogenic type[17] and increases HDL cholesterol level by 15% to 30%. When the baseline HDL cholesterol level is less than 35 mg/dL, the increase in this level is much more pronounced and may reach 50%. Fenofibrate substantially reduces levels of VLDL cholesterol and triglyceride-rich lipoproteins and has a beneficial effect on Lp(a). Its lipid-lowering and antiatherogenic effects have been confirmed by the results of the Diabetes Atherosclerosis Intervention Study (DAIS). This study showed that treatment with micronized fenofibrate, which is about 25% more bioavailable than nonmicronized fenofibrate, significantly corrected the lipid abnormalities typical in patients with type 2 diabetes. Reported reduction was about 10% for total cholesterol level, about 5% for LDL cholesterol level, and about 30% for triglyceride level. The HDL cholesterol level increased by about 8%. More importantly, on the basis of angiographic measurements, DAIS showed that treatment with micronized fenofibrate significantly decreased the progression of focal atherosclerotic lesions by 40% and caused a similar but nonsignificant trend in the reduction of diffuse atherosclerosis.[42] These changes even occurred in patients with lipid levels that many physicians would consider normal. Although the study was not designed to have the power to detect significant differences in clinical end points, fenofibrate-treated patients had a 23% reduction in the combined end point of death, myocardial infarction, angioplasty, and coronary bypass operation compared with the placebo-treated group.[18,43]

Other evidence that fibrate therapy may reduce the risk of cardiovascular events was supplied by the Helsinki Heart Study, which included 135 patients with diabetes. In this primary prevention study, the 5-year incidence of major CHD events in diabetic patients without CHD who were treated with gemfibrozil was reduced by 68% vs the placebo-treated group. However, this difference did not reach statistical significance because of the small numbers of patients in the analysis of the subgroup with diabetes.[18] The utility of gemfibrozil in secondary CHD event prevention was also demonstrated in the Veterans Affairs Cooperative Studies Program HDL-Cholesterol Intervention Trial (VA-HIT), in which 627 patients, or 25%, had diabetes. In this study, the cardiovascular event rate was reduced by 24% in gemfibrozil-treated patients with type 2 diabetes vs the placebo-treated group.[1]

Fenofibrate therapy has been shown to increase levels of two important components of HDL cholesterol. Increases from baseline levels of apolipoprotein A-I and apolipoprotein A-II of 5% to 16% and 20% to 29%, respectively, have been observed after micronized fenofibrate therapy. These increases are significantly greater than those produced by statins in most trials, especially in patients with mixed dyslipidemia and low baseline HDL cholesterol levels. Moreover, in a Canadian trial that compared micronized fenofibrate therapy with gemfibrozil therapy, the fenofibrate-treated group experienced a significantly greater increase in apolipoprotein A-I than the gemfibrozil-treated group.[42] Additional clinical trial data on the effectiveness of fibrate therapy, including reductions in the cardiovascular event rate reported from subgroup analyses of patients with type 2 diabetes, are provided in Table 8-3. Dosing and administration of fibrates are presented in Table 8-2.

Finally, in patients with type 2 diabetes, gemfibrozil has been reported to increase or to have no significant effect on LDL cholesterol levels.[18] However, gemfibrozil therapy has also been shown to increase LDL particle size in inverse proportion to the degree of reduction in triglyceride level. Fenofibrate would be expected to have similar effects, and both agents should also enhance clearance of postprandial lipoproteins,[1] which is an important consideration in patients with type 2 diabetes because of the atherogenicity of postprandial remnant particles.[18]

Adverse effects. Fibrates are generally well tolerated. Their most common adverse effects are gastrointestinal disturbances such as nausea, dyspepsia, diarrhea, and abdominal pain. Less common side effects include headache, rash (reported in less than 2% of patients), and pruritus. When used in patients with combined hyperlipidemia, fibrates may slightly increase the risk of gallstones and occasionally cause abnormal liver function test results. Because of these adverse effects, they are generally contraindicated in patients with gallstones or liver dysfunction. However, by decreasing triglyceride levels, fibrates can sometimes reverse abnormalities of liver function associated with fatty infiltration of the liver. Although they do not cause deterioration in glycemic control in patients with diabetes, they may cause myopathy, which has been reported in as many as 5% of treated patients,[6] particularly patients with impaired renal function. Risk of myopathy increases when fibrates are combined with statins or nicotinic acid. As a result, laboratory assessment of side effects, including periodic liver and renal function testing and measurement of creatine kinase levels, is recommended.[1,4,17]

Clofibrate has been found to increase the risk of developing peripheral vascular disease, intermittent claudication, pulmonary embolism, thrombophlebitis, angina pectoris, and arrhythmias. WHO study results first published in 1978 indicated that long-term use of clofibrate may increase mortality from noncardiovascular causes (malignancy, complications after cholecystectomy, pancreatitis). However, the Coronary Drug Project report of 1975 did not reach this conclusion, although it did indicate that clofibrate use greatly increases the risk of cholelithiasis and cholecystitis requiring surgery, a finding that was confirmed in the WHO study.[34] Because of these findings, and because other fibrates have not been shown to increase the risk of vascular disease and do not increase the risk of cholelithiasis as much as clofibrate does, clinical use of clofibrate has decreased.

Drug interactions. Patients taking some fibrates and coumarin anticoagulants have experienced bleeding and increased clotting times; therefore, the dosage of anticoagulant should be decreased in these patients to keep prothrombin time at optimal levels, and frequent assessment of prothrombin time is recommended until this laboratory value stabilizes. Concomitant treatment with statins and fibrates, particularly gemfibrozil and fenofibrate, should be avoided unless the benefit is likely to outweigh the increased risk of myopathy. Interactions between fibrates, which are primarily excreted by the kidneys, and potentially nephrotoxic drugs, such as cyclosporine, may also pose problems. As a result, the benefits of using fibrates with potentially nephrotoxic immunosuppressants should be weighed against the risks, and the lowest effective doses should be used.[2,44]

Contraindications and precautions. Results of animal studies showed fibrates to be embryocidal and teratogenic at high doses. Fibrates should therefore be used during pregnancy only if the potential benefit justifies the potential risk to the fetus. Because of their potential to promote tumor growth in animals, fibrates should not be used by nursing mothers. The safety and efficacy of fibrates have not been established in pediatric patients. Patients with impaired renal function, including elderly patients, may be at greater risk of adverse reactions to fibrates.[44]

Resins

The bile acid sequestrants, or ion exchange resins, decrease LDL cholesterol levels and slightly increase HDL cholesterol levels. However, they can induce hypertriglyceridemia[6] and often cause gastrointestinal side effects. As a result, they have not been extensively used in treating patients with type 2 diabetes.[18] Two of these drugs, cholestyramine (Questran®, Questran Light®) and colestipol hydrochloride (Colestid®), have been in extensive clinical use for more than 20 years.[17] A third and possibly better-tolerated drug in this class, colesevelam hydrochloride (WelChol®), recently received FDA approval.[6]

Indications. Treatment with resins is indicated when the primary dyslipidemia is an elevated LDL cholesterol level and the response to maximum statin therapy is inadequate or contraindicated. However, because resins can increase triglyceride levels, their use is not recommended if the patient's triglyceride level exceeds 120 mg/dL.[1] As monotherapy, treatment with resins is most appropriate for women who are pregnant or planning a pregnancy, children with familial hypercholesterolemia, and patients with modestly elevated LDL cholesterol levels who desire to or must avoid systemic lipid-lowering medications.[17]

Mechanism of action. These drugs do not act systemically. Instead, they bind bile acids in the intestinal lumen and block their normal reabsorption in the ileum, which leads to increased fecal excretion of bile acids. The ability of resins to reduce LDL cholesterol levels reflects depletion of the hepatic bile acid pool and resultant increase in the synthesis of bile acids from cholesterol. This increase leads to increased hepatic cholesterol biosynthesis, increased expression of LDL receptors on hepatocyte membranes, and enhanced clearance of LDL.[17]

Effectiveness. When used in moderate doses, resins can reduce LDL cholesterol by 15% to 20% and increase HDL cholesterol by 3% to 8% while producing a mild increase in triglyceride levels in patients without previous hypertriglyceridemia. However, because resins increase VLDL production, they should not be used as monotherapy in patients with combined hyperlipidemia.[17] Dosing and administration of resins are presented in Table 8-2.

Adverse effects. Widespread use of cholestyramine and colestipol hydrochloride has been limited by their adverse effects, which are primarily poor palatability and gastrointestinal side effects such as constipation, worsening of hemorrhoids, bloating, nausea, dyspepsia, and reflux esophagitis. Newer formulations of these agents, such as colestipol tablets or finer-grained bulk cholestyramine, enhance compliance by enhancing palatability, and initiating therapy at low doses and instructing patients to take these agents with meals can minimize adverse effects.[17] However, resins may interfere with the absorption of fat-soluble vitamins.[4]

Drug interactions. Because of their ion-exchange-related binding action, resins may bind other charged drugs such as thyroxine, warfarin, digitalis, and, to a lesser extent, fibrates and statins. To minimize such interactions, other agents should be taken either 1 hour before or 3 to 4 hours after resins are taken at mealtime.[17]

Contraindications and precautions. Because resins may induce hypertriglyceridemia, triglyceride levels should be monitored in patients receiving resin therapy.[6]

Nicotinic Acid

The hypolipidemic effects of nicotinic acid, or niacin, have been recognized for more than 40 years, and this agent has been used widely to treat hypercholesterolemia and combined hyperlipidemia[17] because of its excellent lipid-lowering properties.[4] It is the most effective available agent for elevating HDL cholesterol levels, and it decreases triglyceride, LDL cholesterol, and even Lp(a) levels.[1] Nicotinic acid is available in immediate-release or crystalline (Nicolar®) and sustained-release (Niaspan®) forms.[17] Although nicotinic acid decreases insulin sensitivity and may therefore worsen glycemic control,[4] acipimox, a nicotinic acid derivative, does not appear to exert this effect.[18]

Indications. In patients with type 2 diabetes, nicotinic acid is typically used as a second-line agent in high-risk patients at dosages that do not exceed 1 g daily.[1] Because nicotinic acid therapy can cause hyperglycemia, it may be particularly inappropriate for patients whose blood glucose levels are poorly controlled.[6]

Mechanism of action. The hypolipidemic effects of nicotinic acid are dose dependent and mediated by its ability to reduce lipolysis in adipose tissue, inhibit hepatic synthesis and secretion of apolipoprotein B-containing lipoproteins, reduce synthesis of Lp(a), and alter HDL metabolism in a manner that increases plasma levels of HDL particles.[17]

Effectiveness. In one dose-titration study, after 26 weeks of crystalline nicotinic acid therapy, reductions in LDL cholesterol levels and Lp(a) of 21% and 35%, respectively, were reported. The largest reductions were seen in patients with the highest baseline levels of these lipids. In addition, HDL cholesterol levels increased by 32%.[17] The positive correlation between reductions in LDL cholesterol and Lp(a) concentrations observed in this study further indicates that niacin reduces the level of Lp(a) via a reduction in Lp(a) synthesis.[17]

Nicotinic acid is reported to have near-maximum HDL-cholesterol-raising effects at a dosage of 1.5 g daily.[4] In a dose-titration study of 2 g of extended-release nicotinic acid daily, the LDL cholesterol level decreased by 15%, and Lp(a) and triglyceride levels decreased by 28%.

The beneficial effects of nicotinic acid therapy on atherosclerosis have been shown in several clinical and angiographic trials in which it has been used as part of lipid-lowering therapy in patients with hypercholesterolemia.[17] Dosing and administration of the various formulations of nicotinic acid are presented in Table 8-2.

Adverse effects. The most common adverse effect of niacin is cutaneous flushing, which can be minimized by initiating therapy at low doses, slowly titrating the dose, and instructing the patient to take the drug with meals. Other side effects include paresthesias, abdominal discomfort, stomach irritation, pruritus, dry skin, nausea, hepatitis, and, rarely, blurred vision.[4,17] Flushing and paresthesias can be minimized by ingesting aspirin or nonsteroidal anti-inflammatory agents 30 minutes before taking nicotinic acid.[4]

Drug interactions. Nicotinic acid potentiates the effects of antihypertensive agents,[6] and concomitant administration of these medications may require adjustment of their dosage.

Contraindications and precautions. Because it may worsen hyperglycemia, nicotinic acid therapy is relatively contraindicated in patients with type 2 diabetes. Nicotinic acid is also contraindicated in patients with a history of hyperuricemia or gout, peptic ulcer disease, or liver dysfunction because it may worsen these conditions. As a result, blood glucose, uric acid, and hepatic enzyme levels should be monitored regularly in patients with type 2 diabetes who are receiving nicotinic acid therapy.[17] An increase in hepatic enzyme levels to more than three times the upper limit of normal should trigger immediate discontinuation of nicotinic acid therapy.[4] Timed-release nicotinic acid may be hepatotoxic at dosages that exceed 2 g daily. For this reason, and because various forms of niacin are available over the counter, patients taking the crystalline form should be advised to avoid changing their nicotinic acid formulation. Nicotinic acid may also elevate levels of homocysteine, an amino acid associated with increased cardiovascular disease risk. As a result, baseline and periodic assessment of homocysteine levels every 4 to 5 months after a stable dose has been reached is recommended.[17]

Ezetimibe

Ezetimibe (Zetia®) is a new type of cholesterol-lowering agent that selectively reduces the absorption of cholesterol by more than 50%.

Indications. Ezetimibe is indicated as monotherapy and in combination with a statin for therapy of primary hypercholesterolemia to reduce total cholesterol, LDL, and apolipoprotein B and as monotherapy for treatment of homozygous sitosterolemia.[35]

Mechanism of action. Ezetimibe acts in the brush border of the small intestine to inhibit cholesterol transport across the intestinal wall. It is primarily metabolized by the small intestine and liver by glucuronidation and excreted through the urine and bile. Its plasma half-life is approximately 22 hours. It can be administered with or without food.

Effectiveness. Alone or in combination with a statin, ezetimibe effectively lowers total cholesterol, LDL, apolipoprotein B, and triglycerides and raises HDL. Its maximal effect is achieved within 2 weeks of initiation of therapy.[35] Dosing and administration of ezetimibe are provided in Table 8-2.

Adverse effects. Adverse effects that were reported in clinical trials with a significantly higher incidence than placebo included back pain and arthralgia in monotherapy and back pain and abdominal pain in combination with a statin. The percentages in all cases were 4% or less.

Drug interactions. Ezetimibe potentiates the effect of the HMG-CoA reductase inhibitors ('statins') and exhibits true synergism with these agents: the effect of both combined exceeds the added effects of each alone. This potentiation is not achieved by an alteration in statin bioavailability or plasma levels. Ezetimibe does not impair the absorption of fat-soluble vitamins or oral contraceptives, nor does it reduce adrenal steroidogenesis. It does not affect levels or activity of cytochrome P-450 enzymes and does not alter the effect of drugs metabolized through these enzymes. The administration of gemfibrozil or fenofibrate increases the oral bioavailability of ezetimibe by 65% to 70%, while cholestyramine administration decreases it by about the same amount.

Contraindications and precautions. Plasma levels in persons older than 65 years may be twice as high as in those younger than 65. Women exhibit slightly higher plasma levels than men, but no racial differences have been described. Ezetimibe is not recommended in patients with moderate or severe hepatic dysfunction, in whom plasma levels are unpredictable and may be six times higher than in patients with normal liver function. Plasma levels may be increased by 50% in patients with moderately severe renal insufficiency. Elevations of serum transaminases were three to four times more frequent when ezetimibe was coadministered with a statin than with statin therapy alone.[36] Therefore, liver function tests should be performed when ezetimibe is added to ongoing statin treatment. Ezetimibe does not appear to independently add to the risk of rhabdomyolysis or myopathy versus statin alone.[36] It is not recommended for coadministration with fibrates because of lack of clinical data.[35]

Combination Lipid-lowering Agent Therapy

Combination therapy with two or sometimes three lipid-lowering agents is appropriate for adults with severe hypercholesterolemia or combined hyperlipidemia. Combination therapy with low doses of drugs with complementary mechanisms of action may be safer and better tolerated than high doses of a single agent and therefore can also be used in patients with more moderate hypercholesterolemia. Because their mechanism of action complements that of the statins and nicotinic acid, resins can be integral to many combination therapies, particularly for patients with severe primary hypercholesterolemia. Combining a fibrate with a statin is conceptually attractive for treating patients who require reduction in LDL cholesterol and triglyceride levels and an increase in HDL cholesterol levels, but this combination has been associated with increased risk of myopathy and, rarely, rhabdomyolysis.[17] In particular, the combination of gemfibrozil with a statin, especially lovastatin, has been reported to increase the risk of myopathy.[18] Because fibrates and statins do not raise each other's plasma concentrations, the reasons for this increased risk are unclear. However, the myopathy appears to result from an underlying disorder in muscle metabolism that becomes symptomatic during combination therapy. Once-daily fenofibrate given in the morning combined with an evening dose of a short-acting statin can reduce the risk of producing simultaneously elevated plasma levels of both the fibrate and the statin. When such treatment is attempted, its efficacy and safety should be carefully monitored while low doses of statin are added. This combination was well tolerated in 80 patients with combined hyperlipidemia and showed beneficial effects on all lipoprotein parameters.[17]

Combination therapy also allows the use of resins at less-than-maximal doses, which are better tolerated.[4] In patients with severe primary hypercholesterolemia, resins may complement higher doses of statins, and studies of lovastatin, pravastatin, or simvastatin combined with colestipol hydrochloride or cholestyramine have produced reductions in LDL cholesterol levels of 45% to 64%. Triple therapy with a statin plus cholestyramine or colestipol hydrochloride and nicotinic acid may be required to treat adults with heterozygous familial hypercholesterolemia, but referral to a lipid specialist to manage such therapy is strongly advised. A statin plus nicotinic acid may be effective in treating patients who cannot tolerate cholestyramine or colestipol hydrochloride but is associated with increased risk of hepatotoxicity and requires careful monitoring.[17] Combining statins with nicotinic acid is an extremely effective means of treating diabetic dyslipidemia and is associated with some of the largest increases in HDL cholesterol levels. However, this combination may significantly worsen hyperglycemia and should therefore be used with extreme caution. Low doses of nicotinic acid (less than 2 g/d) and frequent monitoring of blood glucose levels[2] and hepatic enzyme and creatine kinase levels are recommended.[1]

Lipopheresis

Patients with severe hypercholesterolemia, such as those with the homozygous familial form of the disease, may benefit from LDL apheresis therapy. Two LDL apheresis systems are available: the Kaneka Liposorber LA-15® system, in which disposable dextran sulfate columns selectively bind VLDL, LDL, and Lp(a) from plasma as it passes over the columns, and the B. Braun heparin-induced extracorporeal LDL precipitation (HELP®) system, which involves extracorporeal precipitation of these subfractions. These devices have been approved by the FDA for use in patients with severe hypercholesterolemia, which is defined as an LDL cholesterol level of more than 300 mg/dL in patients without evidence of CHD or a level greater than 200 mg/dL in patients with CHD. Patients who meet these criteria and qualify for LDL apheresis therapy should be referred to a qualified lipid specialist with access to this technology. Each LDL apheresis treatment takes 3 to 4 hours and reduces LDL cholesterol levels by 70% to 80%. Even when combined with pharmacologic therapy, the procedure must be repeated every 2 weeks in patients with severe heterozygous familial hypercholesterolemia and every 7 to 10 days in patients with the homozygous form of this disease. However, such therapy has shown clinical benefit in these patients.[17]

References

1. Best JD, O'Neal DN: Diabetic dyslipidemia: current treatment recommendations. *Drugs* 2000;59:1101-1111.

2. American Diabetes Association: Position statement: management of dyslipidemia in adults with diabetes. *Diabetes Care* 2003;26:S83-S86. Available at: http://care.diabetesjournals.org/cgi/content/full/26/suppl_1/s83.

3. Rath MR: *Eradicating Heart Disease.* San Francisco, Health Now, 1993, pp 42-44.

4. Fineberg SE: The treatment of hypertension and dyslipidemia in diabetes mellitus. *Prim Care* 1999;26:951-964.

5. Goldberg IJ: Diabetic dyslipidemia: causes and consequences. *J Clin Endocrinol Metab* 2001;86:965-971.

6. Marcus AO: Lipid disorders in patients with type 2 diabetes. Meeting the challenges of early, aggressive treatment. *Postgrad Med* 2001;110:111-114, 117-118, 121-123.

7. Steiner F: Lipid intervention trials in diabetes. *Diabetes Care* 2000;23(suppl 2):B49-B53.

8. Executive Summary of the Third Report of the National Cholesterol Education Program (NCEP) Expert Panel on Detection, Evaluation, and Treatment of High Blood Cholesterol in Adults (Adult Treatment Panel III). *JAMA* 2001;285:2486-2497.

9. Jeppesen J, Hein HO, Suadicani P, et al: Triglyceride concentration and ischemic heart disease: an eight-year follow-up in the Copenhagen Male Study. *Circulation* 1998;97:1029-1036.

10. Fontbonne A, Eschwege E: Insulin-resistance, hypertriglyceridaemia and cardiovascular risk: The Paris Prospective Study. *Diabete Metab* 1991;17(1 pt 2):93-95.

11. Assmann G, Schulte H, Von Eckardstein A: Hypertriglyceridemia and elevated lipoprotein(a) are risk factors for major coronary events in middle-aged men. *Am J Cardiol* 1996;77:1179-1184.

12. Austin MA, Hokanson JE, Edwards KL: Hypertriglyceridemia as a cardiovascular risk factor. *Am J Cardiol* 1998;81(4A):7B-12B.

13. American Diabetes Association: Position statement: evidence-based nutrition principles and recommendations for the treatment and prevention of diabetes and related complications. *Diabetes Care* 2003;26:S51-S61. Available at: http://care.diabetesjournals.org/cgi/content/full/26/suppl_1/s51.

14. Hallikainen MA, Uusitupa MI: The effects of 2 low-fat stanol ester-containing margarines on serum cholesterol concentrations as part of a low-fat diet in hypercholesterolemic subjects. *Am J Clin Nutr* 1999;69:403-410.

15. Jones PJ, Ntanios FY, Raeini-Sarjaz M, et al: Cholesterol-lowering efficacy of a sitostanol-containing phytosterol mixture with a prudent diet in hyperlipidemic men. *Am J Clin Nutr* 1999;69:1144-1150.

16. Miettinen TA, Puska P, Gylling H, et al: Reduction of serum cholesterol with sitostanol-ester margarine in a mildly hypercholesterolemic population. *N Engl J Med* 1995;333:1308-1312.

17. Illingworth DR: Management of hypercholesterolemia. *Med Clin North Am* 2000;84:23-42.

18. Papadakis JA, Milionis HJ, Press M, et al: Treating dyslipidaemia in non-insulin-dependent diabetes mellitus—a special reference to statins. *J Diabetes Complications* 2001;15:211-226.

19. Zock PL, Katan MB: Butter, margarine and serum lipoproteins. *Atherosclerosis* 1997;131:7-16.

20. Wheeler ML: Nutrition management and physical activity as treatments for diabetes. *Prim Care* 1999;26:857-868.

21. Schectman G, Kaul S, Kissebah AH: Effect of fish oil concentrate on lipoprotein composition in NIDDM. *Diabetes* 1988;37:1567-1573.

22. Malasanos TH, Stacpoole PW: Biological effects of omega-3 fatty acids in diabetes mellitus. *Diabetes Care* 1991;14:1160-1179.

23. American Diabetes Association: Position statement: physical activity/exercise and diabetes mellitus. *Diabetes Care* 2003;26:S73-S77. Available at: http://care.diabetesjournals.org/cgi/content/full/26/suppl_1/s73.

24. Jeppesen J, Zhou MY, Chen YD, et al: Effect of glipizide treatment on postprandial lipaemia in patients with NIDDM. *Diabetologia* 1994;37:781-787.

25. Simonson DC, Kourides IA, Feinglos M, et al: Efficacy, safety, and dose-response characteristics of glipizide gastrointestinal therapeutic system on glycemic control and insulin secretion in NIDDM. Results of two multicenter, randomized, placebo-controlled clinical trials. The Glipizide Gastrointestinal Therapeutic System Study Group. *Diabetes Care* 1997;20:597-606.

26. DeFronzo RA: Pharmacologic therapy for type 2 diabetes mellitus. *Ann Intern Med* 1999;131:281-303.

27. Bell DS, Ovalle F: Metformin lowers lipoprotein(a) levels [letter]. *Diabetes Care* 1998;21:2028-2029.

28. Mudaliar S, Henry RR: New oral therapies for type 2 diabetes mellitus: the glitazones or insulin sensitizers. *Annu Rev Med* 2001; 52:239-257.

29. Malinowski JM, Bolesta S: Rosiglitazone in the treatment of type 2 diabetes mellitus: a critical review. *Clin Ther* 2000;22:1151-1168.

30. Ahmann AJ, Riddle MC: Oral pharmacological agents. In Leahy JL, Clark NG, Cefalu WT, eds. *Medical Management of Diabetes Mellitus.* New York, Marcel Dekker, 2000, pp 267-283.

31. Parulkar AA, Pendergrass ML, Granda-Ayala R, et al: Nonhypoglycemic effects of thiazolidinediones. *Ann Intern Med* 2001;134:61-71.

32. Langtry HD, Markham A: Fluvastatin: a review of its use in lipid disorders. *Drugs* 1999;57:583-606.

33. Nissen D, ed: *2002 Mosby's Drug Consult.* St. Louis, MO, Mosby, 2002.

34. U.S. Pharmacopeial Convention, Inc: U.S. Pharmacopeia Dispensing Information, Volume II-Drug Information for Health Care Professional. Greenwood Village, CO, MICROMEDIX Thomson Healthcare, 2002.

35. Zetia (ezetimibe) Annotated Prescribing Information. North Wales, PA, Merck/Schering-Plough Pharmaceuticals Inc., 2002.

36. Gagne C, Bays H, Weiss SR, et al: Efficacy and safety of ezetimibe added to ongoing statin therapy for treatment of patients with primary hypercholesterolemia. *Am J Cardiol* 2002;90: 1084-1091.

37. Yki-Jarvinen H: Management of type 2 diabetes mellitus and cardiovascular risk: lessons from intervention trials. *Drugs* 2000;60:975-983.

38.   Koskinen P, Manttari M, Manninen V, et al: Coronary heart disease incidence in NIDDM patients in the Helsinki Heart Study. *Diabetes Care* 1992;15:820-825.

39.   Diabetes Atherosclerosis Intervention Study Investigators: Effect of fenofibrate on progression of coronary-artery disease in type 2 diabetes: the Diabetes Atherosclerosis Intervention Study, a randomised study. *Lancet* 2001;357:905-910.

40.   Downs JR, Clearfield M, Weis S, et al: Primary prevention of acute coronary events with lovastatin in men and women with average cholesterol levels: results of AFCAPS/TexCAPS. *JAMA* 1998;279:1615-1622.

41.   Zocor Package Insert. Whitehouse Station, NJ, Merck & Co, 2001.

42.   Despres J-P: Increasing high-density lipoprotein cholesterol: an update on fenofibrate. *Am J Cardiol* 2001;88(suppl):30N-36N.

43.   Steiner G: Treating lipid abnormalities in patients with type 2 diabetes mellitus. *Am J Cardiol* 2001;88(suppl):37N-40N.

44.   Tricor Package Insert. North Chicago, IL, Abbott Laboratories, 2001.

Chapter 9

Nephropathy in Diabetes: New Insights

Definition, Incidence, and Consequences

Diabetic nephropathy is defined as the persistent presence of more than 300 mg of albumin in the urine for 24 hours.[1,2] Albuminuria must be present in the absence of urinary tract infection, other kidney or renal tract disease, or heart failure.[3] Diabetic nephropathy affects up to 35% of patients with type 1 diabetes. In patients with type 2 diabetes, the cumulative incidence of nephropathy after at least 25 years of diabetes is 25% to 60%, depending on race.[1,4] In general, all type 1 diabetes patients with nephropathy also have retinopathy, while only 50% to 70% of type 2 diabetes patients do.[3]

Diabetic nephropathy accounts for 25% to 44% of all cases of end-stage renal disease (ESRD) and is the leading cause of ESRD in the United States, Europe, and Japan.[4] Patients with diabetes and hypertension have a fivefold to sixfold greater risk of ESRD than patients with hypertension alone.[5] In fact, because the prevalence of type 2 diabetes is increasing and patients with type 2 diabetes are surviving longer, patients with type 2 diabetes now comprise the largest, fastest-growing group requiring renal replacement therapy.[1] Diabetic nephropathy confers a high risk of not only ESRD, but also cardiovascular morbidity and mortality.[4] In addition, because ESRD patients with diabetic nephropathy often have concomitant coronary artery and cerebrovascular disease, their mortality and morbidity are greater than those of patients with ESRD from other causes.[2] A World Health Organization study found an all-cause mortality ratio of 2.8 in type 2 diabetes patients with marked proteinuria after a mean of 9.4 years, and even microalbuminuria considerably increased mortality risk. After 10 years, the hazard ratios for mortality in type 2 diabetes patients with microalbuminuria ranged from 1.5 to 2.3, and survival rates in these patients were about 30% to 40% vs 55% to 60% for patients with normoalbuminuria.[1]

Clinical Course and Natural History

In its early stages, diabetic nephropathy has no clinical signs or symptoms.[3] The course of nephropathy in type 2 diabetes can be arbitrarily divided into three stages: (1) no nephropathy to incipient nephropathy, indicated by progression from a normal urinary albumin excretion rate (UAER) (less than 30 mg/d) to microalbuminuria; (2) incipient nephropathy to established nephropathy, indicated by progression from microalbuminuria to macroalbuminuria (more than 300 mg/d); and (3) established nephropathy to ESRD.[6] Once nephropathy is established, the rate of decrease in the glomerular filtration rate (GFR) ranges from 4 to 22 mL/min/yr.[1] Although microalbuminuria progresses to nephropathy in 20% to 40% of patients with type 2 diabetes without medical intervention, only about 20% have ESRD 20 years after diagnosis of nephropathy.[7]

Proteinuria is preceded by changes in renal function such as hyperfiltration, hyperperfusion, and increased capillary permeability to macromolecules. These changes are accompanied by renal hypertrophy, including glomerular basement membrane thickening, glomerular hypertrophy, and mesangial expansion leading to glomerulosclerosis and tubulointerstitial fibrosis.[1,2] As the mesangium expands, it impinges on the glomerular capillary loops and filtration surface area to impede glomerular function.[8] In addition, glomerular podocytes progressively slough off the glomerular basement membrane as a result of apoptosis and do not regenerate.[9] These changes correlate with proteinuria.[9] Hypertension or increased glomerular perfusion pressure correlates with mesangial changes.[10] Angiotensin II, transforming growth factor-β (TGF-β), and hyperglycemia contribute to mesangial and podocyte pathology.[11]

Hypertension results from renal disease in type 1 diabetes. It is common in type 2 diabetes regardless of renal disease status[8] and is found in 30% of patients at diabetes diagnosis.[12] It frequently precedes onset of type 2 diabetes by years or even decades, and preexisting hypertension strongly predicts risk of proteinuria after type 2 diabetes develops.[13] Because confounding conditions such as essential hypertension are common in type 2 diabetes, microalbuminuria is a weaker indicator of diabetic nephropathy and predictor of its progression in patients with type 2 diabetes than in patients with type 1 diabetes.[14] In patients without diabetes, microalbuminuria is a marker for renal disease and vascular injury in the presence of hypertension and a predictor of diabetes.[15]

Risk Factor Assessment and Management

Epidemiologic studies have identified several risk factors for the development and progression of microalbuminuria in patients with type 2 diabetes. In addition to obesity, hyperglycemia, hyperinsulinemia, and hypertension,[6] they include duration of diabetes; age at diagnosis; male sex; and genetic predispositions such as race, familial disease clusters, and angiotensin-converting enzyme (ACE) polymorphisms. Initial UAER, poor glycemic control, mean arterial blood pressure greater than 94 mm Hg, retinopathy, dyslipidemia, and smoking also heighten the risk of nephropathy. Those older than 50 years at diabetes diagnosis have a higher prevalence of microalbuminuria than those younger than 40 years at diagnosis. In some studies, the male-to-female incidence ratio for ESRD was as high as 5:1. The cumulative incidence of nephropathy also differs by race; it is about 20% in European patients and 50% in Pima Indians and Japanese patients.[1] Native Americans, Asians, Hispanics (especially Mexican Americans), and African Americans have a much higher risk of ESRD than non-Hispanic whites.[7] Among Pima Indians with type 2 diabetes, proteinuria was three times more common in patients whose parents both had proteinuria than in patients whose parents did not.[1] Moreover, cardiovascular events and hypertension in first-degree relatives were the single most powerful predictors of early microalbuminuria in patients with recent-onset type 2 diabetes. These findings, as well as familial clustering of nephropathy, indicate that the disease has a strong genetic component.[13]

In patients with type 2 diabetes, a high-normal UAER was the most important risk factor for nephropathy, suggesting that even relatively normal UAERs reflect the pathological processes that cause diabetic kidney disease. In addition, baseline and annual increase in UAER are important risk factors for the progression of microalbuminuria to overt nephropathy.[1] Hyperglycemia has been established as an important risk factor for the onset of microalbuminuria, and no risk threshold exists.[13] Maintaining glycated hemoglobin (Hb A_{1c}) below 7.5% has been shown in many studies to reduce the risk of developing microalbuminuria, and those who developed microalbuminuria or progressed from it to macroalbuminuria had higher Hb A_{1c} levels.[1] Moreover, in patients with overt nephropathy, mean Hb A_{1c} has been shown to correlate with loss of renal function.[12] Intensive glycemic control (Hb $A_{1c} \leq 7\%$) in patients with newly diagnosed type 2 diabetes reduced the rate of progression from normoalbuminuria to microalbuminuria in the United Kingdom Prospective Diabetes Study (UKPDS), even though it did not reduce risk of progression from microalbuminuria to proteinuria.[1] However, a Japanese study of patients with type 2 diabetes showed that intensive insulin therapy prevented progression not only from normoalbuminuria to microalbuminuria, but also from microalbuminuria to macroalbuminuria. Three or more insulin injections daily resulted in less new or progressive nephropathy during 6 years than one or two injections daily (7.7% vs 28%).[12]

Elevated systemic blood pressure is also a risk factor for the development and progression of microalbuminuria, and mean arterial pressure greater than 94 mm Hg predicts microalbuminuria progression more strongly than hyperglycemia does. Once microalbuminuria appears, blood pressure rises about 2 to 3 mm Hg annually, and nocturnal decrease in blood pressure (dipping) is commonly impaired. As a result, the prevalence of hypertension is 40% in those with microalbuminuria and 80% in those with overt nephropathy, compared with 20% in those with normoalbuminuria.[1] Hypertension clearly accelerates loss of renal function in patients with overt nephropathy.[12]

Some studies have shown that hyperlipidemia is an independent risk factor for microalbuminuria, although small studies of hypercholesterolemic type 2 diabetes patients with elevated UAER did not find less albuminuria and decline in GFR with statin therapy.[1] Renal disease results in accumulation of intact or partly metabolized triglyceride-rich complex apo B-containing lipoproteins that are associated with the progression of small atherosclerotic lesions and may be responsible for lipid nephrotoxicity.[16] As many as 20% of patients with type 2 diabetes have ischemic nephropathy secondary to atherosclerosis of the abdominal aorta with renal artery stenosis or cholesterol microembolism,[13] and diabetic patients with elevated cholesterol or triglyceride levels have faster renal functional decline than patients without such elevations. In the presence of mesangial dysfunction, lipoproteins may accumulate in glomeruli and adversely affect glomerular function.[16]

In patients with type 2 diabetes, smoking is an independent risk factor for nephropathy and is associated with accelerated loss of renal function.[12] Diabetic patients who smoke have a greater risk of developing microalbuminuria and of progressing to ESRD than those who do not smoke. The ability of smoking to accelerate diabetic nephropathy is well established but not widely appreciated.[1,14] Moreover, at least in patients with type 1 diabetes, smoking cessation slows loss of renal function[14] and may reduce the risk of disease progression by 30%.[12] Although smoking cessation has not been proven to have a renoprotective effect in patients with type 2 diabetes, it clearly reduces cardiovascular risk and can be expected to reduce renovascular risk.[1]

Prevention and Treatment
Rationale and Goals

Renoprotective measures should prevent nephropathy and delay its progression.[6] Studies have demonstrated that, although the onset and course of diabetic nephropathy can be mitigated considerably by several interventions, these measures have their greatest effect when begun early in the course of the disease.[7] Tight glycemic control using intensive insulin therapy in patients with type 2 diabetes has decreased the frequency of developing microalbuminuria by 57% and of developing macroalbuminuria by 70%.[3] Aggressive control of hypertension also prevents nephropathy in patients in whom microalbuminuria has not yet developed. Maximizing the angiotensin-converting enzyme inhibitor (ACEI) dose can substantially decrease or even reverse confirmed microalbuminuria.

Intensive multifactorial treatment appears to prevent overt nephropathy in type 2 diabetes patients with microalbuminuria. In a 4-year trial, such treatment was shown to slow progression of microalbuminuria to overt nephropathy to a statistically significant degree compared with conventional treatment. The treatment goals for the intensive therapy group and the conventional therapy group were Hb A_{1c} <6.5% and <7.5%, blood pressure <140/85 mm Hg and <160/95 mm Hg, total cholesterol

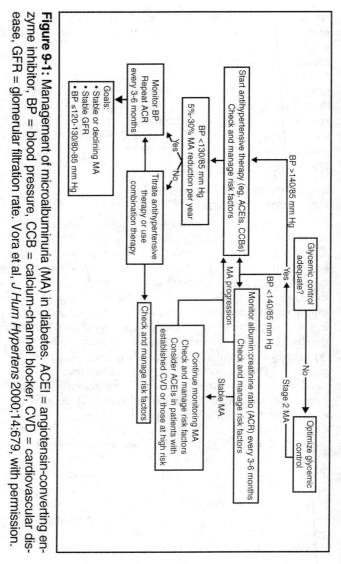

Figure 9-1: Management of microalbuminuria (MA) in diabetes. ACEI = angiotensin-converting enzyme inhibitor, BP = blood pressure, CCB = calcium-channel blocker, CVD = cardiovascular disease, GFR = glomerular filtration rate. Vora et al, *J Hum Hypertens* 2000;14:679, with permission.

<5 mm/L and <6.5 mmol/L, high-density lipoprotein cholesterol >1.1 mmol/L and >0.9 mmol/L, and triglyceride <1.7 mmol/L and <2.2 mmol/L, respectively. Intensive therapy included the ACEI captopril (Capoten®) 50 mg twice daily, irrespective of blood pressure, and, in patients with ischemic disease, aspirin.[1] Figure 9-1 illustrates an approach to the management of microalbuminuria in patients with type 2 diabetes.

Once macroalbuminuria develops and nephropathy becomes overt, glycemic control is less likely to stabilize or reverse its progression.[3] At this stage, progression to renal failure may depend more on injurious compensatory measures within the nephron than on hyperglycemic injury.[8] Thus, the most important factor in slowing loss of renal function in type 2 diabetes patients with overt nephropathy is aggressive treatment of hypertension, which can halve loss of function compared with that in untreated patients.[3] The National Kidney Foundation recommends a goal blood pressure of less than 125/75 mm Hg for diabetic patients with overt nephropathy.[13] If initial goals can be met and therapy is well tolerated, greater reduction is indicated.[7] Additional decrease in systolic blood pressure to 100 to 110 mm Hg is beneficial,[3] particularly if drug side effects can be avoided. Once persistent proteinuria appears, conventionally treated patients typically survive for a mean of 5 to 7 years, but studies of aggressive antihypertensive therapy have shown that such treatment resulted in a median survival of at least 14 years.[4] In numerous long-term trials in patients who have lost more than 35% of renal function, reducing proteinuria to more than 30% below baseline correlated with marked reduction in renal disease progression. In contrast, in patients with near normal renal function, results of studies exploring such an association have been mixed. Nevertheless, these findings have led to the recommendation that the goal of antihypertensive therapy be to reduce proteinuria as well as decrease blood pressure.[17]

Prevention and Treatment Strategies
General Measures

Patients with diabetic nephropathy should avoid dehydration, which can irreversibly decrease renal function.[3] Smoking cessation markedly reduces nephropathy risk; therefore, all patients with diabetes should be strongly encouraged to stop smoking and to abstain permanently.[13] Use of radiocontrast media or nephrotoxic drugs, overuse of diuretics, and urinary tract infections accelerate the progression of nephropathy to ESRD and should be avoided. However, coronary angiography is often necessary in patients with diabetic nephropathy because of their high incidence of ischemic heart disease. When radiocontrast procedures are warranted, the lowest possible dose of radiocontrast medium should be used. Because dehydration and use of nephrotoxic antibiotics, antifungal agents, or nonsteroidal anti-inflammatory drugs (NSAIDs) increase the risk of radiocontrast-induced renal shutdown, such drugs should be withdrawn well in advance of radiocontrast procedures, which should be preceded by active rehydration and accompanied and followed by high intravenous fluid intake. Renotoxic drugs should be avoided or only used when essential, diuretic dose should be decreased to eliminate only morning and not evening ankle edema, and even minor urinary tract infections should be treated aggressively.[3]

Lifestyle Intervention

Lifestyle changes, including weight loss, exercise, and reduced salt and alcohol intake, should receive special emphasis in patients at high risk of nephropathy.[7] Salt restriction has been shown to not only reduce hyperfiltration, albuminuria, and kidney weight in animal models, but also improve the antiproteinuric effect of ACEIs.[14] In addition, because hyperglycemia and dyslipidemia are risk factors for diabetic nephropathy, and because diet therapy is crucial for controlling these risk factors even when pharmacotherapy is used, consistent use of diet therapy should be stressed. Dyslipidemia is especially common in patients with overt nephropathy,[12] and because these patients and those with microalbuminuria are at greatly increased risk of cardiovascular morbidity and mortality, restricted dietary cholesterol intake is clearly warranted. Preliminary evidence suggests that decreasing cholesterol levels may also decrease proteinuria.[7]

Most patients with diabetes should obtain 10% to 20% of their daily caloric intake from protein.[18] In patients with type 1 diabetes, UAER was found to increase with higher protein intakes, especially in those who consumed more than 20% of their dietary energy as protein. Because high protein intake can accelerate loss of renal function, protein restriction may be indicated in diabetic nephropathy. A low-protein diet (0.6 g/kg body weight daily) can theoretically decrease glomerular hypertension, reduce proteinuria, and retard loss of renal function, although it has no effect on albuminuria or the nephrotic syndrome once hepatic albumin production maximizes at 150% of normal.[3] The Modified Diet in Renal Disease Study did not show a clear benefit from protein restriction, but only 3% of patients in this study had type 2 diabetes, none had type 1, and few experienced renal failure.[7] More recently, meta-analysis has indicated that a low-protein diet does deter the progression of diabetic nephropathy.[3] Combined results of five smaller studies including patients with type 1 diabetes showed that protein consumption ranging from 0.5 to 0.85 g/kg daily significantly reduced the rate of decline in GFR or creatinine clearance or the increase in UAER. Equally compelling data for patients with type 2 diabetes are not available.[14]

The consensus for treating type 2 diabetes patients with overt nephropathy is to prescribe a protein intake of 0.8 g/kg of body weight daily, which is about the Recommended Dietary Allowance for normal adults.[18] Once the GFR begins to decrease, restriction of protein intake to 0.6 g/kg/d may help slow this decrease in selected patients. However, this approach must be balanced against nutrition-related muscle weakness.[18] Protein-restricted meal plans should be designed by a registered dietitian well versed in the comprehensive dietary management of diabetes.[7]

Renoprotective Pharmacotherapies

Reaching blood pressure goals is clearly important for renal protection. Clinical trials suggest that inhibition of the renin-angiotensin system (RAS) may offer additional benefit. ACEIs and angiotensin-receptor blockers (ARBs) have favorable effects on glomerular hemodynamics and proteinuria independent of their primary effect in reducing blood pressure. These effects may stem from their ability to mitigate angiotensin II's profibrotic nonhemodynamic effects and stimulation of aldosterone, which is also profibrotic. The ARB irbesartan (Avapro®) has also been found to prevent nephrin depletion in glomerular podocytes. Nephrin modulates the filtration of proteins across the glomerular barrier. This effect was associated with reduction in albuminuria.[19]

In normotensive type 2 diabetes patients with microalbuminuria, ACEIs can reduce the rate of decrease in GFR and the progression of microalbuminuria to macroalbuminuria.[14] In its diabetes substudy, the Heart Outcomes Prevention Evaluation (HOPE) trial showed that, after 4.5 years, ramipril (Altace®) decreased the rate of progression to overt nephropathy by 24% compared with placebo in type 2 diabetes patients with normoalbuminuria and those with microalbuminuria.[12] In normotensive type 2 diabetes patients with microalbuminuria, 4 to 5 years of treatment with enalapril (Vasotec®) stabilized or reduced albuminuria and preserved renal function in three separate studies of different ethnic populations.[1] As a result, ACEIs have been the preferred agents in treating diabetic patients with incipient nephropathy.[14] ACEIs also appear to be valuable in preventing microalbuminuria. Results of a small preliminary study of hypertensive type 2 diabetes patients with normoalbuminuria found that 3 years of ACEI therapy slightly improved GFR and decreased risk of progression to microalbuminuria. Treatment with enalapril for 6 years decreased UAER and progression to microalbuminuria more effectively than placebo in normotensive type 2 diabetes patients with normoalbuminuria.[10] In this study, enalapril reduced the absolute risk of developing microalbuminuria by 12.5% and significantly retarded loss of renal function as indicated by creatinine clearance measurements.

Although ACEIs reduce mortality in the more advanced stages of nephropathy,[14] their renoprotective benefits for patients with overt nephropathy are less clear. For example, ACEIs reversed glomerular barrier size-selective dysfunction and proteinuria in type 1 diabetes patients with overt nephropathy, but they did not do so in studies of proteinuric patients with type 2 diabetes. Although results of reported studies of antihypertensive therapy in type 2 diabetes patients with overt nephropathy found greater antiproteinuric effects for ACEI regimens than for regimens without ACEIs,[1] with one exception, available studies have not been statistically powerful enough to detect an effect of ACEIs on the decrease in GFR in these patients.[4,12] In addition, the antiproteinuric effect of ACEIs in patients with diabetic nephropathy varies considerably. This variation may result from individual, genetically based differences in the RAS. In particular, patients homozygous for the 289-base pair sequence deletion in the ACE gene may benefit from more aggressive ACE inhibition or combination therapy with ARBs and nondihydropyridine calcium-channel blockers (CCBs).[1] ACEIs are contraindicated in proteinuric patients with type 2 diabetes with renovascular disease,[10] which contributes to hypertension in as many as 40% of these patients[12] and increases the risk of ACEI-related acute renal failure and hyperkalemia. However, hyperkalemia caused withdrawal from these trials in only 1.5% of patients and did not result in fatality,[12] although a crossover study showed that patients randomized to receive an ARB had even less hyperkalemia than those randomized to receive an ACEI.[17]

Results of two recent trials indicate that ARBs are the agents of first choice for preventing nephropathy in patients with type 2 diabetes.[5] Irbesartan and losartan (Cozaar®) recently received approval from the US Food and Drug Administration for an additional indication for use in treating diabetic nephropathy.

The Irbesartan Diabetic Nephropathy Trial (IDNT) compared irbesartan with amlodipine (Norvasc®, Lotrel®) or conventional treatment with agents other than ACEIs, ARBs, or dihydropyridines. In IDNT, irbesartan was superior to conventional therapy in reducing the primary end point, a composite of doubling of serum creatinine level, renal failure, and mortality, even though differences in blood pressure control between groups were negligible or nonexistent.[19] IDNT was part of the Program for Irbesartan Mortality and Morbidity Evaluations (PRIME), which was designed to examine the full spectrum of renal disease and also incorporated the Irbesartan in Patients with Type 2 Diabetes and Microalbuminuria (IRMA) trial.[20] In IRMA, after 2 years, the irbesartan group showed a dose-dependent risk reduction in the primary outcome, which was onset of diabetic nephropathy as indicated by proteinuria; a dose of 300 mg daily reduced this risk by 70%. Moreover, this dose of irbesartan reduced albuminuria by 38% compared with a 2% increase in the placebo group. In addition, regression to normoalbuminuria occurred in 34% of patients in the group receiving irbesartan 300 mg daily vs 21% in the placebo group.[19] The IRMA investigators concluded that irbesartan is renoprotective independent of its antihypertensive effects in hypertensive type 2 diabetes patients with macroalbuminuria. When considered together, the results of these studies confirm that ARB therapy is nephroprotective when used in early and late stages of type 2 diabetic nephropathy.[20]

In a population similar to that studied in IDNT, the Reduction of Endpoints in NIDDM with the Angiotensin II Antagonist Losartan (RENAAL) Trial compared losartan with conventional treatment in a predominantly hypertensive population of type 2 diabetes patients with macroproteinuria and impaired renal function. Many of the patients in this study received dihydropyridine CCBs as part of their conventional treatment. In RENAAL, losartan 50 to 100 mg daily reduced the risk of progression to ESRD by 28%, the risk of doubling of serum creatinine level by 25%, and proteinuria by 35%.[19] Relative risk reduction for the composite end point of doubled creatinine level, ESRD, or death was 16% for losartan vs conventional treatment.[20] Results of a recent dose-escalation study suggest that the optimal dose of losartan appears to be 100 mg daily, which was shown to maximally reduce albuminuria by 49% in type 1 diabetes patients with nephropathy.[4]

Although ACEIs reduce the impact of angiotensin II, they do not completely eliminate its effects. However, combining an ACEI and an ARB can do so while still exploiting the positive effects of bradykinin stimulation by the ACEI and further reducing levels of the profibrotic hormone aldosterone. Moreover, long-term use of an ACEI plus an ARB may result in less glomerular and interstitial fibrosis than use of an ACEI alone by further attenuating the effects of angiotensin II.[21] Results of studies in type 2 diabetes patients with microalbuminuria or overt nephropathy suggest that combining an ACEI and an ARB enhances their antihypertensive and antiproteinuric effects and is well tolerated.[4] For example, in the Candesartan and Lisinopril Microalbuminuria (CALM) study of hypertensive patients with type 2 diabetes, candesartan (Atacand®) plus lisinopril (Prinivil®; Zestril®) was associated with not only better blood pressure control, but also a trend toward reduction in UAER when compared with monotherapy with either agent.[19]

Like ACEIs and ARBs, nondihydropyridine CCBs are also renoprotective independent of their ability to reduce systemic blood pressure. They appear to reduce intraglomerular capillary pressure and thereby prevent mesangial expansion and glomerulosclerosis. In three different meta-analyses, nondihydropyridine CCBs were found to reduce albuminuria and further decrease GFR in patients with established diabetic nephropathy. These findings were confirmed by the results of two studies in type 2 diabetes patients with established nephropathy who were followed up for at least 5 years. In these studies, long-acting verapamil (Calan® SR) or diltiazem (Cardizem® SR) slowed the progression of established renal disease as much as an ACEI.[21] Additive antiproteinuric effects have been observed from combining a nondihydropyridine CCB with an ACEI, which appears to potentiate the renoprotective effect of the ACEI. For example, trandolapril (Mavik®) plus verapamil produced greater renoprotection in type 2 diabetes patients with nephropathy than either agent alone despite comparable blood pressure control among treatment groups. Such combinations also generally produce fewer side effects than either agent used alone.

The complex pathophysiology of hypertension in diabetic nephropathy usually requires more than one agent for adequate control. Inhibiting the RAS in patients with type 2 diabetes and evidence of nephropathy by using an ARB as first-line therapy is recommended, although an ACEI may be useful.[22] They may be combined with a nondihydropyridine CCB and/or a diuretic when necessary to reach blood pressure goals and reduce albuminuria.[1] Both of these classes of antihypertensives have been shown to increase the antiproteinuric effects of ACEIs. Moreover, combining an ACEI, an ARB, a diuretic, and a nondihydropyridine CCB with a statin and antiglycemic treatment to reach a goal of Hb A_{1c} <7.5% resulted in remission (UAER <1 g/24 h and no greater loss of renal function than that associated with aging) in 14 of 20 patients with chronic nephropathy and persistent, nephrotic-range proteinuria. All three patients with type 2 diabetes in this uncontrolled study experienced remission.[12]

Oral glucose-control agents such as some sulfonylureas and metformin (Glucophage®, Glucophage® XR), are metabolized or cleared by the kidneys and may accumulate to toxic levels in patients with poor renal function. As a result, metformin therapy is contraindicated in patients with renal failure. Insulin is also cleared by the kidney, so insulin doses may decrease as renal failure progresses. In contrast, the thiazolidinediones (TZDs) (pioglitazone, Actos®; rosiglitazone, Avandia®) are cleared by the liver and therefore may be particularly useful in these patients. In addition to counteracting insulin resistance, TZDs, or peroxisome proliferator-activated receptor-γ (PPAR-γ) ligands, exert antihypertensive and antiproteinuric effects in diabetic patients. Their antihypertensive mechanism appears to result from improved insulin sensitivity or direct beneficial effects on vascular tone. Because TZDs mitigate extracellular matrix expansion induced by TGF-β, they may be of particular benefit in diabetic nephropathy. They also reduce albuminuria in animals, and, in studies of patients with type 2 diabetes, they decreased UAER more than other antiglycemic agents did. These findings, along with the finding that PPAR is expressed on mesangial cells, suggest that TZDs have direct glomerular effects.[23]

Classes of antihypertensive agents other than ACEIs, ARBs, and nondihydropyridine CCBs have not been clearly demonstrated to protect the kidney beyond the effects produced by blood pressure lowering. In the UKPDS, captopril and atenolol (Tenormin®) had similar cardiovascular protective effects and effects on the kidney, although there were fewer patients with nephropathy.[12] α-Blockers have neutral effects on proteinuria despite their antihypertensive effect,[17] and dihydropyridine CCBs may worsen proteinuria and accelerate progression of nephropathy[12] unless they are combined with an ACEI. Although less progression of nephropathy without reduction in proteinuria was reported with dihydropyridine CCB therapy in patients with early diabetic nephropathy, once renal disease is established, these agents should not be used without an ACEI.[17]

Statins may also exert renoprotective effects unrelated to their other benefits in patients with type 2 diabetes. For example, meta-analysis of 13 controlled trials involving 253 diabetic patients showed that statins decreased proteinuria and preserved GFR in patients with chronic renal disease, and these effects were not entirely explained by reduction in serum cholesterol.[12] In addition, lowering cholesterol with lovastatin (Mevacor®) and lowering triglyceride with gemfibrozil (Lopid®) have been shown to retard the progression of diabetic nephropathy.[14] High-dose vitamin E (1,800 IU daily) has been shown to reduce mean creatinine clearance from 186 to 130 mL/min/1.73 m^2 after 4 months of treatment and may be of particular benefit in patients who respond poorly to ACEIs.[24]

Treatment of Advanced Nephropathy

Once macroalbuminuria develops, ESRD almost inevitably results. Substantial decline in GFR or a GFR <60 mg/cc/min warrants a nephrology referral.[7] As nephropathy progresses, serum creatinine, blood pressure, edema, congestive heart failure, and serum electrolytes, especially potassium and bicarbonate, should be carefully monitored. Treatment of ESRD is required when uremic symptoms such as pruritus, nausea, vomiting, muscle cramps, refractory edema, hyperkalemia, or acidosis develop. In patients with type IV metabolic acidosis, oral sodium bicarbonate or sodium citrate improves acidosis and hyperkalemia, although the increase in sodium load may require an increased dose of diuretic. Because ACEIs, ARBs, and NSAIDs worsen hyperkalemic metabolic acidosis, they should be discontinued if acidosis cannot otherwise be controlled. In addition, wide fluctuations in glycemic control accentuate hyperkalemia in type IV acidosis and should be avoided. Although uremia-related insulin resistance is well documented, hypoglycemia from decreased renal insulin degradation is a greater problem, and insulin dose usually must be reduced at this stage.[8] Another complication of advanced renal disease, osteodystrophy, is typically treated with sodium and phosphate restriction and phosphate binders.[7]

Renal Replacement Therapy

Once serum creatinine approaches 4 mg/dL, renal replacement therapy should be examined. Although dialysis or transplantation is usually required when serum creatinine reaches 8 to 10 mg/dL in patients without diabetes, patients with diabetes are less able to tolerate uremic symptoms and generally require renal replacement therapy well before this level is reached. Diabetic patients are candidates for all three types of renal replacement therapy: hemodialysis, peritoneal dialysis, and transplantation.[8]

Hemodialysis

Although renal transplantation produces the greatest subjective benefits of all three renal replacement therapies,[8] dialysis is often required in type 2 diabetes patients with ESRD, in whom transplantation is rarely an option.[3] Diabetic patients generally tolerate hemodialysis well, and when blood pressure is well controlled between treatments, retinopathy does not accelerate. However, subjective improvement in peripheral and autonomic neuropathy is not as great after initiation of dialysis as it is after transplantation, and hemodialysis has many other disadvantages. For example, the use of heparin in hemodialysis may cause vitreous and other hemorrhages. However, injected or oral heparin exerts a renoprotective effect by replenishing depleted levels of heparin sulfate and other proteoglycans underproduced by mesangial cells in diabetic nephropathy. Although experimental, heparin therapy reverses related proteinuria and loss of anionic charge in the basement membrane and inhibits mesangial cell proliferation and glomerulosclerosis, thereby stabilizing the mesangium. Hemodialysis also requires an arteriovenous shunt,[3] but constructing a well-functioning fistula in diabetic dialysis patients can be difficult because of vascular disease. Therefore, a fistula or Gore-Tex graft should be placed several months before initiation of dialysis. Temporary or tunneled catheters can cause infection, thrombosis, and inadequate hemodialysis. Hemodialysis worsens neuropathy, accelerates atherosclerosis, and has a high mortality rate. It may also cause digital ischemia and gangrene.

Continuous ambulatory peritoneal dialysis (CAPD) overcomes many of the disadvantages of hemodialysis. Instead of using heparin or requiring vascular access, this method delivers dialysate intraperitoneally into the portal circulatory system. Although the high glucose concentrations in peritoneal dialysate may worsen hyperglycemia, addition of insulin minimizes this problem, and peritoneal dialysis is generally well tolerated in diabetic patients. Moreover, when insulin is injected into the portal rather than the systemic circulatory system, its action becomes more like that of endogenous insulin, thereby enhancing glycemic control.[8] The main complication of CAPD is acute peritonitis, which occurs with the same frequency in patients with diabetes as in those without.[3] Because anemia often develops in patients during dialysis, this therapy has not offered patients the same degree of improvement in quality of life as renal transplantation. However, the recent introduction of erythropoietin therapy (epoetin alfa, Procrit®) for nephropathy-related anemia has diminished the difference between these therapies in the resulting quality of life.[8] Furthermore, anemia, which can occur much earlier than the need for dialysis, should be monitored closely and managed aggressively. Referral to a nephrologist should be considered at the first signs of anemia.

Transplantation

Because it offers the greatest sense of well-being and best chance for a productive lifestyle,[8] transplantation is the treatment of choice in patients with ESRD. To avoid complications resulting from ESRD, assessment for renal transplantation should be done when creatinine clearance is <30 mL/min. Transplantation success rates in carefully matched related donors are excellent.[3] In diabetic patients who received renal transplants in the late 1960s and the 1970s, after 10 years, 75% had a functioning graft, and 40% had survived. However, survival is only increased relative to that in dialysis patients in recipients of HLA-identical sibling grafts. The recent introduction of highly effective immunosuppressive agents has increased these survival rates.

The development of laparoscopic organ harvesting procedures has made kidney donation much less traumatic for donors than it was previously. Successful transplantation results in subjective improvement in symptoms of peripheral and autonomic neuropathy in the first 6 to 12 months after the procedure, and advanced retinopathy stabilizes in most transplant patients. However, 5 years after transplantation, almost 20% of patients have lost a limb because of peripheral vascular disease, and cardiovascular disease is a major cause of mortality in these patients.[8] These statistics further accentuate the need to prevent nephropathy or halt its progression early through intensive multifactorial intervention.

References

1.   Vora JP, Ibrahim HA, Bakris GL: Responding to the challenge of diabetic nephropathy: the historic evolution of detection, prevention and management. *J Hum Hypertens* 2000;14:667-685.

2.   Raptis AE, Viberti G: Pathogenesis of diabetic nephropathy. *Exp Clin Endocrinol Diabetes* 2001;109(suppl 2):S424-S437.

3.   Bell DS, Alele J: Dealing with diabetic nephropathy. *Postgrad Med* 1999;105:83-87, 91-94.

4.   Parving HH, Hovind P, Rossing K, et al: Evolving strategies for renoprotection: diabetic nephropathy. *Curr Opin Nephrol Hypertens* 2001;10:515-522.

5. Bakris GL: A practical approach to achieving recommended blood pressure goals in diabetic patients. *Arch Intern Med* 2001; 161:2661-2667.

6. Wesson DE: Can risk factor modification prevent nephropathy in type 2 diabetes mellitus? *Am J Kidney Dis* 2000;36:1054-1056.

7. American Diabetes Association. Position statement: diabetic nephropathy. *Diabetes Care* 2003;26:S94-S98. Available from http://care.diabetesjournals.org/cgi/content/full/26/suppl_1/s94.

8. Daniels BS, Goetz FC: Diabetes and the kidney. In Davidson JK, ed: *Clinical Diabetes Mellitus: A Problem-Oriented Approach.* New York: Thieme Medical Publishers, Inc., 2000, pp 529-537.

9. Pagtalunan ME, Miller PL, Jumping-Eagle S, et al: Podocyte loss and progressive glomerular injury in type II diabetes. *J Clin Invest* 1997;99:342-348.

10. Ruggenenti P, Remuzzi G: Nephropathy of type 1 and type 2 diabetes: diverse pathophysiology, same treatment? *Nephrol Dial Transplant* 2000;15:1900-1902.

11. Leehey DJ, Singh AK, Alavi N, et al: Role of angiotensin II in diabetic nephropathy. *Kidney Int Suppl* 2000;77:S93-S98.

12. Remuzzi G, Schieppati A, Ruggenenti P: Clinical practice. Nephropathy in patients with type 2 diabetes. *N Engl J Med* 2002; 346:1145-1151.

13. Ritz E, Tarng DC: Renal disease in type 2 diabetes. *Nephrol Dial Transplant* 2001;16(suppl 5):11-18.

14. Roshan B, Solomon RJ: Diabetes and nephropathy. In Johnstone MT, Veves A, eds: *Diabetes and Cardiovascular Disease.* Totowa (NJ): Humana Press, 2001, pp 399-410.

15. Mykkanen L, Zaccaro DJ, O'Leary DH, et al: Microalbuminuria and carotid artery intima-media thickness in nondiabetic and NIDDM subjects. The Insulin Resistance Atherosclerosis Study (IRAS). *Stroke* 1997;28:1710-1716.

16. Attman PO: Progression of renal failure and lipids—is there evidence for a link in humans? *Nephrol Dial Transplant* 1998; 13:545-547.

17. Bakris GL, Williams M, Dworkin L, et al: Preserving renal function in adults with hypertension and diabetes: a consensus approach. National Kidney Foundation Hypertension and Diabetes Executive Committees Working Group. *Am J Kid Dis* 2000;36: 646-661.

18. American Diabetes Association: Position statement: evidence-based nutrition principles and recommendations for the treatment and prevention of diabetes and related complications. *Diabetes Care* 2003;26:S51-S61. Available from http://care.diabetesjournals.org/cgi/content/full/26/suppl_1/s51.

19. Jandeleit-Dahm K, Cooper ME: Hypertension and diabetes. *Curr Opin Nephrol Hypertens* 2002;11:221-228.

20. Studney D: Angiotensin blockade in type 2 diabetes: what the new evidence tells us about renal and cardiac complications. *Can J Cardiol* 2002;18(suppl A):3A-6A.

21. Odama UO, Bakris GL: Combination therapy for hypertension and renal disease in diabetes. Chapter 42. In Mogensen CE, ed: *The Kidney and Hypertension in Diabetes Mellitus.* 5th ed. Boston: Kluwer Academic Publishers, 2000, pp 559-573.

22. Hsueh WA: Treatment of type 2 diabetic nephropathy by blockade of the renin-angiotensin system: a comparison of angiotensin-converting-enzyme inhibitors and angiotensin receptor antagonists. *Curr Opin Pharmacol* 2002;2:182-188.

23. Hsueh WA, Nicholas SB: Peroxisome proliferator-activated receptor-γ in the renal mesangium. *Curr Opin Nephrol Hypertens* 2002;11:191-195.

24. Microalbuminuria. In Charles MA: *Diabetes Management: Complication Risk Assessment, Diagnosis, and Therapeutic Options.* Larchmont (NY): Mary Ann Liebert, Inc., Publishers. 2000, pp 83-91.

Chapter 10

Retinopathy of Diabetes: New Horizons

Because early detection, prompt treatment, and consistent follow-up are key aspects of diabetic retinopathy management, clinicians must recognize signs of the disease and rapidly refer patients for laser therapy to limit progression and protect vision. When a patient with diabetes reports blurred vision, careful eye examination is indicated to determine whether referral is appropriate. Referral is clearly indicated when visual acuity is worse than 20/40 or proliferative disease, characterized by the formation of new retinal vessels, is apparent.[1] In addition to recognizing established retinopathy, properly managing systemic factors that fuel it, such as hyperglycemia, anemia, hypertension, and nephropathy, is crucial to prevent this complication from threatening vision in patients with type 2 diabetes.

Prevalence, Incidence, and Progression

At any given time, diabetic retinopathy affects more than 35% of all diabetic patients[2] and, given enough time, eventually affects nearly 100%.[3] However, although retinopathy may be the first sign of type 2 diabetes,[4] patients with type 2 diabetes have a lower prevalence of retinopathy and, typically, less severe disease than patients with type 1 diabetes. Nevertheless, because 90% of all diabetic patients have type 2 diabetes, it accounts for more cases of diabetic retinopathy than type 1 diabetes does.[5]

Analysis of the United Kingdom Prospective Diabetes Study (UKPDS) data on type 2 diabetes patients found that 37% had retinopathy at diagnosis. In the 63% who did not, after 6 years, at least one microaneurysm had developed in 41%, microaneurysms in both eyes had developed in 22%, and retinopathy had progressed in 22%. In addition, after 6 years, the disease had progressed by two standard steps or more in 29% of the patients who had retinopathy at baseline.[6]

Natural History

Although the retina may appear normal on clinical examination even after several years of diabetes, important biochemical and physiologic changes, such as leukocyte adhesion and altered retinal blood flow, can be detected with sophisticated testing.[7] Retinopathy generally has an orderly course beginning with mild nonproliferative abnormalities characterized by increased vascular permeability.[8] As the disease progresses, retinal hemorrhages, microaneurysms, and more severe microvascular abnormalities appear.[7] Such moderate to severe nonproliferative diabetic retinopathy is characterized by vascular closure.[8] The progressive retinal capillary nonperfusion that results from vascular closure causes retinal ischemia, which may increase growth factor levels and may stimulate abnormal proliferation of new vessels[7] on the retina and posterior surface of the vitreous body.[8] The fragile new vessels that characterize such proliferative disease tend to bleed, scar, undergo fibrosis, and exude blood serum components into the retina.[7]

Retinopathy and Blindness
Causes of Vision Loss

Diabetic retinopathy causes vision loss via several mechanisms. Central vision may be diminished by capillary nonperfusion or blurred by thickening and structural distortion of the middle of the most visually acute area of the central retina, the macula. Such blurring is caused by swelling, or macular edema, produced by extravasated fluid from increased vascular permeability. In addition, the new blood vessels that form in proliferative diabetic retinopathy and the contraction of their accompanying fibrous tissue can distort the retina and detach it under force of traction, causing severe, often permanent, vision loss. Furthermore, these new vessels may bleed and cause hematomas in front of the retina or within the vitreous body of the eye. These hematomas may enlarge enough to impede vision by blocking the transmission of light to the retina.[8] In diabetic patients with proliferative retinopathy, these vitreous hemorrhages were found to be the leading cause of severe persistent vision loss, which was reported in 3% of these patients.[1]

Statistics

Blindness is 25 times more common in diabetic patients than in people without diabetes.[2] The Wisconsin Epidemiologic Study of Diabetic Retinopathy (WESDR) found that 1.6% of patients with diabetes onset after 30 years of age, an operational definition of type 2 diabetes, were legally blind, compared with 3.6% of patients with diabetes onset before 30 years of age (type 1 diabetes).[8] Blindness in diabetic patients typically results from proliferative diabetic retinopathy or macular edema. However, it may also result from cataract and glaucoma,[4] which, although not unique to diabetes, are more prevalent in patients with type 2 diabetes than in the general population. Nevertheless, most vision loss in diabetic patients is caused by diabetic retinopathy, which accounts for approximately 8,000 new cases of legal blindness annually and is the leading cause of blindness in the working-age US population (those aged 20 to 74 years).[2] However, in a large, population-based study, although diabetic retinopathy caused legal blindness in 87% of patients with type 1 diabetes, it was a causal factor in only one third of type

Table 10-1: Summary of American Academy of Ophthalmology Preferred Practice Plan for Diabetic Retinopathy: Schedule of Follow-up Examinations

Retinopathy Severity Level	Follow-up (mos)
No retinopathy or microaneurysms only	12
Mild to moderate nonproliferative retinopathy with macular edema	6 to 12
Mild to moderate nonproliferative retinopathy with macular edema that is not clinically significant	4 to 6
Mild to moderate nonproliferative retinopathy with clinically significant macular edema	3 to 4
Severe to very severe nonproliferative retinopathy	3 to 4
Mild to moderate proliferative retinopathy but not high risk	2 to 3
High-risk proliferative retinopathy	3 to 4

Adapted from American Academy of Ophthalmology: Diabetic retinopathy, Preferred practice pattern. San Francisco, CA: American Academy of Ophthalmology; 1998.

2 diabetic patients. This finding reflects the role of cataract, glaucoma, and macular degeneration in inducing vision loss in patients with type 2 diabetes, who, as a group, are generally older than patients with type 1 diabetes.[2] In patients with diabetic retinopathy, cataracts may also contribute to vision loss because their surgi-

cal treatment can accelerate the development of the retinal changes associated with retinopathy progression and can increase the risk of vision loss from laser photocoagulation therapy for diabetic retinopathy.[3]

Screening

Because type 2 diabetes is often already well established by the time it is discovered, diabetic retinopathy is commonly present at diagnosis. As a result, type 2 diabetic patients should have a dilated, comprehensive eye examination by an ophthalmologist or suitably trained optometrist shortly after diagnosis of diabetes. If retinopathy is not found or if only microaneurysms are discovered, annual examinations should follow.[3,5] If retinopathy is more severe or progressing, more frequent examination and fluorescein angiography are warranted so that laser therapy can be started at the most appropriate and effective point in the course of the disease, before substantial and possibly permanent vision loss occurs. In type 2 diabetic patients with severe proliferative diabetic retinopathy, laser therapy can halve the risk of severe vision loss and vitrectomy (ie, removal of the vitreous body). Thus, early referral to an ophthalmologist is particularly important for these patients.[3] Table 10-1 provides the schedule of follow-up examinations recommended by the American Academy of Ophthalmology for each level of severity of retinopathy.

In addition, because pregnancy can increase the risk of onset of diabetic retinopathy or accelerate its progression in patients with diabetes, women with preexisting diabetes who are planning a pregnancy should receive a comprehensive eye examination and counseling regarding these risks. If pregnancy is confirmed in a woman who has not had a recent comprehensive eye examination, an examination should be performed as soon as possible after conception is confirmed. Follow-up examinations should be performed at least once during the pregnancy, depending on the initial findings, and 3 to 6 months postpartum. However, these guidelines do not apply to women in whom gestational diabetes develops because they are not at increased risk of diabetic retinopathy.[3,4]

The undilated pupil allows for only limited retinal examination; therefore, examination of the retina after the pupil has been pharmacologically dilated was previously considered crucial. The pupil could be adequately dilated for examination 10 to 20 minutes after instillation of a few drops of 1% tropicamide and 2.5% phenylephrine hydrochloride solution.[5] However, modern retinal screening cameras provide 80% of the accuracy of a traditional dilated eye examination and can provide rapid screening information from undilated eyes, especially if data are digitally transmitted to a retinal specialist facility.[9] Regular funduscopic examination enables the primary care physician to help the eye care specialist monitor the course of retinopathy and provides an opportunity to stress the importance of optimal diabetes care in preserving vision. Nevertheless, such examination does not substitute for more detailed regular examinations by the ophthalmologist or optometrist.[5]

Risk Factors and Their Management
Duration of Diabetes
A predictably linear relationship exists between development of retinopathy and duration of diabetes, the most important determinant of retinopathy.[2] Once retinopathy develops, its level of severity is closely associated with the duration of diabetes.[3]

Age and Sex
Analysis of the UKPDS data found no effect of age on incidence of diabetic retinopathy, but progression of diabetic retinopathy was more common in older UKPDS patients. Those in the middle tertile (aged 50 to 57 years at study entry) had a relative risk (RR) of 1.6, and those in the top tertile (aged 58 years or older at study entry) had

an RR of 2.1, compared with those in the bottom tertile. Although the incidence of retinopathy was the same in men and women in the UKPDS, multivariate analysis of the UKPDS data showed that women had a lower RR (0.54) of retinopathy progression compared with men.[6]

Hyperglycemia

Both the Diabetes Control and Complications Trial (DCCT) in type 1 diabetic patients and the UKPDS in type 2 diabetic patients established the importance of good glycemic control in slowing the progression and reducing the severity of diabetic retinopathy.[2,8] In the DCCT, after a mean of 6.5 years of follow-up, reaching a mean hemoglobin A_{1c} (Hb A_{1c}) of 7.2% with intensive therapy using three or more insulin injections daily reduced progression of retinopathy or delayed its development by 27%, compared with reaching a mean Hb A_{1c} of 8.9% with conventional therapy using two or fewer injections daily.[2] In patients who had no visible retinopathy at baseline, this reduction in Hb A_{1c} reduced the 3-year risk of developing retinopathy by three fourths, and, in those who did have retinopathy at baseline, reduction in Hb A_{1c} halved the progression rate.[5] Moreover, the Epidemiology of Diabetes Interventions and Complications (EDIC) study found that the ocular benefits of intensive therapy persisted 4 years after the DCCT ended, despite the narrowing of the difference in the level of glucose control between the conventional (median Hb A_{1c} = 8.2%) and the intensive therapy group (median Hb A_{1c} = 7.9%).[10]

In the largest, longest study of type 2 diabetic patients, the UKPDS, improved blood glucose control with intensive therapy reduced microvascular complications by 25%, compared with control achievable with conventional therapy.[8] In the UKPDS, intensive therapy incorporated either insulin or a sulfonylurea, and microvascular end points included vitreous hemorrhage, retinopathy requiring laser therapy, and renal failure.[11]

Moreover, a continuous relationship between the risk of these complications and the degree of glycemia was found in the UKPDS data: every percentage point decrease in Hb A_{1c} resulted in a 35% reduction in risk.[8] These findings were substantiated in a Japanese study of patients with type 2 diabetes. In that study, after 6 years of follow-up, intensive therapy reduced retinopathy onset from 32% to 8% and retinopathy progression from 44% to 19%, compared with conventional therapy.[12] Although these studies show that intensive therapy can preserve vision and reduce the need for laser therapy, they also showed that intensive therapy could not completely prevent retinopathy in the long term.[5]

Like the microvascular complications of hyperglycemia, the benefits of decreasing glycemia take years to appear. Although early studies such as the DCCT showed worsened retinopathy soon after a marked reduction in hyperglycemia, it was not typically associated with vision loss in patients with mild to moderate nonproliferative retinopathy and was outweighed by intensive therapy's long-term benefits. In patients with more severe retinopathy, referral to an ophthalmologist is recommended before intensive insulin therapy is initiated because laser therapy may be indicated before insulin therapy is intensified.[4]

Insulin Dependence

The need for exogenous insulin increases the risk of diabetic retinopathy in type 2 diabetic patients.[4] After a known duration of diabetes of less than 5 years, 40% of those taking insulin had retinopathy compared with 24% of those who were not taking insulin.[5] After 20 years of diabetes, type 2 diabetic patients who require insulin have an approximately 80% risk of any form of diabetic retinopathy and a 40% risk of the more severe, proliferative form. In contrast, those who do not require insulin have only a 20% risk of diabetic retinopathy and a 5% risk of the proliferative form after 20 years of diabetes.[4] Because the severity of diabetic retinopathy correlates with more frequent episodes of hypoglycemia, the association between insulin therapy and retinopathy risk may stem from hypoglycemia as a side effect of insulin therapy.[1] Alternatively, it may indicate that the switch to insulin therapy follows poor glycemic control and more severe disease. However, clinically significant macular edema, a particularly vision-threatening complication of diabetic retinopathy, which swells the central retinal area responsible for acute vision, affects approximately 15% of type 2 diabetic patients after about 20 years of diabetes, regardless of exogenous insulin requirement.[4]

Hypertension

Hypertension can independently cause retinopathy and is particularly prevalent in type 2 diabetes patients. In addition, results of epidemiologic studies indicate that hypertension may promote the development and progression of diabetic retinopathy[11] and is an established risk factor for macular edema.[3] Approximately two thirds of all relevant studies found an association between diabetic retinopathy and diastolic or systolic hypertension or both, although studies of elderly patients with type 2 diabetes have not found much effect of blood pressure on prevalence of retinopathy. Nevertheless, elevated systolic blood pressure may be an especially important promoter of type 2 diabetic retinopathy.[11] Analysis of updated UKPDS data showed that systolic blood pressure was significantly associated with the incidence but not the progression of retinopathy, although the risk of incidence and progression increased from the lowest to the highest tertile of mean blood pressure.[6] The UKPDS also showed that reducing systolic blood pressure by only 10 mm Hg and diastolic blood pressure by 5 mm Hg reduced diabetic microvascular complications by 37% after 8.4 years,[13] mostly owing to less need for laser therapy. Moreover, intensive blood pressure reduction from a baseline of 160/94 mm Hg to 144/82 mm Hg vs to 154/87 mm Hg for conventional antihypertensive therapy reduced retinopathy progression by 34% and risk of moderate loss of vision by 47%. These reductions were independent of the degree of glycemic control.[11]

Hypertension may promote diabetic retinopathy via several mechanisms. At elevated mean arterial pressures, diabetic patients with high blood glucose levels have poor autoregulation of retinal blood flow compared with nondiabetic patients. As a result, in diabetic patients, retinal vascular autoregulation may not adequately mitigate elevated systemic blood pressure. In addition, hypertension may worsen retinal endothelial damage in diabetic patients. Furthermore, retinal vascular endothelial stretch increases expression of vascular endothelial growth factor (VEGF) and its receptors, accounting for progression of retinopathy and some features of diabetic retinopathy that mimic those of hypertensive retinopathy.[11]

Nephropathy and Anemia

Results of extensive epidemiologic studies have indicated that microalbuminuria or proteinuria and retinopathy are related[11] and that the severity of nephropathy correlates with the severity of retinopathy.[2] Common predisposing factors, such as chronic hyperglycemia, duration of diabetes, and hypertension, may account for this relationship. Nonetheless, proteinuria predicts proliferative diabetic retinopathy, and two thirds of type 2 diabetic patients receiving dialysis have some form of retinopathy.[11] Moreover, like hypertensive retinopathy, renal retinopathy can be superimposed on diabetic retinopathy.[3] Therefore, patients with progressive renal dysfunction should be closely monitored for rapid worsening of retinopathy, and rapid progression of retinopathy suggests the need for renal evaluation.[11]

Renal failure often results in anemia, which has been associated with rapid progression of diabetic retinopathy.[11] Moreover, epidemiologic evidence indicates that, next to hyperglycemia, anemia is the second greatest risk factor for the development of diabetic retinopathy.[14] For example, a Finnish study found that retinopathy was twice as likely to be present in patients with a hemoglobin of less than 12 g/dL as in those with a hemoglobin of more than 12 g/dL. Furthermore, the risk of severe disease in retinopathy patients with low hemoglobin levels was five times the risk of severe disease in those with higher hemoglobin levels. In addition, the Early Treatment Diabetic Retinopathy Study (ETDRS) found that low hematocrit was an independent risk factor for high-risk proliferative retinopathy and severe vision loss. In anemic diabetic patients with renal failure, an increase in hematocrit from 29.6% to 39.5%, produced by treatment with erythropoietin (epoetin alfa, Procrit®, Epogen®), resolved macular edema in three of five patients studied, and the rest had improved or stable visual acuity. These findings indicate that appropriate management of anemia may be particularly essential in patients with diabetic retinopathy.[11]

Dyslipidemia

In the WESDR, cholesterol level did not predict severity of retinopathy or macular edema in type 2 diabetic patients.[15] However, the WESDR did find an association between elevated serum lipid levels and more severe retinal hard exudate, and such exudate was found to be a significant risk factor for moderate vision loss.[15] Severe exudate was also associated with decreased visual acuity independent of macular edema in the ETDRS.[16] In addition, the ETDRS found that, in patients with diabetic macular edema, severe hard exudate was the greatest risk factor for subretinal fibrosis, an important factor in the pathophysiology of vision loss.[16] The ETDRS also found that a baseline elevated serum triglyceride level was associated with proliferative diabetic retinopathy characterized by features that confer a high risk of vision loss, also known as high-risk proliferative disease.[17] This association was confirmed in another study, which found a similar association between such retinopathy and low-density lipoprotein (LDL) cholesterol.[18] However, the few, small interventional studies that have been done so far have not found a substantial effect of decreasing elevated serum lipid levels on vision loss in diabetic patients during the limited follow-up periods studied.[11] Nevertheless, the observational findings are compelling enough to recommend decreasing elevated serum lipid levels to reduce the risk of vision loss in patients with diabetic retinopathy.[5]

Alcohol Consumption and Smoking

The WESDR suggested that moderate alcohol consumption does not affect retinopathy prevalence, incidence, or progression in patients with older-onset diabetes. Nevertheless, diabetic patients with retinopathy who drink heavily have increased mortality,[2] and, therefore, heavy alcohol consumption should be discouraged. In contrast, because some studies have found a positive association between smoking and diabetic retinopathy but others have not, the effects of smoking on diabetic retinopathy are less clear. A literature review concluded that the positive association between smoking and retinopathy is less consistent than that between smoking and nephropathy.[11]

Prevention and Treatment Strategies

The data generated by the DCCT, EDIC, and UKPDS support initiating tight glucose control as early as possible and maintaining it as long as possible. In addition, the UKPDS provided more convincing data regarding the benefits of tight blood pressure control than regarding the benefits of intensive blood glucose control. Although rapidly decreasing blood glucose levels can initially worsen moderate nonproliferative retinopathy, possibly via effects on the growth hormone-insulinlike growth factor-I (IGF-I) axis, no data exist to indicate that improving blood glucose control slowly can prevent this effect. Moreover, the long-term ocular benefits of intensive glucose control more than compensate for this initial worsening.[10]

Lifestyle Interventions

Pros and Cons of Exercise

Because regular exercise can often substantially reduce blood glucose and blood pressure levels or maintain pharmacologic reductions in these levels over the long term, a properly designed, individually tailored exercise program is an important component of the diabetes treatment plan. However, some types of exercise appear to place patients with proliferative diabetic retinopathy at increased risk of disease progression or vitreous hemorrhage.[2] Exercise may promote advanced diabetic retinopathy by increasing systolic blood pressure, thereby promoting vitreous hemorrhage, or by decreasing already low tissue oxygen concentrations, thereby promoting progression. In addition, type 2 diabetic patients with retinopathy have an impaired cardiovascular response to exercise. The resulting loss of ocular circulatory autoregulation may allow the retinal arteriolar perfusion pressure to pass the hemorrhagic threshold in abnormal vessels during exercise-induced increases in blood pressure. Passing this threshold could cause vitreous hemorrhage and vision loss in patients with proliferative disease.

However, in general, exercise and physical activity have not been shown to worsen diabetic retinopathy.[11] For example, the WESDR suggested that exercise may be unimportant in determining the course of advanced diabetic eye disease. Another study found no association between physical activity and vitreous hemorrhage: most hemorrhages were found to occur at rest or after awakening.[2] A retrospective study found that 84% of vitreous hemorrhages occurred during activity no more strenuous than walking.[19] In addition, a recent prospective study in patients with type 2 diabetes found that inadequate exercise may be associated with the development of retinopathy.[20] Moreover, in a cross-sectional epidemiologic study of patients with type 1 diabetes, higher levels of physical activity resulted in less risk of proliferative diabetic retinopathy in women but not in men.[21] Also, the more strenuous the activity was, the less likely the women that were studied were to have proliferative diabetic retinopathy. However, further study found that exercise did not prevent proliferative diabetic retinopathy in either sex.[11]

Nevertheless, no study of patients with type 1 diabetes has shown a detrimental effect of exercise on the development of proliferative diabetic retinopathy, and a large epidemiologic study did not report worsening of retinopathy from moderate exercise in these patients. Despite these findings, patients with proliferative diabetic retinopathy should avoid anaerobic exercise and activities that involve straining, jarring, near maximal isometric contractions, or Valsalva maneuvers. Activities to be avoided include high-impact aerobics, jogging, and heavy weight training. Those to be encouraged include stationary cycling and low-intensity rowing, as well as swimming and walking. Even diabetic patients with vision loss should engage in such activities regularly.[11]

Continuous, Low-level Background Phototherapy

Because dark adaptation by rod cells consumes large amounts of oxygen and promotes retinal hypoxia and diabetic retinopathy, using continuous low-level background lighting to prevent full dark adaptation may be a simple and inexpensive, yet powerful way to decrease retinal oxygen demand and slow the progression of diabetic retinopathy. Alternatively, the amount of oxygen demanded by rods during dark adaptation could be reduced by pharmacologically preventing calcium entry or by reducing guanylyl cyclase activity in rods.[14]

Pharmacotherapy

In the UKPDS, all the intensive glucose-control therapies that were investigated, except chlorpropamide (Diabinese®), were associated with a clear reduction in the risk of progression of diabetic retinopathy, compared with conventional therapy.[10] Although the angiotensin-converting enzyme inhibitor (ACEI) lisinopril (Prinivil®, Zestril®) was found to be especially beneficial in slowing retinopathy progression in patients with type 1 diabetes,[4,5] in the type 2 diabetic patients in the UKPDS, the ACEI captopril (Capoten®) and the β-blocker atenolol (Tenormin®) slowed it equally well.[4] These findings indicate that, for slowing the progression of diabetic retinopathy in patients with type 2 diabetes, decreasing blood pressure may be more important than inhibiting ACE.[11] However, although the UKPDS showed that tight blood glucose and blood pressure control substantially reduced the risk of development and progression of diabetic retinopathy in type 2 diabetic patients, it also established that these measures alone cannot completely prevent retinopathy in many patients.[10] As a result, additional strategies for reducing the risk of diabetic retinopathy have been studied.

Thiazolidinediones for Additional Retinoprotection

Along with their antihyperglycemic effect, the thiazolidinediones (TZDs) appear to have an antiangiogenic effect on the ocular cells involved in neovascularization. Because of these effects, they may be particularly effective in inhibiting the progression of diabetic retinopathy.[22] Used in vitro, rosiglitazone (Avandia®) inhibited VEGF-induced migration and proliferation of retinal pigment epithelial cells, as well as retinal endothelial cells and endothelial tube formation. Moreover, as shown by angiography of experimentally induced ocular lesions in animals, rosiglitazone also inhibited retinal neovascularization, and troglitazone inhibited choroidal neovascularization without exerting toxic effects on the adjacent retina. These findings indicate that TZDs could inhibit the progression of diabetic retinopathy as well as the progression of age-related macular degeneration complicated by choroidal neovascularization through direct, nonglycemic effects on ocular cells.[22,23]

Antiplatelet Therapy

Aspirin. Because patients with type 2 diabetes have altered platelet function, the use of aspirin to retard the progression of microvascular angiopathy in diabetic retinopathy has been studied. Although the WESDR was not designed to evaluate the effectiveness of aspirin therapy for diabetic retinopathy, this epidemiologic study found no association between aspirin use and retinopathy severity.[2] In the ETDRS, designed specifically to assess the effect of aspirin on diabetic retinopathy, 650 mg daily had no effect on the progression of retinopathy,[5] macular edema,[11] or risk of vision loss.[5] Nevertheless, other studies of aspirin therapy for diabetic retinopathy have shown a reduced rate of microaneurysm formation in the early stages.[13] Moreover, even though the ETDRS indicated that aspirin may not be effective for diabetic retinopathy, it did provide evidence that aspirin does not increase the risk of vitreous hemorrhage in proliferative diabetic retinopathy.[5] Specifically, the RR of vitreous hemorrhage in aspirin-treated patients with any baseline neovascularization was 1.05, compared with similarly diseased patients who did not take aspirin.[8] Furthermore, in the ETDRS, aspirin therapy was associated with a 17% reduction in cardiovascular morbidity and mortality. Taken as a whole, the ETDRS data indicate that, even if aspirin does not alter the course of diabetic retinopathy, it has no adverse effect on preexisting disease, even at the advanced, proliferative stage, which might counterbalance its cardiovascular benefits. Thus, diabetic retinopathy does not contraindicate the use of aspirin to prevent or treat other diabetic complications.[5]

Dipyridamole and ticlopidine. Like aspirin therapy, antiplatelet therapy with ticlopidine (Ticlid®) or with dipyridamole plus aspirin (Aggrenox®) does not substantially affect the course of diabetic retinopathy. Both the Dipyridamole Aspirin Microangiopathy of Diabetes Study and the Ticlopidine Microangiopathy of Diabetes Study found little difference in retinopathy severity, determined by visual acuity measurement or ophthalmoscopy, between the treatment groups and the control group. However, in these studies, angiographic assessments did find fewer microaneurysms in the aspirin, aspirin plus dipyridamole, and ticlopidine treatment groups than in the control groups. Nevertheless, these small differences were of borderline statistical significance and may not be clinically significant.[5] There are insufficient data regarding the effect of clopidogrel (Plavix®) on retinopathy.

Thrombolysis and risk of vitreous hemorrhage. Although diabetic patients have a poorer outcome after myocardial infarction than nondiabetic patients, they are less likely to receive thrombolytic therapy than nondiabetic patients are. However, no ocular complications have been found in trials of thrombolytic agents after myocardial infarction, which, together, included approximately 9,000 diabetic patients. Although at least one case of vitreous hemorrhage associated with retinopathy after thrombolysis has been reported, the use of fibrinolytic agents has not been associated with an excess number of hemorrhagic complications in diabetic patients. Moreover, in the 35 days after infarction, fibrinolysis was shown to reduce mortality in diabetic patients by 21.7%.[11] Thus, in diabetic patients with myocardial infarction, thrombolytic therapy or fibrinolytic therapy offers cardiovascular benefits without increasing the risk of vitreous hemorrhage. As a result, the American College of Cardiology guidelines state that diabetic retinopathy does not contraindicate thrombolytic therapy for acute myocardial infarction.[1]

Emerging Agents

Aldose reductase inhibitors. Although results of animal studies suggested that aldose reductase inhibition could slow the development of diabetic retinopathy, clinical studies have not yet shown that this approach can reduce progression of retinopathy. In the Sorbinil Retinopathy Trial in type 1 diabetic patients with little or no retinopathy, 3 to 4 years of treatment with the aldose reductase inhibitor sorbinil did not reduce the progression of diabetic retinopathy or neuropathy.[4]

Somatostatin analogs. Although initial clinical trials did not consistently show the effectiveness of somatostatin analogs for diabetic retinopathy, these trials used short-dosing durations, and doses were often too low to suppress growth hormone or IGF-I levels. Other trials in early-stage retinopathy found no change in the course of retinopathy. However, administration of the stabilized somatostatin analog lanreotide in a continuous infusion pump for 4 weeks was more effective. In the 8 of 11 patients with non-high-risk proliferative disease, who completed the dosing schedule, six patients showed no progression, and two patients showed regression. In contrast, diabetic retinopathy progressed in one half of the six patients in the control group.[24]

Visual acuity improved after continuous infusion of the somatostatin analog octreotide (Sandostatin®) for several months in an uncontrolled trial of four patients. In another clinical trial of octreotide, only one of the 22 treated eyes required laser therapy after 12 months of treatment, compared with nine of the 24 eyes in the control group. The investigators in this study also found that advanced proliferative disease was more likely to regress in octreotide-treated patients who were also taking thyroid hormone, a finding supported by research indicating that T_3 upregulates somatostatin expression in neurons and increases pituitary somatostatin receptor expression. More stable somatostatin analogs with longer half-lives and greater receptor selectivity are being developed, and several long-acting, sustained-release depot agents are being clinically evaluated as retinopathy therapies. Further research could produce a new generation of nonpeptide somatostatin analogs that are more selective, stable, and effective in treating abnormal angiogenesis than the agents that have been studied so far.[24]

Antioxidants. Because oxidative stress promotes ocular abnormalities, antioxidants such as vitamin E are hypothesized to decrease the progression of diabetic retinopathy. Although a cross-sectional longitudinal study of type 2 diabetic patients did not find that vitamin C or E or β-carotene could protect against diabetic retinopathy,[11] studies in animal models of diabetes have shown that high-dose vitamin E reduces excess activity of protein kinase C (PKC),[3] an enzyme involved in cellular processes that damage the microvasculature and promote blood leakage.[25] Animal studies have also shown that high-dose vitamin E can normalize retinal blood flow. This finding was confirmed in humans by results of initial clinical studies using 1,800 IU/day of vitamin E in type 1 diabetic patients with diabetes of recent onset and minimal retinopathy.[1,3,11] Nevertheless, whether vitamin E therapy can delay the onset or progression of diabetic retinopathy is unclear.[11]

Other Agents

Although aminoguanidine therapy has not shown therapeutic benefit,[13] clinical trials of advanced glycation end product inhibitors and of antiangiogenic agents, such as VEGF inhibitors,[5] PKC inhibitors, or pigment epithelium derived factor,[7] are being pursued to determine the value of these potentially powerful new treatment approaches. Because VEGF promotes both retinopathy and maculopathy[13] by enhancing vascular permeability,[24] VEGF inhibition may be particularly useful in reducing the risk of both these forms of diabetic eye disease simultaneously.[13]

Intravitreal injection therapy with the anti-VEGF agent EYE001 is being explored for the treatment of diabetic macular edema. In early studies in patients with neovascularization secondary to macular degeneration, EYE001 alone significantly improved vision in 25%, and EYE001 with photodynamic therapy significantly improved vision in up to 60%. Oral treatment with the PKC inhibitor LY333531 is also being explored in patients with diabetic macular edema, as well as in patients with diabetic retinopathy. Intravitreal injection therapy with purified hyaluronidase (Vitrase®), an enzyme that cleaves a component of vitreous gel to promote clearing of vitreous hemorrhage, is also being explored as a diabetic retinopathy treatment. Although hyaluronidase improved visual acuity in a phase III trial, it did not clear the hemorrhage enough to allow diagnosis and treatment of the underlying cause. In an earlier trial, hyaluronidase therapy appeared to stabilize diabetic retinopathy.

Steroid therapy has shown some promise for treating diabetic macular edema. In patients unresponsive to laser therapy, direct injection of triamcinolone acetonide decreased central macular thickness, but the effect lasted only 4 to 6 months, and this treatment may increase intraocular pressure and promote cataract. Intravitreal implants that deliver steroids are also under development, and administration of fluocinolone acetonide with one such implant reduced macular edema, decreased retinopathy, and improved visual acuity in early trials.[25]

Surgery
Laser Photocoagulation Therapy

Laser photocoagulation of the retina is the therapeutic mainstay for established or impending high-risk proliferative diabetic retinopathy or clinically significant macular edema.[11] Two types of laser therapy exist: focal or direct and panretinal or scatter. In focal or direct therapy, which is used for macular edema, only small areas of macular tissue with leakage that contributes to macular thickening are directly treated with moderately intense photoenergy. Treatment is restricted to lesions that are 300 to 3,000 micrometers from the macula's center, and fluorescein angiography is generally used to identify treatable culprit vessels.[3] Focal treatment of areas closer to the center, near the optic disk, is avoided because, although this technique increased risk of hemorrhage, it did not increase the neovascularization regression rate.[4]

In contrast, in panretinal or scatter therapy, 1,500 to 2,000 large laser burns are applied in the midperipheral and posterior retina[5] at the level of the retinal pigment epithelium.[3] Each burn is separated from another by one burn-width to produce a polka-dotted pattern. The macula, optic nerve, and major vessels, as well as areas of preretinal hemorrhage, are carefully avoided.[2,3] Panretinal therapy, which is also known as grid therapy, is used for established or impending retinal neovascularization.[4] Although the mechanism by which panretinal therapy exerts its effect is unclear, it is believed to work by closing leaking vessels and, thus, preventing the release of vasoactive factors. However, other findings indicate that its effectiveness results mainly from its ability to reduce retinal oxygen demand[14] by destroying ischemic and hypoxic areas of the retina.[1]

In general, laser surgery is done in the office, often during topical or retrobulbar anesthesia.[2] Because argon laser therapy confers less risk of decreased visual field and acuity than xenon laser therapy, the argon laser is the preferred instrument for laser therapy.[4] Therapy is carefully titrated to the condition of each retina. No postoperative restrictions are required. However, more than one session may be needed if neovascularization does not sufficiently regress or if it increases, if new areas of neovascularization form, or if new vitreous hemorrhage develops.[2] Sessions are spaced 1 to 2 weeks apart, and follow-up evaluation is generally done about 3 months after the procedure. Although regression of neovascularization is the most desirable treatment response, stabilization or no more new vessel growth may be acceptable if follow-up is adequate.[3]

Side effects may include mild loss of visual acuity and constriction of the peripheral visual field.[2] Risk of angle-closure glaucoma or worsening of macular edema can be minimized by spreading treatments over several sessions.[1] Scotomas from focal laser burns are a common side effect,[4] and diminished color vision and delayed dark adaptation, which may make night driving difficult, are rare side effects.[1] However, the procedure generally has a favorable risk-to-benefit profile in eyes at high risk for severe vision loss.[2]

Effectiveness. The current standard of care for the use of laser therapy in diabetic retinopathy offers clear proof of the value of evidence-based medicine in clinical practice. Extensive, rigorous trials provided detailed data on the prevalence, progression, and risk to vision of diabetic retinopathy, as well as its response to treatment.[11] These trials have established that laser therapy can reduce risk of blindness from retinopathy by as much as 95% if given at the appropriate disease stage, although it is somewhat less effective (60% to 70%) in preventing blindness from maculopathy.[13] Nevertheless, although laser therapy can reduce the risk of further vision loss, it generally cannot restore lost visual acuity.[8]

The methods for assessing the severity of retinopathy to determine whether laser treatment is indicated and for delivering laser energy to the retina, as well as the recommended schedules for disease monitoring and treatment follow-up, have been solidly established by two major, randomized, multicenter clinical trials.[11] The Diabetic Retinopathy Study (DRS) in 1976 showed that panretinal therapy halved the 5-year risk of severe vision loss (acuity 5/200 or worse) from proliferative diabetic retinopathy. Moreover, the DRS found that extensive neovascularization, especially when it approached or affected the optic disk or caused vitreous hemorrhage, elevated the risk of severe vision loss from proliferative disease to 26% if untreated, compared with 7% if these features were not present. However, panretinal therapy reduced the risk conferred by these features to 11%.[4]

Table 10-2: Levels of Diabetic Retinopathy*

Nonproliferative Diabetic Retinopathy (NPDR)	Characteristics
Mild NPDR	At least one microaneurysm Characteristics not met for more severe DR
Moderate NPDR	Hemorrhages and/or microaneurysms (H/Ma) of a moderate degree (ie, ≥ standard photograph 2A)** and/or Soft exudates (cotton wool spots), venous beading (VB), or intraretinal microvascular abnormalities (IRMA) definitely present and Characteristics not met for more severe DR
Severe NPDR	One of the following: • H/Ma ≥ standard photograph 2A in four retinal quadrants • Venous beading in ≥ two retinal quadrants (see standard photograph 6B)** • IRMA in ≥ one retinal quadrant ≥ standard photograph 8A** • Characteristics not met for more severe DR
Very severe NPDR	Two or more lesions of severe NPDR No retinal neovascularization

DR = diabetic retinopathy

* Based on ETDRS definitions in *Ophthalmology* 1991;98;786-806.

Proliferative Diabetic Retinopathy (PDR)

	Characteristics
Early PDR	New vessels definitely present Characteristics not met for more severe DR
High-risk PDR	One or more of the following: • Neovascularization on the optic disk (NVD) ≥ standard photograph 10A (ie, 1/4 to 1/3 disk area) • Any NVD with vitreous or pre-retinal hemorrhage Neovascularization elsewhere on the retina (NVE) ≥1/2 disk area with vitreous or preretinal hemorrhage

Clinically Significant Macular Edema (CSME)

Any one of the following lesions:

- Retinal thickening at or within 500 μm (1/3) optic disk diameter from the center of the macula
- Hard exudates at or within 500 μm from the center of the macula with thickening of the adjacent retina
- A zone or zones of retinal thickening ≥ one optic disk area in size, any portion of which is at or within one optic disk diameter from the center of the macula

** Standard photographs refer to the Modified Airlee House Classification of Diabetic Retinopathy (see ETDRS report no. 12, published in *Ophthalmology* 1991;98:823-833).

Table 10-3: Recommended General Management of Diabetic Retinopathy

	Risk (%) of Progression	
Level of DR	PDR-1 yr	High-risk PDR-5 yrs
Mild NPDR	5	15
No ME		
ME		
CSME		
Moderate NPDR	12-27	33
No ME		
ME		
CSME		
Severe NPDR	52	60
No ME		
ME		
CSME		
Very severe NPDR	75	75
No ME		
ME		
CSME		
PDR < high risk		75
No ME		
ME		
CSME		
High-risk PDR		
No ME		
ME		
CSME		

NPDR = nonproliferative diabetic retinopathy, PDR = proliferative diabetic retinopathy, FA = fluorescein angiography, PRP = panretinal photocoagulation, F/U = follow-up,

Evaluation		Laser Treatment		
Color Photo	FA	Scatter PRP	Focal	F/U (mos)
No	No	No	No	12
Yes	Occ	No	No	4-6
Yes	Yes	No	Yes	2-4
Yes	No	No	No	6-8
Yes	Occ	No	Occ	4-6
Yes	Yes	No	Yes	2-4
Yes	No	Rarely	No	3-4
Yes	Occ	OccAF	Occ	2-3
Yes	Yes	OccAF	Yes	2-3
Yes	No	Occ	No	2-3
Yes	Occ	OccAF	Occ	2-3
Yes	Yes	OccAF	Yes	2-3
Yes	No	Occ	No	2-3
Yes	Occ	OccAF	Occ	2-3
Yes	Yes	OccAF	Yes	2-3
Yes	No	Yes	No	2-3
Yes	Yes	Yes	Usually	1-2
Yes	Yes	Yes	Yes	1-2

ME = macular edema, CSME = clinically significant macular edema, mos = months, Occ = occasionally, OccAF = occasionally after focal

The findings of the DRS were elaborated by the ETDRS in which 70% of the study patients had type 2 diabetes. The ETDRS showed that, when combined with panretinal therapy, focal therapy for clinically significant macular edema roughly halved the 5-year risk of moderate vision loss, reducing it to less than 15% from almost 30%.[3] Moreover, focal therapy can increase the chance that vision will improve, decreases vision-threatening exudates, and reduces the chance that macular edema will persist.[1,2] The ETDRS also explored the effects of timing of therapy. As a result, it determined that if panretinal therapy is applied early, just before or after high-risk proliferative diabetic retinopathy has developed, it can reduce the 5-year risk of severe vision loss more than deferred treatment can (2.6% for early vs 3.7% for deferred treatment).[4]

Furthermore, the ETDRS established the types of nonproliferative lesions that confer a high risk of vision loss when they complicate untreated proliferative diabetic retinopathy. These lesions include hemorrhages, microaneurysms, venous caliber abnormalities, such as venous loops, tortuosity, and beading, which indicate severe retinal hypoxia, and intraretinal microvascular abnormalities, which include shunt vessels, or enlarged hypercellular capillaries that appear dilated and telangiectatic and form near occluded areas.[3] In addition to these lesions, cotton-wool spots indicate microischemia of nerve fiber layers and also signal worsening retinopathy.[1] Table 10-2 provides the characteristics used to distinguish between nonproliferative and proliferative diabetic retinopathy and to determine the level of disease severity and the risk of vision loss it confers. Nonproliferative disease is generally less severe and vision-threatening than proliferative disease, although macular edema can develop at any stage and intensifies the risk of vision loss.[3]

Timing. Correct staging of diabetic retinopathy and identification of high-risk characteristics in proliferative disease guide proper timing of follow-up evaluation and laser therapy. Table 10-3 provides recommendations for the management of diabetic retinopathy on the basis of disease stage and the risk it confers.[3] When high-risk proliferative disease is found, prompt panretinal therapy is indicated. Treatment before high-risk proliferative disease develops can halve the risk of severe vision loss and the need for more invasive therapy, especially in type 2 diabetic patients. Moreover, because panretinal therapy may worsen macular edema, early focal therapy is especially necessary for even clinically insignificant macular edema in patients with proliferative disease, who will probably require panretinal therapy soon.

Severe nonproliferative diabetic retinopathy, also called preproliferative diabetic retinopathy, has high-risk features and confers a 10% to 50% risk that proliferative disease will develop within 1 year.[2] In patients with non-high-risk proliferative or severe nonproliferative disease, rapidity of progression, concomitant illnesses that promote progression, such as hypertension and nephropathy, and compliance with follow-up should be considered in deciding when laser surgery is appropriate.[3] However, because mild to moderate nonproliferative disease poses a much lower risk of severe vision loss than more severe disease does, reduction of this already low risk with early laser therapy does not compensate for the side effects of laser therapy.[4]

Because laser therapy is most effective at the proper stage of the disease, before vision loss can occur, motivating symptom-free patients to pursue regular examinations is paramount. To ensure adequate disease monitoring and motivate patients to obtain it, patients should be educated about the course of the disease and the effectiveness of initiating therapy before symptoms appear.[3] This need is especially crucial considering that only approximately 60% of all US diabetic retinopathy patients who need laser therapy receive it and that inadequate care costs more than $275 million and 72,180 person-years of sight in the United States annually.[11]

Vitrectomy

Some vitreous or preretinal hemorrhages may make applying laser therapy from outside of the eye impossible.[2] In these cases, vitrectomy may be indicated because it facilitates endolaser therapy, the application of laser energy within the eye. Vitrectomy may also be indicated when laser therapy applied from outside of the eye fails to reverse or stabilize neovascularization, despite additional treatment sessions, and when such neovascularization threatens vision.[3] During vitrectomy, which is always done in an operating suite using general or retrobulbar anesthesia, the vitreous gel is removed to allow operation on the posterior of the eye. Small instruments are inserted into the eye at the pars plana to cut the vitreous, suction out the vitreous gel, and replace it with aqueous fluid. Once this has been accomplished, vitreous hemorrhages that do not clear or fibrous tissue that exerts traction, which threatens the macula's center, can be removed and areas of detachment flattened.[4]

Vitrectomy is generally recommended if tractional macular detachment is present or if severe vitreous hemorrhage has not cleared in 4 to 6 months. Other indications for vitrectomy include combined tractional and rhegmatogenous (ruptured) retinal detachment, progressive fibrovascular proliferation, dense premacular hemorrhage, macular edema with premacular traction,[2] neovascularization of the iris (rubeosis iridis) with vitreous hemorrhage, and cataract with proliferative diabetic retinopathy.[1] Side effects of vitrectomy may include pain; ocular phthisis, or wasting degeneration of the eye; and severe vision loss with complete absence of light perception.[2]

The Diabetic Retinopathy Vitrectomy Study (DRVS) found that early vitrectomy substantially benefited patients with severe, active proliferative diabetic retinopathy who still had relatively good visual acuity.[26] However, although vitrectomy performed soon after vision loss caused by severe vitreous hemorrhage provided substantial benefits in early-onset diabetes, it did not do so in later-onset diabetes.[26] These findings indicate that vitrectomy may be relatively ineffective in type 2 diabetic patients with vision loss, presumably because they are older and usually have less severe retinopathy.[27] The DRVS also established that, in patients with severe fibrovascular proliferation, early pars plana vitrectomy was more likely to result in better vision and less likely to result in poor vision than deferred vitrectomy.[26,28] However, because surgical techniques have improved considerably since the DRVS was completed and endolaser therapy has become available for use during vitrectomy, its current benefits are even greater than those found in the DRVS.[3] Success rates vary depending on the surgical indication and its severity. For all indications combined, the chance of improvement in vision after vitrectomy for diabetic retinopathy is 67%.[29,30]

References

1. Wipf JE, Paauw DS: Ophthalmologic emergencies in the patient with diabetes. *Endocrinol Metab Clin North Am* 2000;29:813-829.

2. Holekamp NM, Meredith TA: Diabetic eye disease. In: Davidson JK, ed. *Clinical Diabetes Mellitus: a Problem Oriented Approach.* 3rd ed. New York, NY: Thieme Medical Publishers, Inc.; 2000:513-528.

3. Aiello LP, Cavallerano J: Diabetic retinopathy. In: Johnstone MT, Veves A, eds. *Contemporary Cardiology: Diabetes and Cardiovascular Disease.* Totowa, New Jersey: Humana Press; 2001: 385-398.

4. Ferris FL III, Davis MD, Aiello LM: Treatment of diabetic retinopathy. *N Engl J Med* 1999;341:667-678.

5. Chew EY, Murphy RP: Diabetic eye disease. In: Taylor SI, ed. *Current Review of Diabetes.* Philadelphia, PA: Current Medicine, Inc.; 1999:61-70.

6. Stratton IM, Kohner EM, Aldington SJ, et al: UKPDS 50: risk factors for incidence and progression of retinopathy in Type II diabetes over 6 years from diagnosis. *Diabetologia* 2001;44:156-163.

7.   Aiello LP: Diabetic retinopathy: an eye toward the future. Conference Coverage of the 62nd Scientific Sessions of the American Diabetes Association. WebMD [Web site]. Available at: http://www.medscape.com/viewartcle/438360. Accessed December 11, 2002.

8.   American Diabetes Association. Position Statement: Diabetic retinopathy. *Diabetes Care*. 2003;26:S99-S102. http://care.diabetesjournals.org/cgi/content/full/26/suppl_1/s99.

9.   Gomez-Ulla F, Fernandez MI, Gonzalez F, et al: Digital retinal images and teleophthalmology for detecting and grading diabetic retinopathy. *Diabetes Care* 2002;25:1384-1389.

10.   Spranger J, Pfeiffer AF: New concepts in pathogenesis and treatment of diabetic retinopathy. *Exp Clin Endocrinol Diabetes* 2001;109:S438-S450.

11.   Aiello LP, Cahill MT, Wong JS: Systemic considerations in the management of diabetic retinopathy. *Am J Ophthalmol* 2001;132:760-776.

12.   Ohkubo Y, Kishikawa H, Araki E, et al: Intensive insulin therapy prevents the progression of diabetic microvascular complications in Japanese patients with non-insulin-dependent diabetes mellitus: a randomized prospective 6-year study. *Diabetes Res Clin Pract* 1995;28:103-117.

13.   Broadbent DM: Diabetic eye disease: how can it be prevented? *Practitioner* 2000;244:696-700, 702.

14.   Arden GB: The absence of diabetic retinopathy in patients with retinitis pigmentosa: implications for pathophysiology and possible treatment. *Br J Ophthalmol* 2001;85:366-370.

15.   Klein BE, Moss SE, Klein R, et al: The Wisconsin Epidemiologic Study of Diabetic Retinopathy. XIII. Relationship of serum cholesterol to retinopathy and hard exudate. *Ophthalmology* 1991;98:1261-1265.

16.   Fong DS, Segal PP, Myers F, et al: Subretinal fibrosis in diabetic macular edema. ETDRS report number 23. Early Treatment Diabetic Retinopathy Study Research Group. *Arch Ophthalmol* 1997;115:873-877.

17.   Davis MD, Fisher MR, Gangnon RE, et al: Risk factors for high-risk proliferative diabetic retinopathy and severe visual loss: Early Treatment Diabetic Retinopathy Study report #18. *Invest Ophthalmol Vis Sci* 1998;39:233-252.

18.   Kostraba JN, Klein R, Dorman JS, et al: The epidemiology of diabetes complications study. IV. Correlates of diabetic background and proliferative retinopathy. *Am J Epidemiol* 1991;133:381-391.

19.   Anderson B Jr: Activity and diabetic vitreous hemorrhages. *Ophthalmology* 1980;87:173-175.

20.   Rasmidatta S, Khunsuk-Mengrai K, Warunyuwong C: Risk factors of diabetic retinopathy in non-insulin dependent diabetes mellitus. *J Med Assoc Thai* 1998;81:169-174.

21.   Cruickshanks KJ, Moss SE, Klein R, et al: Physical activity and proliferative retinopathy in people diagnosed with diabetes before age 30 yr. *Diabetes Care* 1992;15:1267-1272.

22.   Murata T, Hata Y, Ishibashi T, et al: Response of experimental retinal neovascularization to thiazolidinediones. *Arch Ophthalmol* 2001:119:709-717.

23.   Murata T, He S, Hangai M, et al: Peroxisome proliferator-activated receptor-gamma ligands inhibit choroidal neovascularization. *Invest Ophthalmol Vis Sci* 2000;41:2309-2317.

24.   Davis MI, Wilson SH, Grant MB: The therapeutic problem of proliferative diabetic retinopathy: targeting somatostatin receptors. *Horm Metab Res* 2001;33:295-299.

25.   Singerman L, Miller DG: Diabetic retinopathy and DME drug trials advance. Review of Ophthalmology [Web page]. Jobson Publishing, New York. October 15, 2002. Available at: http://www.revophth.com/index.asp?page=1_204.htm. Accessed January 31, 2003.

26.   Early vitrectomy for severe proliferative diabetic retinopathy in eyes with useful vision. Results of a randomized trial—Diabetic Retinopathy Vitrectomy Study Report 3. The Diabetic Retinopathy Vitrectomy Study Research Group. *Ophthalmology* 1988; 95:1307-1320.

27.   Early vitrectomy for severe vitreous hemorrhage in diabetic retinopathy. Four-year results of a randomized trial. Diabetic Retinopathy Vitrectomy Study Report 5. *Arch Ophthalmol* 1990;108:958-964.

28.   Early vitrectomy for severe proliferative diabetic retinopathy in eyes with useful vision. Clinical application of results of a randomized trial—DRVS report no. 4. The Diabetic Retinopathy Vitrectomy Study Research Group. *Ophthalmology* 1988;95:1321-1334.

29. Michels RG: Vitrectomy for complications of retinopathy. *Arch Ophthalmol* 1978;96:237-246.

30. Thompson JT, de Bustros S, Michels RG, et al: Results of vitrectomy for proliferative diabetic retinopathy. *Ophthalmology* 1986;93:1571-1574.

Chapter 11

Neuropathy: Types and Treatment

Although poorly understood,[1] diabetic neuropathy is the most common complication of diabetes and the most common form of neuropathy in the developed world. Often disabling, it can greatly reduce quality of life,[2] particularly in the elderly. One study of patients aged 70 to 75 years found that diabetic patients with neuropathy did worse than patients without neuropathy on tests of walking speed, static and dynamic balance, and coordination,[3] indicating a decrease in ambulatory ability that can lead to falls and serious injuries such as hip fracture. Diabetic neuropathy may also lead to premature death. For example, diabetic autonomic neuropathy confers a 25% to 50% risk of death in 5 to 10 years. Complications of diabetic neuropathy result in the greatest morbidity and mortality of any diabetic complication and account for more hospital admissions than all other diabetic complications combined. The most important consequence of somatic diabetic neuropathy is foot ulceration, which often leads to gangrene and is responsible for 50% to 75% of all nontraumatic amputations.

Neuropathy increases amputation risk 1.7-fold when it is uncomplicated, 12-fold if it also causes deformity, and 26-fold if it has caused ulceration. It is the major contributor to 87% of the 65,000 amputations performed annually in the United States. However, at least half the amputations that result from diabetic neuropathy are preventable,[2] which indicates that prompt diagnosis and adequate care and follow-up of this condition are important.

Prevalence

Definitions of neuropathy and the diagnostic procedures used to identify it vary greatly.[1] Excluding nondiabetic neuropathy may be difficult,[4] and diabetic neuropathy itself encompasses a wide range of abnormalities. These factors make developing precise estimates of the prevalence of diabetic neuropathy challenging. Such estimates have been further confounded by the increasing prevalence of neuropathy with greater duration of diabetes,[3] greater age,[4] and poorer glycemic control.[5] Therefore, the reported prevalence of diabetic neuropathy has ranged from 10% to 90%[2] and even as high as 100% when sensitive tests are used in asymptomatic patients.[6]

In one of the largest published series, a prospective study of 4,400 patients from 1947 through 1973, before electrophysiologic testing became available, the reported prevalence of clinically detectable neuropathy ranged from 12% at diagnosis to 50% after 25 years of diabetes.[2] Subsequent research suggests that most diabetic patients will develop some degree of neuropathy if diabetes duration is long enough and if the most sensitive neurophysiologic testing methods are used.[7] For example, in the 1990s, three European clinic-based studies found a remarkably consistent prevalence of symptomatic neuropathy ranging from 22.5% to 28.5%.[4] This estimate was confirmed in a later clinic study. However, although only 25% of patients in that study reported symptoms, neuropathy was diagnosed in 50% of patients by using ankle jerk, vibration perception, or other simple tests, and results of sophisticated testing of autonomic function or peripheral sensation indicated neuropathy in almost 90%.[2] Based on electrophysiologic findings, a prevalence of 40% was found for patients with type 2 diabetes after

10 years of diabetes,[7] and population-based studies indicate that about 50% of patients with type 2 diabetes have neuropathic deficits.[4] Another series found a neuropathy prevalence of 66% in all patients with diabetes, using a definition based on symptoms, signs, and results of quantitative sensory and autonomic testing and nerve conduction studies.[3]

Most studies include patients with type 1 and type 2 diabetes, but unlike type 1 diabetes, neuropathy may be present at diagnosis of type 2 diabetes. This difference may complicate the extrapolation of prevalence figures for the general population with diabetes to patients with type 2 diabetes in particular. The Finnish prospective study and the United Kingdom Prospective Diabetes Study (UKPDS) found a 5% to 10% prevalence of neuropathy at diagnosis of type 2 diabetes.[4] These findings are in accord with those of the 1947 to 1973 study of patients with diabetes, which reported a 7.5% prevalence at diabetes diagnosis.[6] Several reports have found no difference in the general prevalence of diabetic peripheral neuropathy based on type of diabetes; reported median prevalence for both types was about 32%.[1] Although prevalence estimates vary greatly and may be confounded by a variety of factors, they indicate that the diagnosis of neuropathy is being missed in many patients with diabetes. This poor capture rate results because most cases of diabetic neuropathy are asymptomatic until complications ensue and because many clinicians do not adequately examine their patients' feet for the signs of neuropathy.[6]

Types, Clinical Presentations, and Natural Histories

Diabetic neuropathy is not a single, homogeneous clinical entity. Instead, it is a variety of syndromes that may be superimposed, including subclinical neuropathy, indicated by abnormal results of electrodiagnostic and quantitative sensory testing; diffuse vs focal neuropathy; and

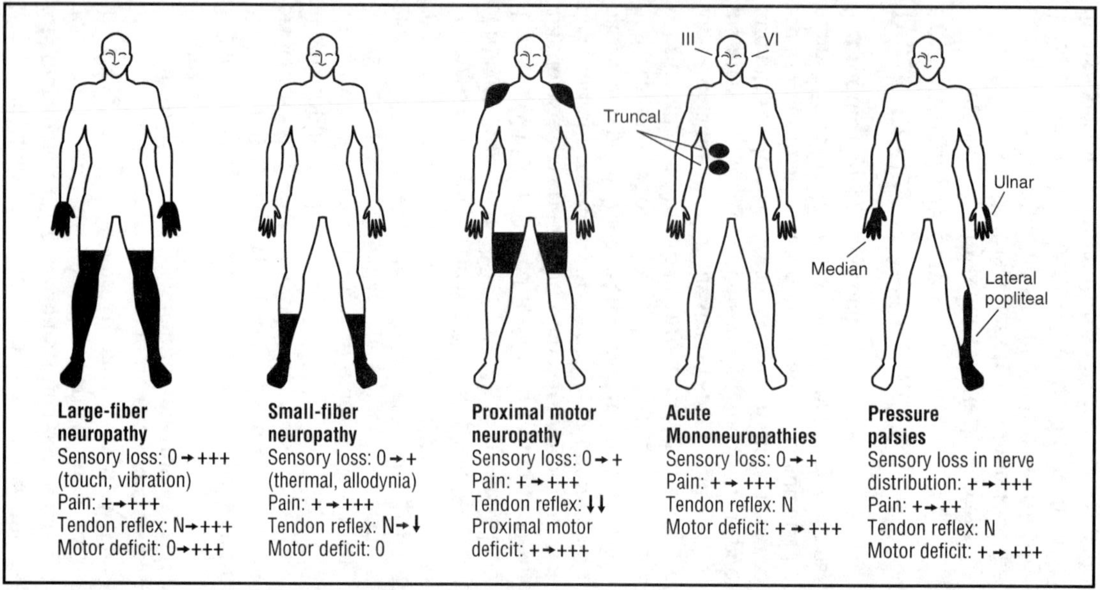

Figure 11-1: Different clinical presentations of diabetic neuropathy. Reprinted with permission from Vinik et al, *Diabetologia* 2000;43:960 ©Springer-Verlag GmbH & Co. N = normal.

Large-fiber neuropathy
Sensory loss: 0 → +++
(touch, vibration)
Pain: + → +++
Tendon reflex: N → +++
Motor deficit: 0 → +++

Small-fiber neuropathy
Sensory loss: 0 → +
(thermal, allodynia)
Pain: + → +++
Tendon reflex: N → ↓
Motor deficit: 0

Proximal motor neuropathy
Sensory loss: 0 → +
Pain: + → +++
Tendon reflex: ↓ → +++
Proximal motor deficit: + → +++

Acute Mononeuropathies
Sensory loss: 0 → +
Pain: + → +++
Tendon reflex: N
Motor deficit: + → +++

Pressure palsies
Sensory loss in nerve distribution: + → +++
Pain: + → ++
Tendon reflex: N
Motor deficit: + → +++

Truncal

III

VI

Median

Ulnar

Lateral popliteal

Table 11-1: Stage 1 and 2 Investigations of Peripheral Neuropathy

Stage 1

Urine—Glucose, protein

Hematology—Full blood count, erythrocyte sedimentation rate, vitamin B_{12}, folate

Biochemistry—Fasting blood glucose concentration, renal function, liver function, thyroid stimulating hormone

Stage 2

Neurophysiologic tests—Assessment of distal and proximal nerve stimulation

Biochemistry—Serum protein electrophoresis, serum angiotensin-converting enzyme

Immunology—Antinuclear factor, antiextractable nuclear antigen antibodies (anti-Ro, anti-La), antineutrophil cytoplasmic antigen antibodies

Other—Chest radiography

Hughes, *BMJ* 2002;324:467, reprinted with permission from the BMJ Publishing Group.

symmetric vs asymmetric neuropathy.[6] Neuropathy can be acute or chronic. Some types affect small-fiber myelinated or unmyelinated nerves, others affect large-fiber nerves, and some affect both. Autonomic, sensory, or motor nerves may be affected; in many patients, all three nerve types are affected. Sensory and autonomic neuropathy are closely correlated.[2] Figure 11-1 depicts the various clinical presentations of some of the more common forms of diabetic neuropathy, and Table 11-1 provides recommendations on staged testing to pinpoint the cause of neuropathy.

Table 11-2: Causes of Acute, Severe, Generalized Peripheral Neuropathy

Causes	Predominantly Motor	Mixed	Predominantly Sensory
Guillain-Barré syndrome	+	+	−
Vasculitis	−	+	−
Diabetes mellitus	−	+	+
Drugs*	−	+	+
Porphyria	+	−	−
Diphtheria	−	+	−
Paraneoplastic neuropathy	−	+	+
Acute idiopathic sensory neuropathy	−	−	+
Critical illness	+	+	−

*For example, nitrofurantoin, vincristine, cisplatin, and reverse transcriptase inhibitors.

Hughes, *BMJ* 2002;324:467, reprinted with permission from the BMJ Publishing Group.

Distal Symmetric Polyneuropathy

The most common type of diabetic neuropathy is distal symmetric polyneuropathy. Population-based and clinic-based studies estimate that 23% to 43% of diabetic patients have this type of neuropathy,[8] and some prevalence estimates are as high as 70%.[5] Because many patients are asymptomatic, the diagnosis is best made by detection of diminished pain sensation in the legs. Symptoms may range from complete insensitivity to severe, burning pain; stabbing and shooting sensations; uncomfortable hot and cold feelings; and allodynia (painful touch). Although symptoms fluctuate, they can produce extreme discomfort and distress and worsen at night, even causing hypersensitivity to bed coverings.[4] Paresthesias may also be felt, and the feet are usually more affected than the hands.[5] Paresthesias affect the toes first, followed by the legs, and then may eventually spread up the arms, beginning with the fingers. Rarely, in severe cases, neuropathy may affect the anterior chest and abdomen and spread laterally around the torso. Initially, small-fiber unmyelinated nerves are affected, but later, large-fiber nerves often become affected as well. Small-fiber damage causes loss of pain and temperature sensation and may lead to foot ulcers and injury.[6] Neuropathic joint degeneration (Charcot's joint) may occur.[5] Degeneration of large-fiber nerves causes loss of vibratory and proprioceptive sensation. Severe cases of sensory nerve degeneration may cause defective muscular coordination (ataxia) from postural loss.[5,6] Table 11-2 lists possible causes of acute distal symmetric polyneuropathy with their general symptom profiles.

Although the symptoms of diabetic distal symmetric polyneuropathy are predominantly sensory, in some cases, signs are both sensory and motor.[4] Motor involvement is usually minor, affecting only the distal extremities. However, the resulting foot deformity disrupts weight bearing, further contributing to callus and ulcer formation.[6] In severe cases, sensory loss occurs in all limbs in a 'stocking-and-glove' distribution, and motor deficits are extensive.[4] The eight-point Michigan Neuropathy Screening Instrument (Figure 11-2) can aid in the assessment of signs and symptoms of distal symmetric polyneuropathy.[3]

In addition to the chronic form, there is a rare, acute form of this condition that lasts less than 6 months. It often appears when diabetes worsens or, conversely, when treatment with glucose-control agents is begun and gly-

Michigan Neuropathy Screening Instrument

Pt. Name: _____
Pt. Identification #: _____
Date: _____

B. Physical assessment (To be completed by health professional)

1. Appearance of feet

Right

a. Normal ☐ 0 Yes ☐ 1 No

b. If no, check all that apply:

Deformities ☐
Dry skin, callus ☐
Infection ☐
Fissure ☐
Other ☐
specify: _____

Left

a. Normal ☐ 0 Yes ☐ 1 No

b. If no, check all that apply:

Deformities ☐
Dry skin, callus ☐
Infection ☐
Fissure ☐
Other ☐
specify: _____

	Right			**Left**		
2. Ulceration	Absent ☐ 0		Present ☐ 1	Absent ☐ 0		Present ☐ 1
3. Ankle reflexes	Present ☐ 0	Present/ Reinforcement ☐ 0.5	Absent ☐ 1	Present ☐ 0	Present/ Reinforcement ☐ 0.5	Absent ☐ 1
4. Vibration perception at great toe	Present ☐ 0	Decreased ☐ 0.5	Absent ☐ 1	Present ☐ 0	Decreased ☐ 0.5	Absent ☐ 1
5. Monofilament	Normal ☐ 0	Reduced ☐ 0.5	Absent ☐ 1	Normal ☐ 0	Reduced ☐ 0.5	Absent ☐ 1

Signature: _____   Total score _____ /10 Points

Figure 11-2: Michigan Neuropathy Screening Instrument. ©1994 American Diabetes Association (ADA) from *Diabetes Care* 1994;17:1281-1289, reprinted with permission from ADA.

cemic control improves, a condition often referred to as 'insulin neuritis.'[4,5] This syndrome occurs primarily in men and affects patients with type 2 or type 1 diabetes. Although the episodes of pain that characterize this form of diabetic neuropathy can be severe and disabling enough to disrupt basic activities like sitting at a desk, the condition is self-limiting and responds to simple symptomatic treatment. It may be associated with profound weight loss and severe depression in a condition known as diabetic neuropathic cachexia,[2] which tends to resolve spontaneously in 6 to 10 months.[5]

Amyotrophy

In patients with type 2 diabetes, particularly those older than 60 years, amyotrophy, or proximal motor neuropathy, may be superimposed on distal symmetric polyneuropathy. When it occurs alone, it may be called diabetic lumbosacral plexopathy, diabetic femoral neuropathy, or Bruns-Garland syndrome and is slightly more common in men.[5] It presents as deep, jabbing upper leg pain, then as weakness and wasting of the proximal leg muscles. Although it initially occurs on one side in 75% of cases, it sometimes affects both sides asymmetrically.[4,6] The pain typically affects the anterior thigh or leg and the lumbar region, but it may also affect the posterior thigh, calf, entire leg, foot, hip, buttock, and/or perineum. These symptoms and signs are associated with decreased or absent patellar reflex and mild sensory loss over the anterior thigh and tend to worsen at night.[5] Appearance of symptoms is followed by proximal muscle weakness that causes an inability to rise from the sitting position.[2] Over the course of a few weeks, the symptoms spread from the proximal to the distal leg and to the opposite side. The cervical nerve roots are affected in 30% to 50% of cases, causing a 30-lb to 40-lb weight loss before other symptoms begin.

Onset of amyotrophy may be insidious, but in most patients, it is abrupt.[5] Recovery is gradual in most cases[4] and may take 1 to 18 months (mean 3 to 6 months). Im-

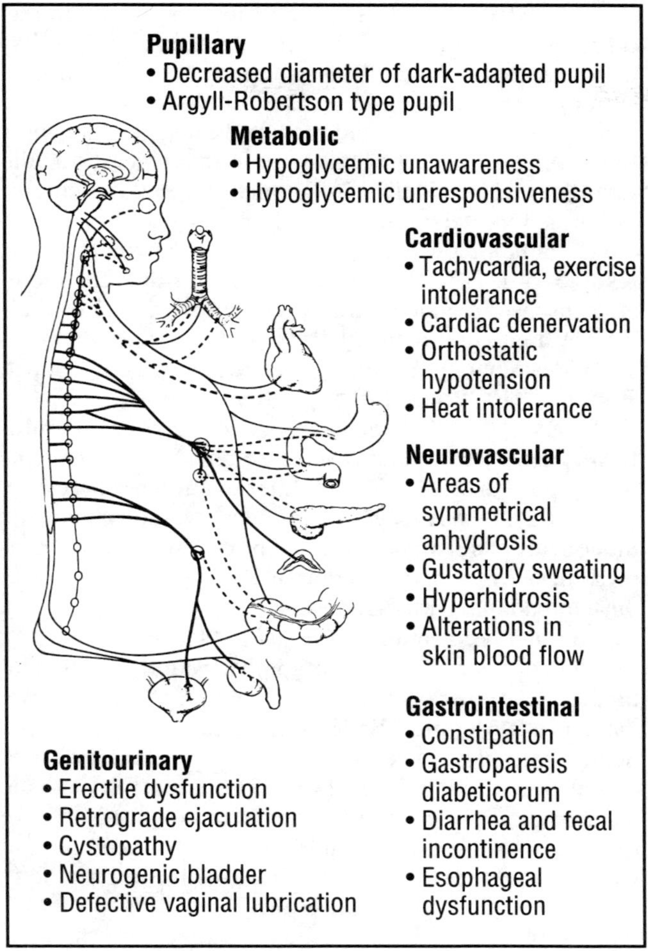

Pupillary
- Decreased diameter of dark-adapted pupil
- Argyll-Robertson type pupil

Metabolic
- Hypoglycemic unawareness
- Hypoglycemic unresponsiveness

Cardiovascular
- Tachycardia, exercise intolerance
- Cardiac denervation
- Orthostatic hypotension
- Heat intolerance

Neurovascular
- Areas of symmetrical anhydrosis
- Gustatory sweating
- Hyperhidrosis
- Alterations in skin blood flow

Gastrointestinal
- Constipation
- Gastroparesis diabeticorum
- Diarrhea and fecal incontinence
- Esophageal dysfunction

Genitourinary
- Erectile dysfunction
- Retrograde ejaculation
- Cystopathy
- Neurogenic bladder
- Defective vaginal lubrication

Figure 11-3: Clinical manifestations of autonomic neuropathy. Sympathetic fibers are shown in gray, parasympathetic in black, preganglionic as solid lines, and postganglionic as dashed lines. Adapted from Vinik et al, *Cleve Clin J Med* 2001;68:930.

proved glycemic control and physiotherapy are the recommended treatments. Elevated sedimentation rate may be found. Although diabetes itself may trigger an inflammatory response,[5] in many cases, amyotrophy seems to result from several immune-mediated causes that are more frequent in diabetic patients than in the general population. These causes include inflammatory vasculitis, chronic inflammatory demyelinating polyneuropathy, and monoclonal gammopathy. If immune-mediated, symptoms can resolve in days with immunotherapy. In immune-mediated disease, demyelination predominates, and patients have a high cerebrospinal fluid protein content and increased lymphocyte count.[2]

Focal or Multifocal Neuropathies

About 10% of diabetic neuropathies are focal or multifocal. These neuropathies typically affect older patients with type 2 diabetes. Although the pain they cause may be severe, they have a good prognosis.[4] Subtypes include mononeuropathies and entrapment or compression neuropathies, which have a combined prevalence of 3% to 36% in patients with diabetes.[5]

Entrapment and compression neuropathies

One common form of entrapment neuropathy, carpal tunnel syndrome, occurs twice as frequently in diabetic patients as in people without diabetes. In one study of patients with mild diabetic neuropathy and no symptoms of carpal tunnel syndrome, 23% of patients fulfilled the electrodiagnostic criteria for carpal tunnel syndrome. In that study, carpal tunnel syndrome was more common in women, shorter patients, and those with a higher body mass index, possibly because increased fat deposits affect the median nerve.[5] Diabetes may increase the incidence of entrapment neuropathies associated with repetitive injury and inflammation or external pressure by altering the movement of materials from the cell body to the distal nerve endings and back again, a process called axonal transport. Entrapment neuropathy may also result

Table 11-3: Differential Diagnosis of Diabetic Autonomic Neuropathy

- Idiopathic orthostatic hypotension (Shy-Drager syndrome—orthostatic hypotension, pyramidal and cerebral signs, including tremor, rigidity, hyper-reflexia, ataxia, and urinary and bowel dysfunction)

- Panhypopituitarism

- Pheochromocytoma

- Chagas' disease

- Amyloidosis

- Hypovolemia caused by poor glycemic control or diuretics

- Effects of insulin

- Complications from vasodilators (nitrates, calcium-channel blockers, hydralazine)

- Complications from sympathetic blockers (methyldopa, clonidine, prazosin, guanethidine, phenothiazine, tricyclic antidepressants)

- Orthostatic hypotension caused by alcoholic neuropathy

- Congestive heart failure

- Other causes of diarrhea, constipation, and gastrointestinal dysfunction

- Other causes of genitourinary and erectile dysfunction

- Other causes of pedal edema

- Hypoglycemic unresponsiveness and unawareness occurring with intensive glycemic control

- The Argyll-Robertson pupil of syphilis

Reprinted with permission from Vinik et al, *Cleve Clin J Med* 2001;68:932.

Table 11-4: Screening for and Treating Diabetic Autonomic Neuropathy

1. Tight Glycemic Control

For all diabetic patients: maintain aggressive control of blood glucose, hemoglobin A_{1c}, blood pressure, and lipids with pharmacologic therapy and lifestyle changes

2. Screening

- Begin screening at the time of diagnosis of type 2 diabetes
- Ask about symptoms
- Examine for signs
- Test for heart-rate variability
  - Expiration:inspiration ratio
  - Response to Valsalva maneuver
  - Response to standing
- If negative: repeat yearly
- If positive: apply appropriate diagnostic tests, treat symptoms

Reprinted with permission from Vinik et al, *Cleve Clin J Med* 2001;68:936.

3. Treatment

Symptoms	Tests	Treatments
Cardiac	Multigated angiography, thallium scan, iodine-123 metaiodobenzylguanidine scan	Angiotensin-converting enzyme inhibitors, β-blockers, antioxidants, aldose reductase inhibitors
Postural hypotension	Measure standing and supine blood pressure, measure catecholamines	Supportive garments, clonidine, midodrine, octreotide
Gastrointestinal	Emptying study, barium study, endoscopy, manometry, electrogastrogram	Prokinetic agents, antibiotics, bulking agents, tricyclic antidepressants, pancreatic extracts
Sexual dysfunction	Penile-brachial pressure index, nocturnal penile tumescence	Sex therapy, psychological counseling, sildenafil, prostaglandin E_1 injection, device or prosthesis
Bladder dysfunction	Cystometrogram, post-voiding sonography	Bethanechol, intermittent catheterization
Sudomotor (sweating) dysfunction	Quantitative sudomotor axon reflex, sweat test, skin blood flow	Scopolamine, glycopyrrolate, botulinum toxin, vasodilators

4. Follow-up

Monitor every year for response to treatment

because diabetes changes intraneural circulation or joint and connective tissue and increases neural water content, resulting in edema and increasing pressure in the confined space enclosing the nerve.[2] Other, less common compression neuropathies affect the radial nerve at the wrist, the ulnar nerve at the elbow (cubital tunnel syndrome), the lateral cutaneous nerve of the thigh (meralgia paresthetica), or the peroneal nerve at the knee.[4,5]

Cranial nerve palsies

Mononeuropathies unrelated to entrapment or compression occur primarily in older patients, are painful, and have a rapid onset and a self-limiting course of 6 weeks[2] to 6 months.[6] They may result from vascular obstruction and resolve as adjacent fascicles assume the function of the infarcted ones.[2] However, microinfarcts within the nuclei of affected nerves have been demonstrated and may instead be the cause.[4] Such mononeuropathies often affect the cranial nerves. The most common is a painful third-nerve palsy[5] with diplopia and ptosis.[4] In this variant of third-nerve palsy, the contractile response of the pupil to light is typically spared. The second most frequently affected cranial nerve in patients with diabetes is the fourth, and the third most frequently affected is the sixth.[6]

Other focal neuropathies

Other diabetic focal neuropathies include truncal radiculoneuropathy, characterized by severe, intermittent, aching or burning pain; a girdlelike sensation around the chest or abdomen; and, sometimes, motor deficits that appear as unilateral bulging of abdominal muscles. These symptoms may be accompanied by profound weight loss at their onset and by lancinating or stabbing sensations and may result from ischemia or inflammation. In most patients, this condition lasts at least 4 months and resolves spontaneously. It is distinct from truncal neuropathy, which is characterized by spreading sensory deficits in the distribution of the thoracic intercostal nerves and is often associated with autonomic neuropathy.[5]

Autonomic Neuropathy

Autonomic neuropathy can affect any system in the body (Figure 11-3) and can occur as early as the first year after diagnosis of type 2 diabetes, when it can often be detected at the subclinical stage with quantitative functional testing.[9] Its major manifestations include dysfunction of the gastrointestinal, genitourinary, and cardiovascular systems, and its consequences can be serious. Autonomic neuropathy can sometimes cause respiratory failure[2] and is an independent risk factor for stroke. The 5-year mortality in patients with diabetic autonomic neuropathy is three times that of diabetic patients without it. Death often results from nephropathy and heart disease. Diabetic autonomic neuropathy is linked to increased urinary albumin excretion and may contribute to kidney damage. Table 11-3 lists possible causes of autonomic neuropathy that must be excluded before diabetic autonomic neuropathy can be diagnosed. Recommendations for screening and testing for symptoms of diabetic autonomic neuropathy are provided in Table 11-4.

Cardiac autonomic neuropathy

Cardiac autonomic neuropathy occurs in 22% of patients with type 2 diabetes, and borderline cardiac autonomic neuropathy occurs in an additional 12%.[9] It initially appears as increased heart rate from vagal denervation, then as decreased heart rate from sympathetic denervation, and finally as a fixed heart rate suggesting almost complete denervation.[4] In patients with diabetes, abnormal heart rate variability has been reported to result in a 5.5-year mortality of 27% vs 5% in those with normal variability. Lack of heart rate variability during deep breathing or exercise confers a high risk of coronary heart disease, regardless of the presence of diabetes.[9] Tests used to diagnose cardiovascular autonomic neuropathy are described in Table 11-5.

Cardiac autonomic neuropathy may result in sudden death, congestive heart failure, and silent myocardial in-

Table 11-5: Diagnostic Tests for Cardiovascular Autonomic Neuropathy

Resting heart rate

>100 beats/minute is abnormal

Beat-to-beat heart rate variation

- The patient should abstain from drinking coffee overnight
- Test should not be performed after overnight hypoglycemic episodes
- When the patient lies supine and breathes 6 times per minute, a difference in heart rate of less than 10 beats/minute is abnormal
- An expiration:inspiration R-R ratio >1.17 is abnormal

Heart rate response to standing

- The R-R interval is measured at beats 15 and 30 after the patient stands
- A 30:15 ratio of less than 1.03 is abnormal

Heart rate response to Valsalva maneuver

- The patient forcibly exhales into the mouthpiece of a manometer, exerting a pressure of 40 mm Hg for 15 seconds
- A ratio of longest to shortest R-R interval of less than 1.2 is abnormal

Reprinted with permission from Vinik et al, *Cleve Clin J Med* 2001;68:934.

farction[2] and has been linked to decreased survival post-infarction. Painless ischemia, which confers a greater risk of mortality after infarction, occurs in 38% of patients with autonomic neuropathy, compared with 5% of those with-

Systolic blood pressure response to standing

- Systolic blood pressure is measured when the patient is lying down and 2 minutes after the patient stands
- A decrease in excess of 12-15 mm Hg is abnormal

Diastolic blood pressure response to isometric exercise

- The patient squeezes a handgrip dynamometer to establish his or her maximum
- The patient then squeezes the grip at 30% maximum for 5 minutes
- An increase of less than 16 mm Hg in the contralateral arm is abnormal

Electrocardiography

- A QTc of more than 440 ms is abnormal
- Depressed very low frequency peak or low-frequency peak indicates sympathetic dysfunction
- Depressed high-frequency peak indicates parasympathetic dysfunction
- Lowered low-frequency/high-frequency ratio indicates sympathetic imbalance

Neurovascular flow

Noninvasive laser Doppler measures of peripheral sympathetic responses to nociception

---

out such neuropathy. Asymptomatic infarction was reported in nearly 40% of diabetic patients in the Framingham study. The mortality after such an infarction is 47%, compared with 35% for a painful infarction.[9]

Orthostatic hypotension

Dysautonomic efferent sympathetic denervation impairs vasoconstriction in the cutaneous and splanchnic vascular beds, often producing postural[4] or orthostatic hypotension, defined as a decrease in systolic blood pressure of more than 30 mm Hg upon standing. Other causes of postural hypotension related to autonomic neuropathy include impaired baroreceptor function, poor cardiovascular reactivity, and volume depletion. Symptoms of orthostatic hypotension include dizziness, weakness, faintness, visual impairment, pain in the back of the head, and loss of consciousness. Eating and insulin injection often provoke symptoms, which precede and are frequently confused with hypoglycemic symptoms. Insulin may worsen dysautonomic hypotension by increasing capillary permeability, resulting in mild intravascular depletion. Advanced autonomic neuropathy can exaggerate these effects.[9]

Other cardiovascular effects

Conversely, autonomic neuropathy may cause paradoxical supine hypertension[2] and disturb the normal circadian pattern of blood pressure variation, resulting in nocturnal hypertension and an early morning decrease in blood pressure. Because of this disturbance, as well as altered sympathovagal balance and reduced nocturnal vagal activity, patients with autonomic neuropathy are more likely to have an infarction at night than in the morning. The reverse is true in patients with normal autonomic function. By impairing sympathetic and parasympathetic responses that augment cardiac output and redirect blood flow to skeletal muscle, autonomic neuropathy decreases exercise tolerance.[9] It may also result in impaired blood flow in the capillaries, which decreases neurovascular flow, thereby worsening neuropathy.

Impaired blood flow can cause heat intolerance by disrupting the microvessels in the smooth skin of the palms, soles, and face, which contain numerous arteriovenous thermoregulatory shunts. Disruption of capillary blood flow can also interfere with the skin's nutrient supply.[9] Dysautonomic sudomotor abnormalities decrease sweating in the lower body and often make the skin of the legs cold and dry,[5] resulting in fissures and cracks that allow microbes to enter and cause infected ulcers and gangrene.[2] To compensate for decreased lower body sweating, particularly as heat intolerance increases, sweating of the face and trunk becomes excessive. Autonomic abnormalities also cause sweating of the face immediately after eating (gustatory sweating).[5]

Hypoglycemic unawareness and unresponsiveness

Autonomic neuropathy may impair catecholamine release, thereby reducing hypoglycemic symptoms and causing patients to not eat when necessary. Hypoglycemic unresponsiveness may result when autonomic impairment blunts short-term release of glucagon and epinephrine and long-term release of growth hormone and cortisol, thereby deranging glucose counterregulation during increased insulin activity and fasting.[9] Together, these defects hamper the patient's efforts to maintain the adequate and consistent control of blood glucose levels required to keep neuropathy from progressing.

Gastrointestinal and urogenital autonomic neuropathy

The incidence of gastrointestinal symptoms in patients with diabetes is as high as 75%. Symptoms of increased or decreased gastric motility may coexist and may result from the effects of diabetes on the sympathetic and parasympathetic nervous systems. Derangement of extrinsic parasympathetic and sympathetic innervation and of intrinsic enteric innervation may also affect gastric secretion and absorption. In one tertiary care center, half of diabetic patients had gastroparesis, and 30% had nausea and vomiting.[5] Emesis of undigested food consumed many hours or even days earlier may occur. Episodes of nausea and vomiting may last days to months or occur in cycles. Other symptoms of gastric autonomic neuropathy include early satiety, bloating, epigastric pain, and anorexia.[9]

Whereas vagal dysfunction causes gastric stasis, disorders of visceral sensory fibers may alter perception of gastric distention.[5] Although uncommon in diabetic patients, dysphagia, retrosternal discomfort, or heartburn may result from impaired esophageal motility caused by autonomic neuropathy. In contrast, constipation, the most common gastrointestinal complication of diabetic autonomic neuropathy, affects almost 60% of patients with diabetes. Atony of the large bowel and rectum and megacolon may result. Alternating episodes of constipation and diarrhea may also occur.[9] Diarrhea is reported in 8% to 22% of patients with diabetes[5] and is more frequent in those with autonomic neuropathy. In such patients, diarrhea may result from intestinal hypermotility caused by diminished sympathetic inhibition or from bacterial overgrowth, pancreatic insufficiency, steatorrhea, or bile-salt malabsorption. It is usually characterized by intermittent episodes that last several hours to several days and may cause as many as 30 bowel movements within 24 hours and fecal incontinence.[9] It often occurs at night after a long history of diabetes and places patients at risk of malabsorption, anemia, and hypoalbuminemia.[5]

Bladder dysfunction may occur from neurogenic abnormality in the detrusor muscle[4] or, in the absence of impaired motor function, from damage to afferent fibers that decreases bladder sensation. When sensation is decreased, the bladder can expand to three times its normal size without producing discomfort. Voiding frequency decreases, complete voiding becomes impossible, and risk of urinary tract infection increases. Dribbling and overflow incontinence commonly result.[9] In many male patients with diabetes, bladder dysfunction is associated with erectile dysfunction, which is often the first manifestation of autonomic neuropathy. Autonomic dysfunction may also result in retrograde ejaculation, diminished ejaculatory force, or loss of ejaculatory effort[5] and related impairment of reproductive capacity.[9]

Diagnostic Assessment and Related Testing

The diagnosis of diabetic neuropathy is one of exclusion, and other causes of neuropathy must first be ruled out, based on information and recommendations for screening and testing such as those listed in Tables 11-1 through 11-5. Diagnosis of neuropathy relies heavily on careful history taking, which may be assisted by a questionnaire.[2] Sensory evaluation should focus on symptoms that concern patients most, such as prickling, tingling, sensation of electrical shock, burning, aching, and throbbing.[3] In addition to pain assessment, light touch, vibration, and position sense should be evaluated.[1] Touch sensitivity is commonly measured by using tactile circumference discrimination testing or monofilament testing.[3] Although testing with a 10-g monofilament can predict foot ulceration, as can Achilles reflex assessment, use of a 1.0-g monofilament increases sensitivity in detecting early neuropathy from 60% to 90%. Vibration perception should be measured with a 128-Hz tuning fork.[2] Motor examination should evaluate muscular strength and reflexes.[1]

Comorbidities and Risk Factors

Thickening of the vascular basement membrane in the nerves, eyes, and kidneys often develops simultaneously in patients with diabetes, and neuropathy, retinopathy, and nephropathy often coexist. Intensive glycemic control decreased the incidence of all these microvascular complications in patients with type 1 diabetes in the Diabetes Control and Complications Trial. In that trial, the effects of intensive insulin therapy with multiple daily injections or an insulin pump were compared with those of conventional therapy with two daily insulin injections in two cohorts, one with no retinopathy and one with mild retinopathy. After 5 years, in the first cohort, incidence of neuropathy was 3% for intensive therapy vs 10% for conventional therapy, and in the second cohort, neuropathy incidence was 7% for intensive therapy vs 16% for conventional therapy.[7] Thus, reduction in mean blood glucose level from 230 mg/dL to 155 mg/dL reduced the 5-year risk of clinically detectable neuropathy in patients with retinopathy at study entry by 56%, compared with about 16% for controls.[6] Moreover, it reduced the risk of autonomic dysfunction by 53%.[9] These results are difficult to extrapolate to patients with type 2 diabetes, especially older ones,[7] but hyperglycemia is clearly implicated in the development of diabetic neuropathy in these patients. This association is indicated by the ability of treatment aimed at achieving near-normoglycemia to slow deterioration in nerve conduction velocities and improve vibration perception after 9 years of follow-up in the UKPDS.[1,10]

In addition to poor glycemic control, the chief risk factors for diabetic autonomic neuropathy include greater age, longer duration of diabetes, higher body mass index, and female sex.[9] In the Pittsburgh epidemiologic study, hypertension and high low-density lipoprotein (LDL) levels were also associated with diabetic autonomic neuropathy. However, the Finnish prospective neuropathy study of patients with type 2 diabetes found that although female sex and fasting insulin level were related to cumulative incidence of parasympathetic neuropathy, neither of these variables predicted sympathetic neuropathy.

Hypertension and dyslipidemia are closely linked with diabetic polyneuropathy as well as diabetic autonomic neuropathy. Analysis of European data showed a notable association between systolic and diastolic blood pressure, cholesterol and triglyceride levels, and neuropathy.[4] Other factors that may increase the risk of neuropathy in diabetic patients include exposure to neurotoxins such as heavy metals and pesticides, smoking, alcohol consumption,[1] adverse medication side effects, and genetic predispositions.[7]

Pathophysiology-Targeted Therapies
Risk Factor Management

Because the pathogenesis of diabetic neuropathy is multifactorial, multiple metabolic and vascular abnormalities must be addressed simultaneously. This need was cogently illustrated by the Steno trial in patients with type 2 diabetes, in which comprehensive risk factor management reduced the odds ratio for developing autonomic neuropathy to 0.32 compared with usual care. Treatment included glucose-control agents, antihypertensives such as angiotensin-converting enzyme inhibitors (ACEIs) and calcium-channel blockers, lipid-lowering agents, aspirin, and antioxidants.[2] In particular, because near-normoglycemia has prevented neuropathy in many patients and slowed the deterioration of nerve function in others, tight glucose control is the paramount goal in treating any diabetic patient with neuropathy. However, in patients with painful symptoms, several years of improved control may be required to reduce the pain.[10] The inability of tight glucose control to completely prevent neuropathy indicates that addressing other contributing factors is crucial.[1]

Many vasoactive agents used for hypertension and ischemia, such as prazosin (Minipress®) and nifedipine (Adalat®, Procardia®), can increase nerve blood flow. Albuterol (Proventil®, Volmax®) and doxazosin (Cardura®) also do so through their effects on nitric oxide (NO). In experimentally induced diabetes, lisinopril (Prinivil®, Zestril®) improved nerve blood flow, and two preliminary clinical trials showed small but significant improvement in results of electrophysiologic and quantitative sensory tests after 12 weeks of lisinopril. A clinical trial of trandolapril (Mavik®) found significant improvement in neural amplitude, latency, and conduction velocity after 12 months of therapy.[4] In diabetic patients with autonomic neuropathy, quinapril (Accupril®) increased parasympathetic activity and improved heart rate variability.[11]

In animal studies, a member of the angiotensin-receptor blocker (ARB) drug class also improved nerve blood flow. Combining an ARB and an endothelin-1 blocker in low doses improved nerve blood flow and conduction velocity more than the additive response expected from either drug alone, indicating synergism between these drug classes.[4] In addition, to prevent small-vessel occlusion, platelet aggregation inhibitors such as aspirin are indicated for the long-term treatment of diabetic neuropathy.[7] Weight loss; decreased consumption of alcohol, fat, and cholesterol; lipid-lowering therapy; smoking cessation; and avoidance of heavy metals, pesticides, and other neurotoxins can also help manage neuropathy.

Emerging and Experimental Agents
Aldose reductase inhibitors

Despite the success of aldose reductase inhibitors (ARIs) in ameliorating neuropathy in diabetic animals, results of clinical trials have been mixed, possibly because of the small size and short duration of these trials. In many trials, ARIs may not have been sufficiently potent or given at high enough doses to have an effect. Doses of the ARI zenarestat that cause more than 80% suppression of nerve sorbitol level were required to show effectiveness. In most trials, treatment may have been initiated after irreversible structural changes developed and therefore too late in the course of neuropathy to have an effect.[3] Large multicenter trials are now assessing whether ARI treatment will prevent neuropathy if given early enough.[7]

Although ARIs caused a multifold increase in nerve regeneration, the regenerating fibers did not mature,[1] and some ARIs have unacceptable toxicity and related side effects that prevent their clinical use.[3] Sorbinil, the first agent extensively studied, was associated with toxic epidermal necrolysis in two patients.[10] Similar toxicity problems have ended clinical trials of another experimental agent, the advanced glycation end product inhibitor aminoguanidine, despite its ability to improve nerve blood flow, conduction velocity, vascular permeability, and structural parameters in experimental diabetes.[2]

Some clinical trials have shown that ARIs can improve neuropathy. In a 1-year trial of tolrestat in patients with distal symmetric polyneuropathy, results of tests of autonomic function and vibration perception improved in treated patients compared with deterioration in most variables measured in placebo-treated patients (P <0.05).[2] However, development of tolrestat was discontinued because of potential hepatotoxicity.[10] A similarly long trial of zenarestat found dose-dependent improvement in the density of nerve fibers, particularly small unmyelinated ones, as well as increased nerve conduction velocity,[2] but development of zenarestat was halted because of potential nephrotoxicity.[10] Zopolrestat improved impaired cardiac ejection fractions[2] but did not improve nerve fiber density enough for continued development.[10] Many new ARIs are being developed and studied,[2] including fidarestat, a more potent ARI. Whether ARIs are effective and safe enough to be used in the long-term treatment of diabetic neuropathy has not yet been determined.[10]

Because aldose reductase inhibition alone may be insufficient to counteract metabolic derangement from multiple biochemical abnormalities, combining ARIs with antioxidants may be critical in halting the progression of diabetic neuropathy.[2] Several antioxidants have shown effectiveness in neuropathy. Probucol protected against decreased nerve conduction velocity, endoneurial blood flow, and oxygen tension in diabetic animals, and the free radical scavenger glutathione partially prevented diabetic neuropathy in experimental diabetes. By suppressing the formation of free radicals, the transition metal chelators deferoxamine and trientine improved nerve blood flow and conduction velocity in diabetic rats.[1,4]

Protein kinase C-β inhibitors

A specific inhibitor of PKC-β, LY333531, improved diabetic peripheral neuropathy as assessed by neurologic examination, clinician assessment, quantitative sensory testing, and electrophysiologic nerve function measurement after 1 year of therapy. The most common reported side effect was diarrhea, although the agent was generally well tolerated and showed no effects on glycemic control or hepatic, renal, or bone marrow function.[12]

γ-Linolenic acid

γ-Linolenic acid (GLA) is metabolized into an important constituent of nerve cell membranes and is a substrate for the formation of prostaglandin E, which preserves nerve blood flow. In diabetes, conversion of GLA is impaired, which may contribute to the pathogenesis of diabetic neuropathy.[2] Dosages of 360 to 480 mg daily resulted in improved nerve conduction velocity, thermal threshold, and symptoms in several clinical trials.[1] A multicenter trial found improvement in GLA patients and large deteriorations in placebo patients that were not consistent with the stable neuropathy found in other trials after 1 year; lack of balance in patient distribution across sites may have contributed to the results.[10] Short-term treatment with a related agent, intravenous lipoprostaglandin, has improved nerve conduction velocity and vibratory threshold without serious adverse effects.[1]

α-Lipoic acid

α-Lipoic or thioctic acid is present in food such as potatoes and broccoli[13] and is synthesized by the liver.[2] It is a potent free radical scavenger, enhances glucose uptake in muscle, and increases insulin sensitivity in patients with type 2 diabetes.[1] It also improves blood flow,[10] can reduce somatic and autonomic neuropathy in diabetes,[2] and has been approved in Germany for the treatment of diabetic neuropathy.[13] In German studies, high-dose oral therapy reduced painful symptoms, presumably via an antioxidant action.[4] In the United States, α-lipoic acid is being studied extensively as an agent to treat diabetic neuropathy as well as an antidiabetic agent.[2] Animal studies have shown that α-lipoic acid prevents nerve dysfunction, increases nerve blood flow, promotes nerve regeneration, and improves nerve conduction velocity. In a study of patients with type 2 diabetes with symptomatic diabetic neuropathy, daily infusion therapy at doses of 600 or 1,200 mg during a 3-week period improved symptom scores remarkably vs placebo.[13] These results indicated that α-lipoic acid was more beneficial than intensified glycemic control. However, the study's validity is questionable because many protocol violators were withdrawn from analysis.[10] Moreover, 7 months of infusion therapy did not further improve the results obtained after 3 weeks of such therapy. A 2-year trial in patients with diabetic polyneuropathy showed small but statistically significant improvement in nerve conduction velocity but no difference in disability scores between treatment and control groups.[1] Cardiac autonomic neuropathy was slightly improved in a 4-month placebo-controlled study using an 800-mg dose. Thus, although the literature supports α-lipoic acid therapy for diabetic neuropathy, additional studies are needed.[13] A 4-year phase III trial of the effects of oral therapy on progression of diabetic polyneuropathy has been under way in North America and Europe.[10] Combining α-lipoic acid with other emerging therapies may improve results. For example, in experimental diabetes, combination therapy with conjugates of lipoic acid and GLA had statistically significant effects on electrophysiologic parameters, nerve blood flow, and neurotrophins that were greater than those produced by either therapy alone.[4]

Neurotrophic therapy

Although an early phase II trial of recombinant nerve growth factor therapy was associated with sensory improvement, phase III studies did not confirm this finding.[1] Development of another neurotrophin, NT3, was halted after it failed to improve vibration perception threshold.[10] These negative findings have dampened enthusiasm for neurotrophic therapy for diabetic neuropathy.[2] Moreover, administering neurotrophic factors is difficult and causes hyperalgesia and pressure allodynia at the injection site.[1] However, prosaptide, a synthetic form of prosaposin, a naturally occurring neurotrophin present in human milk and cerebrospinal fluid, was effective in animal studies and reduced the pain of diabetic polyneuropathy in a phase II study. Other treatments being developed include stimulation of neurite outgrowth, activation of protective receptors with immunophilin ligands, and inhibition of abnormal excitatory activity.[10]

Targeted therapy for specific types of neuropathy

Because amyotrophy may be an autoimmune disease, immunosuppressant treatment agents such as prednisone, azathioprine (Imuran®), intravenous immunoglobulin, and plasmapheresis have been tried with some success, although their effectiveness has not yet been proven in clinical trials.[2,3] Carpal tunnel syndrome may respond to rest, antiinflammatory agents, and splinting in a neutral position. If this approach is ineffective and weakness and severe symptoms ensue, surgical decompression via sectioning of the volar carpal ligament may be indicated.[2] Decompression gives excellent relief of sensory symptoms and recovery of useful two-point discrimination in about 95% of cases, a rate similar to that for patients without diabetes. Diabetic patients with cubital tunnel syndrome also benefit as much as nondiabetic patients from anterior submuscular transposition of the ulnar nerve with musculofascial lengthening; 77% obtain excellent symptom relief, and 55% recover normal grip strength. Decompression of the four medial ankle tunnels relieved pain in 86% of diabetic patients with decreased foot sensation caused by tarsal tunnel syndrome and produced recovery of useful two-point discrimination in 72%. In 43 patients who had such decompression on one lower limb only, none had an ulcer or amputation of the treated limb after 4.5 years, whereas 7 had ulcers and 2 had amputations on the untreated limb (P <0.002).[14]

Foot Care and Follow-up

Because foot complications develop in 25% of patients with diabetes at some point in the course of the disease, good preventive foot care is crucial. Use of a decision pathway in which patients are stratified into one of four risk categories (normal, insensate, insensate and deformed, or history of ulcer)[8] based on results of foot screening for protective sensation can reduce hospital admissions, emergency department visits, and amputation rates.[3] Risk factors for foot disease include history of ulcer, presence of bony deformity and callus, and ischemia. These risk factors can be assessed in about 90 seconds by asking whether the patient has had foot ulcers, visually inspecting the feet, palpating the dorsalis pedis and posterior tibial pulses, and assessing sensate perception by applying the 10-g nylon monofilament to at least five sites on each foot. Patients with healthy feet should receive foot care advice and a brochure and be reexamined annually. Those with at-risk feet should be referred to a podiatrist for more detailed education, investigation, and quarterly follow-up. Patients with ulcers, blisters, bleeding into a callus, cellulitis, or acute ischemia should be referred to a podiatrist or multidisciplinary foot-care team immediately (preferably the same day) for appropriate debridement and dressing, antibiotics, and, after healing, rapid mobilization using special footwear. The relapse rate in patients who wore such footwear was 26% compared with 83% in nonusers. Thorough screening, proper education, and a multidisciplinary treatment approach can reduce amputation rates by 40% or more.[8]

Adequate self-care of feet includes several components. To reduce the risk of ulcers, patients should inspect their feet daily for cuts, sores, and blisters and seek medical care for such trauma immediately. They should also inspect their shoes daily for pebbles, embedded pins or nails, or other hazardous foreign objects. To avoid trauma from footwear, they must wear shoes that fit properly and have adequate support.[2] Walking barefoot should be strictly avoided.[8] Patients should wash and thoroughly dry their feet daily, particularly the areas between the toes, which they should powder. Creams should be used on dry,

Table 11-6: Selected Treatments for Painful Diabetic Neuropathy

Agent	Recommended Daily Dose Range
Amitriptyline (Elavil®)	10-150 mg
Nortriptyline (Aventyl®, Pamelor®)	30-150 mg
Venlafaxine (Effexor®)	37.5-75 mg
Bupropion (Wellbutrin®)	150-300 mg
Carbamazepine (Carbatrol®, Tegretol®)	100-1,000 mg
Gabapentin (Neurontin®)	400-3,600 mg
Lamotrigine (Lamictal®)	200-400 mg
Mexiletine (Mexitil®)	450-900 mg
Calcitonin	100 U

Table data were obtained from references 2, 3, 7, and 10.

cracked skin, and nails should be cut transversely. Padded socks should be worn and changed daily.[2] Patients should avoid immersing their feet in scalding water, walking on hot sand, putting their feet too close to radiators or fires, or otherwise incurring heat injury.[8]

Dosing Instructions and Precautions

Should be given at bedtime; initial dose is 10 mg with low titration upward based on level of morning sedation; side effects may become intolerable at 50-60 mg daily

Should be given at bedtime; initial dose is 10 mg with slow titration upward based on level of morning sedation

Give in divided doses; slowly titrate dose upward

Give in divided doses; slowly titrate dose upward

Divide into three daily doses; regular electrocardiographic monitoring is required to detect possible arrhythmia

May provide complete relief

Symptom Management by Neuropathy Type
Pain Management

At any given time, at least 10% of patients with diabetic polyneuropathy have pain. This pain can be highly variable and is often debilitating and difficult to control, but it is treatable. Specific treatments based on the nature of the pain are often advocated. However, many patients have a mixture of painful symptoms and respond to nonspecific treatment.[10] Deep muscle pain may respond to nonsteroidal anti-inflammatory agents (NSAIDs). If these agents prove ineffective, muscle relaxants may be tried.[1] Other available agents for pain management include opioids and anticonvulsants, antiarrhythmics, and antidepressants, which, although developed for other indications, also have analgesic effects. In clinical trials of these agents, about 60% to 70% of carefully selected patients achieved at least moderate (50%) pain reduction; the response rate in clinical practice is probably lower. As a result, patients should be informed that complete elimination of pain is rare with any agent and that not every patient responds to therapy. To avoid side effects, treatment must generally be initiated at low doses and slowly increased on a weekly basis until pain control is achieved, side effects become intolerable, or the maximum dose is reached. Responses may vary considerably between patients, and side effects can be unpredictable. Clinicians should inform patients that a trial-and-error approach is required. Sequential monotherapy may be necessary, and combination therapy may work when monotherapy fails.[10] Table 11-6 lists some of the more commonly used agents for painful diabetic neuropathy with recommended doses and dosing instructions, although none of these is FDA-labeled for this indication.

Antidepressants

Tricyclics, which act by blocking uptake of norepinephrine or serotonin and increasing their pain-inhibiting action in the brain, are often the first choice. Their analgesic effect is independent of their antidepressant activity. Although they do not reverse numbness, they are sometimes effective in reducing pain at night, thereby improving sleep and daytime functioning.[7] However, their side effects, such as somnolence, are substantial.[10] Side effects related to their anticholinergic action include orthostatic hypotension and urinary retention.[1] Other side effects include arrhythmia, increased hip fracture risk, weight gain, dry mouth, blurred vision, acute angle-closure glaucoma, constipation, and delirium. Their analgesic potency is comparable, and if one agent fails, another should be tried. Amitriptyline (Elavil®) is frequently the first choice,[10] but switching to nortriptyline (Aventyl®, Pamelor®) can reduce anticholinergic effects in patients who are troubled by them. Imipramine (Tofranil®) is recommended for deep burning or prickling pain. If antidepressants are ineffective when used as monotherapy, the antiarrhythmic mexiletine (Mexitil®) may be added and can be replaced with the anticonvulsant carbamazepine (Carbatrol®, Tegretol®) if poorly tolerated.[1] Venlafaxine (Effexor®) is sometimes effective for diabetic polyneuropathy. Although trazodone (Desyrel®) and fluoxetine (Prozac®) were found ineffective in some trials, results have been inconsistent.[10] Serotonin reuptake inhibitors may also be effective. Bupropion (Wellbutrin®), an aminoketone antidepressant and norepinephrine and dopamine reuptake inhibitor, was effective in sustained-release form at a dose of 150 to 300 mg daily in a study of patients with generalized peripheral neuropathy. Reported side effects of bupropion in the 12% of patients with diabetic neuropathy were mild.[3]

Anticonvulsants

If antidepressants prove ineffective or cause side effects, anticonvulsants may be used, although they tend to be less effective.[1] Anticonvulsants that are also effective analgesics include carbamazepine and gabapentin (Neurontin®). Carbamazepine may act by binding voltage-dependent sodium channels, thereby maintaining neuronal firing at a moderate rate.[10] It is particularly effective for shooting pain,[2] but side effects such as headache, drowsiness, ataxia, diplopia, agranulocytosis, hepatotoxicity, and Stevens-Johnson syndrome limit its use, and many patients do not tolerate a high enough dose to produce analgesia. Gabapentin is much better tolerated and has been shown effective for painful diabetic polyneuropathy and to improve mood, sleep, and overall well-being. As a result, it is often the drug of first choice. Its mechanism of action is unknown. Side effects include drowsiness, ataxia, anergy, facial swelling, and dizziness.[10] Lamotrigine (Lamictal®), which stabilizes the neural membrane by blocking activation of voltage-sensitive sodium channels and inhibits the presynaptic release of glutamate, relieved the pain of diabetic neuropathy at doses of 200 to 400 mg daily and was well tolerated.[3] Topiramate (Topamax®) was effective in a preliminary study. Despite the questionable blinding in this study, the results stimulated a larger US trial of topiramate for diabetic neuropathy. Results of this trial are pending. Adequate data on the effectiveness of other anticonvulsants for diabetic polyneuropathy are lacking. Pregabalin was effective for diabetic polyneuropathy but is not yet available.[10]

Antiarrhythmics

Although antiarrhythmics such as mexiletine can relieve the pain of diabetic polyneuropathy, they can induce arrhythmias, particularly in patients with coronary artery disease,[10] and thus require regular electrocardiographic monitoring,[1] which makes them relatively unattractive for use in patients with diabetes. Mexiletine has local anesthetic properties and is similar to lidocaine in structure and action. These agents treat pain caused by hyperexcitability of superficial free nerve endings. Although mexiletine blocks voltage-gated sodium channels, the mechanism by which it relieves pain in diabetic polyneuropathy is unknown.[10] Mexiletine has proven particularly effective for lancinating or burning pain.[1] A slow infusion of lidocaine can relive intractable pain for 3 to 21 days and is most useful in severe, self-limiting types of neuropathy. If such treatment is successful, therapy can be continued with oral mexiletine.[2]

Opioids

Some patients benefit from opioids, although many fail to respond and addiction risk is high. Tramadol (Ultram®)

was effective for painful diabetic polyneuropathy in both long-term and short-term studies, and oxycodone is being studied for its usefulness for this indication. Side effects include nausea, constipation, headache, and somnolence.[10]

Other Agents

For a deep, dull, gnawing ache that does not respond to other therapies, continuous intravenous insulin infusion is occasionally effective in 48 hours and can then be discontinued. Dextromethorphan may exert an analgesic effect in diabetic neuropathy by blocking the excitatory glutaminergic N-methyl-D-aspartate receptor in the spinal cord. Calcitonin 100 U daily produced nearly complete symptom relief in 39% of patients with painful diabetic neuropathy in a small placebo-controlled study after 2 weeks of therapy. Phenytoin (Dilantin®) is not recommended because it lacks efficacy and suppresses insulin secretion, which may cause diabetic coma.[2]

Although dose titration can be difficult, topical clonidine (Catapres®) or phentolamine can resolve the sympathetic-mediated burning, lancinating, and dysesthetic pain that occurs during ongoing nerve damage and is often accompanied by hyperalgesia and allodynia.[2] Other topical agents include capsaicin, which depletes substance P and possibly other neurotransmitters from sensory nerve terminals.[10] This depletion reduces or stops transmission of painful stimuli from peripheral nerves to the higher nervous system centers. Because capsaicin cream (0.075%) desensitizes patients to thermal, chemical, or mechanical stimuli, it is particularly useful for hyperesthesia.[1] Symptoms initially worsen with application and are relieved within 2 to 3 weeks.[2] Capsaicin should not be used for more than 8 weeks.[1] The patient must wear gloves and be careful to avoid touching the eyes or genitals when applying the cream. Like acupuncture, transcutaneous nerve stimulation can be helpful, particularly if electrodes are placed on the most sensitive areas to provide maximum relief.[2]

Table 11-7: Pharmacologic Therapies for Diabetic Autonomic Neuropathy

Indication	Drug and Dosage
Orthostatic hypotension	9-α-fluorohydrocortisone 0.5-2 mg/day
	Clonidine 0.1-0.5 mg at bedtime
	Octreotide 0.1-0.5 μg/kg/day
Gastroparesis	Metoclopramide 10 mg 30-60 min before meals and at bedtime
	Domperidone 10-20 mg 30-60 min before meals and at bedtime
	Erythromycin 250 mg 30 min before meals
	Levosulpiride 25 mg three times a day
Diarrhea	Metronidazole 250 mg three times a day for at least 3 weeks
	Clonidine 0.1 mg two or three times a day
	Cholestyramine 4 g one to six times a day
	Loperamide 2 mg four times a day
	Octreotide 50 μg three times a day
Cystopathy	Bethanechol 10 mg four times a day
	Doxazosin 1-2 mg two or three times a day
Erectile dysfunction	Sildenafil 50 mg 1 hour before sexual activity, once only per day

Reprinted with permission from Vinik et al, *Cleve Clin J Med* 2001;68:938.

Side Effects
Congestive heart failure, hypertension
Hypotension, sedation, dry mouth
Injection site pain, diarrhea
Galactorrhea, extrapyramidal symptoms

Galactorrhea

Abdominal cramps, nausea, diarrhea, rash
Galactorrhea

Orthostatic hypotension

Toxic megacolon
Aggravation of nutrient malabsorption

Hypotension, headache, palpitations

Headache, flushing, nasal congestion, dyspepsia,
musculoskeletal pain, blurred vision; interacts with
nitrate-containing drugs (hypotension and fatal
cardiac events may result)

Managing Diabetic Autonomic Neuropathy

Tight glucose control substantially reduces the prevalence of autonomic dysfunction and is crucial in preventing autonomic neuropathy from developing and in slowing its progression if it is already established.[9] Other management strategies include pharmacologic therapies for specific symptoms of diabetic autonomic neuropathy, which are listed in Table 11-7 with their indications, dosages, and side effects.

Cardiovascular Symptom Management

Early cardiac autonomic neuropathy has a reversible metabolic component.[2] Tight glucose control can reverse deterioration in heart-rate variability after only 1 year of therapy, although response depends on the baseline level of dysfunction.[9] Short-term insulin treatment can reduce loss of beat-to-beat variability, a mortality risk factor, by 33%.[2] In addition, in patients with mild microalbuminuria, ACEI therapy increased heart-rate variation and decreased mortality. Cardioselective or lipophilic β-blockers may modulate the effects of diabetic autonomic dysfunction by acting on the central nervous system or by acting peripherally to oppose sympathetic stimuli and restore balance between the parasympathetic and sympathetic systems.[9] Because decreased plasma free fatty acid levels may improve cardiac autonomic function and decrease risk of sudden death, medications that decrease levels of these acids, including insulin, may be beneficial.[3] In multicenter trials, α-lipoic acid slowed or reversed the progression of cardiovascular autonomic neuropathy if given early enough in the course of the disease. Aldose reductase inhibitors may also reverse the progression of cardiovascular autonomic neuropathy.[9]

Patients with orthostatic hypotension should be warned to get out of bed slowly, avoid hot baths, and inject insulin while lying down.[9] Elevating the head of the patient's bed 6 to 10 inches can prevent sodium and water loss and supine hypertension.[5] Wearing a total body stocking more effectively increases venous return from the periphery than leg compression alone.[15] Patients should put on and take off compressive garments while lying down.[2] Prostaglandin inhibitors such as NSAIDs may also be helpful. Increasing salt intake to 10 to 20 g daily[5] or using 9-α-fluorohydrocortisone therapy may offer benefit, but these agents do not improve symptoms before the onset of edema, which may cause hypertension or congestive heart failure.[9] Metoclopramide (Reglan®) is useful in patients with dopamine excess or increased sensitivity to dopamine.[2] Clonidine can address α_2-adrenoceptor deficiency, but because it may paradoxically increase blood pressure in some patients, it should be initiated at small doses and increased gradually.[9] Yohimbine (Aphrodyne®) may be effective in patients with α_2-adrenoceptor excess. Patients with increased β-adrenoceptors respond to propranolol (Inderal®). Midodrine (ProAmatine®), an α_1-adrenoceptor agonist, or dihydroergotamine with caffeine may help if other measures fail.[2] Subcutaneous octreotide (Sandostatin®) given in the morning may be useful in patients with refractory orthostatic hypotension after eating.[2] However, because the effectiveness of these measures varies with orthostatic tolerance, methods of raising blood pressure dynamically are useful. Simply drinking a few 8-ounce glasses of water can quickly increase systolic blood pressure in patients with severe neurogenic orthostatic hypotension by increasing sympathetic activity. Erythropoietin (Epogen®, Procrit®) has also been effective for orthostatic hypotension in anemic patients with diabetes and may raise standing blood pressure by improving vasomotor tone via increased norepinephrine levels, enhanced hemoglobin binding to NO, increased vascular sensitivity to angiotensin II, or a direct pressor effect on vascular smooth muscle cells.[16]

The severity and frequency of gustatory sweating can be reduced with the antimuscarinic glycopyrrolate (Robinul®).[2] Consumption of spicy foods and cheeses may be linked to such sweating and should be avoided. Patients with hypoglycemic unawareness who use an insulin pump should use boluses of less than the calculated amount. If such patients are receiving intensive glucose control therapy, they should use small boluses of long-acting insulin.[9] Injection of botulinum toxin A (Botox®) can stop excessive axillary and palmar sweating by blocking release of acetylcholine, which mediates sympathetic neurotransmission in sweat glands. Treatment was otherwise well tolerated, but it decreased finger pinch strength by 40%.[16]

Gastrointestinal and Urinary Symptom Management

Patients with gastroparesis should eat 4 to 6 small meals daily and reduce dietary fat content to less than 40 g daily.[9] Consuming liquid meals[5] or a gluten-free diet may be helpful.[2] Fiber intake should be restricted to prevent development of bezoars. Improved blood glucose control can improve gastric motor function. Prokinetic agents such as domperidone (Motilium®), metoclopramide, and levosulpiride can be used, but tolerance develops after a few doses, and effectiveness decreases with use. Periodic withdrawal restores the response to these agents.[9] The antibiotic erythromycin affects the motilin receptor, promotes gastric contraction, shortens gastric emptying time, and can be given in liquid or suppository form.[2] Jejunostomy may be required in severe cases to allow the stomach to rest and gastric function to recover. Initial treatment of diabetic diarrhea should correct fluid and electrolyte imbalances and improve nutrition. Although antidiarrheal agents such as loperamide (Imodium®) and diphenoxylate can reduce the number of stools, they should be used with care because they have been associated with toxic megacolon.[9]

Recently, clinical studies have been initiated with an implantable peristaltic stimulator which delivers a series of electrical pulses to the intestinal wall that stimulate contraction waves (Enterra®). Some patients have experienced dramatic relief and the studies are ongoing.

Antibiotics can address bacterial overgrowth.[9] Metronidazole (Flagyl®, Protostat®) therapy appears most effective, and 3 weeks of treatment is recommended. Bile salt chelation with cholestyramine 4 mg three times daily mixed with fluid may relieve gastric irritation from bile retention.[2] Clonidine can improve diarrhea by reversing adrenergic dysfunction. If diarrhea is resistant to these treatments, octreotide may be used. Constipation can be treated with regular exercise, adequate hydration, fiber consumption, sorbitol, and lactulose. More severe symptoms may require intermittent use of saline or osmotic laxatives. Patients with bladder dysfunction should be advised to palpate their bladder and urinate when it is full. Massaging or pressing the abdomen above the pubic bone can initiate urinary flow. Parasympathomimetics like bethanechol (Urecholine®) may help but often do not empty the bladder completely. Doxazosin can induce long-term relaxation of the sphincter, and self-catheterization is a useful approach with a low risk of infection.[9]

References

1. Sugimoto K, Murakawa Y, Sima AA: Diabetic neuropathy—a continuing enigma. *Diabetes Metab Res Rev* 2000;16:408-433.

2. Vinik AI, Park TS, Stansberry KB, et al: Diabetic neuropathies. *Diabetologia* 2000;43:957-973.

3. Simmons Z, Feldman EL: Update on diabetic neuropathy. *Curr Opin Neurol* 2002;15:595-603.

4. Malik RA, Tesfaye S, Ward JD: Vascular changes and diabetic neuropathy. In: Johnstone MT, Veves A, eds. *Contemporary Cardiology: Diabetes and Cardiovascular Disease.* Totowa, NJ, Humana Press, 2001. pp 411-430.

5. Wein TH, Albers JW: Diabetic neuropathies. *Phys Med Rehabil Clin N Am* 2001;12:307-320.

6. Greene DA, Stevens MJ, Feldman EL: Diabetic neuropathy: scope of the syndrome. *Am J Med* 1999;107:2S-8S.

7. Gominak S, Parry GJ: Diabetic neuropathy. *Adv Neurol* 2002; 88:99-109.

8. Gadsby R: Managing patients with diabetic neuropathy. *Practitioner* 2001;245:748-752.

9. Vinik AI, Erbas T: Recognizing and treating diabetic autonomic neuropathy. *Cleve Clin J Med* 2001;68:928-944.

10. Bril V: Status of current clinical trials in diabetic polyneuropathy. *Can J Neurol Sci* 2001;28:191-198.

11. Malik RA: Can diabetic neuropathy be prevented by angiotensin-converting enzyme inhibitors? *Ann Med* 2000;32:1-5.

12. Litchy W, Dyck P, Tesfaye S, et al: Diabetic peripheral neuropathy (DPN) assessed by neurological examination (NE) and composite scores (CS) is improved with LY333531 treatment. Poster presented at: 62nd Scientific Sessions of the American Diabetes Association; June 14-18, 2002; San Francisco, CA. Poster 800-P.

13. Morelli V, Zoorob RJ: Alternative therapies: Part I. Depression, diabetes, obesity. *Am Fam Physician* 2000;62:1051-1060.

14. Dellon AL: Preventing foot ulceration and amputation by decompressing peripheral nerves in patients with diabetic neuropathy. *Ostomy Wound Manage* 2002;48:36-45.

15. Denq JC, Opfer-Gehrking TL, Giuliani M, et al: Efficacy of compression of different capacitance beds in the amelioration of orthostatic hypotension. *Clin Auton Res* 1997;7:321-326.

16. Low PA: Autonomic neuropathies. *Curr Opin Neurol* 2002;15:605-609.

Chapter 12

Erectile Dysfunction: New Treatment Options

Erectile dysfunction (ED), the persistent inability to achieve and/or maintain an erection sufficient for sexual intercourse, is a common complication of type 2 diabetes. Erectile dysfunction causes anxiety, depression, and loss of self-esteem and self-confidence, and it may not only compromise quality of life but also impede adequate diabetic self-care and worsen outcomes.[1] Erectile dysfunction is often an early symptom of type 2 diabetes, cardiovascular disease, or both. It may be the presenting disorder in as many as 12% of diabetic patients.[2] In one sonographic study, patients with severe arteriogenic ED had a 16% risk of severe asymptomatic ischemic heart disease.[3] Treating ED can reduce cardiovascular mortality. In a UK study, ED treatment reduced cardiovascular mortality by 30% in a group with a large percentage of diabetic patients.[4] Thus, asking patients about their level of sexual satisfaction is a crucial part of the diagnostic work-up. Once ED has been diagnosed, managing it appropriately is an important part of comprehensive care for type 2 diabetic patients of all ages, especially the elderly.

Prevalence

As many as 30 million men in the US may have some degree of ED,[5] and diabetic patients are at much greater risk than the general population. The Massachusetts Male Aging Study (MMAS) of men aged 40 to 70 years, first surveyed in the late 1980s, found a 28% overall prevalence of ED in patients with diabetes, most of whom probably had type 2 diabetes.[6] This prevalence was about three times that of the general study population (9.6%).[7] Additional analysis indicated that, whereas the crude incidence rate of ED for white men in the United States is about 26 cases per 1,000 men per year, the age-adjusted risk of ED is nearly 51 cases per 1,000 men per year for diabetic patients.[2] Estimates of the prevalence of ED in all diabetic men range from 35% to 75%, and the disease occurs in at least one half of them within 10 years of diagnosis of diabetes.[2] As a result, at least 40% of men with ED have diabetes.[1]

Causes

Erectile dysfunction in diabetic patients often has organic and psychogenic components. Even if the initiating factor is not psychological, once organic ED occurs, the performance anxiety and depression that it produces further diminish erectile function by reducing erotic focus or sensory awareness or both, which thereby reinforces the condition.[1,8] Anxiety and depression can cause or worsen relationship problems and prevent adequate stimulation, while further reinforcing ED.[9] Thus, more than 80% of cases of ED include both a psychogenic and an organic component.[4] In diabetic patients, ED usually has vascular and neurogenic components and, possibly, a hormonal component as well. For instance, some studies have shown increased urinary and decreased total and free testosterone levels in diabetic patients with ED, which suggests that the condition may, in part, result from primary gonadal dysfunction. However, most other studies have not confirmed this association.[7] Vascular causes may include an inefficient veno-occlusive mechanism or impaired blood flow into the penis, caused by atherosclerosis.[1] The same processes that cause peripheral vascular disease affect the penile arteries and result in ED.[9] Penile arterial narrowing and arteriolar closure and resultant penile hypotension and cavernous arterial insufficiency have been found in diabetic patients.[7] However, microvascular changes in corporal smooth muscle and endothelial integrity may be the primary cause of ED in diabetic patients.[1,7] Diabetic patients also commonly have somatic and autonomic nerve dysfunction. Because the most vulnerable autonomic nerves are the long parasympathetics innervating the pelvic organs, ED is the most common, and often the first, sign of diabetic autonomic neuropathy. In addition to peripheral autonomic nerve damage, diabetic patients may also have disturbed erectile neuroregulation from abnormal local levels of nitric oxide synthase (NOS) activity, vasoactive intestinal polypeptide (VIP), prostaglandins, endothelins, and other neuromediators.[7] Finally, medications contribute to ED in as many as 36% of cases,[4] and diabetic patients commonly take many classes of medications implicated in causing ED to manage or prevent comorbidities.

Risk Factors

Considerable overlap exists between the comorbidities of diabetes and the risk factors for ED. Vascular disease, hypertension, peripheral neuropathy, and obesity are all more common in diabetic patients than in nondiabetic individuals, and each condition is an ED risk factor.[1] By some estimates, atherosclerotic vascular disease accounts for nearly one half of all ED cases in men older than 50 years,[8] and studies have found a significant correlation between ED and the number of occluded coronary vessels.[3] In the MMAS, ED prevalence in patients with treated heart disease was 39%, and, in treated hypertensive patients, the prevalence was 15%, compared with 9.6% for the entire cohort.[6] Other sources indicate an ED prevalence of 17% in untreated hypertensive patients and of 25% in treated ones,[4] and as many as 40% of hypertensive patients may have ED.[9] The MMAS also found a link between ED and low levels of high-density lipoprotein cholesterol,[8] a feature of diabetic dyslipidemia. However, it did not find a link between total cholesterol level and ED,[6] although other studies have done so.[2] One such study found that 60% of ED patients had abnormal cholesterol levels, and more than 90% had penile arterial disease.[8] In particular, elevated levels of lipoprotein(a), as well as fibrinogen, are linked to ED.[3] Other diabetic comorbidities associated with ED include autonomic neuropathy or polyneuropathy, depression, renal failure, and chronic infection.[2] Erectile dysfunction occurs in 40% of depressed patients, a percentage that, in the long term, increases to 65% in those taking antidepressants.[4]

Other ED risk factors include age; trauma; pelvic or spinal surgery; herniated disc; Peyronie's disease; hypogonadism; consumption of alcohol,[1,8] marijuana, codeine, meperidine (Demerol®), or heroin; and cigarette smoking.[2] In the MMAS, ED prevalence in diabetic patients increased from 15% at 30 years of age to 55% at 60 years of age,[6] and cigarette smoking intensified the ED risk from cardiovascular disease and medication.[2]

Because ED is associated with type 1 and type 2 diabetes, increased glucose levels, rather than the underlying cause of diabetes, appear to account for ED in both types.[10] In patients with type 1 diabetes, a higher Hb A_{1c} confers a greater risk of ED.[6] In patients with type 2 diabetes, this link is supported by the United Kingdom Prospective Diabetes Study (UKPDS), which found a direct relation between Hb A_{1c} and major causes of ED, such as cardiovascular disease and neuropathy. However, although tight glycemic control can prevent or delay the onset of neuropathic ED, by the time ED is diagnosed, neuropathy may be too well established to respond to improved glycemic control.[10]

Diagnosis and Evaluation

Because ED is so common in diabetic patients, they should be adequately assessed for it during office visits. If, for at least 3 months, the patient has repeatedly been unable to attain or maintain an erection sufficient for satisfactory sexual performance, the condition fits the clini-

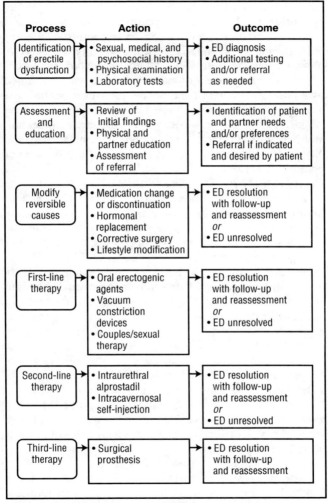

Figure 12-1: The process of care treatment algorithm for erectile dysfunction (ED). Levine, *Am J Med* 2000;109: 3S-12S, with permission from Excerpta Medica, Inc.

cal criteria for ED. Although the nature of the ED may not influence the choice of treatment, adequate evaluation is important to identify comorbid conditions that require management and to determine whether testosterone therapy may be indicated.[7] A goal-directed approach, which uses the process of care model that was developed by a multidisciplinary expert panel to determine the most appropriate treatment for each patient, should be pursued (Figure 12-1). This protocol guides the medical, sexual, and psychosocial history-taking process and focuses the physical examination and laboratory testing to uncover potentially serious or life-threatening causes of ED.[8]

History and Physical Examination

The sexual history should distinguish between ED, low libido, and ejaculatory or orgasmic disturbance.[8] Questioning should review the phases of the sexual cycle; assess desire, arousal, erection, orgasm, ejaculation, and resolution; and uncover any sexual pain (Table 12-1).[5] Whereas low libido may be a defensive reaction to frustration[6] or may indicate depression or androgen deficiency, arousal problems may indicate anxiety.[5] Problems in reaching orgasm during coitus may indicate that erection cannot be maintained long enough.[6] If ED is present, its nature and onset; the frequency, duration, and quality of erections; the presence or absence of morning or nocturnal erections; and the patient's ability to achieve sexual satisfaction should all be explored.

Clinicians can encourage patients to report ED by providing brochures on sexual health in the waiting room, by setting up patient-focused displays on erectile function in the examining room, or by wearing lapel buttons that encourage the patient to discuss ED. Clinicians can encourage patients who report ED to elaborate on the problem by nodding, by rephrasing their statement, or by requesting additional information. If the patient does not report ED on his own, carefully directed questions may encourage him. Open-ended questions such as "Are you sexually active?" may be suitable for patients between 40 and 50 years of age who have no ED risk factors.[5] If the answer is simply yes, a follow-up question, such as "Are you satisfied with your sexual function?" or "Do you have difficulty achieving or maintaining an erection?" can uncover ED without seeming intrusive.[8] In contrast, permission-giving questions may be more appropriate for patients older than 50 years or those with risk factors. With this communication technique, the statement "A lot of diabetic patients have erection problems" precedes the question "Is getting or keeping an erection a problem for you as well?" This approach makes the patient feel less exceptional and, therefore, more comfortable in revealing a problem.[5] Written questionnaires, such as the extensively validated, five-item International Index of Erectile Functions (IIEF) or Sexual Health Inventory for Men (SHIM) (Table 12-2), can also uncover ED and aid discussion of sexual issues.[8] However, to ensure that low IIEF scores indicate severe ED, the questionnaire should be supplemented by questions about desire and opportunity.[5]

The history and physical examination results give important clues to the chief cause or causes of ED. Psychogenic ED comes on suddenly after a stressful event and may come and go depending on the sexual partner or situation. Patients with psychogenic ED often have normal erections during masturbation or while sleeping and after waking.[7] Psychometric test results can indicate psychiatric or relationship problems that may underlie psychogenic ED. In particular, mood disorder questionnaires, such as the Beck Depression Inventory or the Centers for Epidemiologic Studies-Depression Scale,[9] can uncover depression that may underlie or perpetuate ED.[6]

Organic neurogenic ED is indicated by inability to masturbate, postural hypotension, bladder dysfunction, decreased sweating on the lower limbs, diminished penile or testicular sensation, and absence of cremasteric reflex.[7] This reflex retraction of the testes can be assessed by stroking

Table 12-1: Screening for Erectile Dysfunction (ED): Evaluating the Phases of the Male Sexual Cycle

Sexual Phase	Question
Desire	"Do you still feel in the mood, feel desire, have sexual thoughts or fantasies?"
Arousal	"Do you have trouble getting or keeping an erection?"
	"Do you wake up with an erection?"
	"Can you get an erection with self-stimulation?"
Orgasm	"Do you feel you ejaculate (come) too quickly?"
	"Do you ever have difficulty reaching orgasm or ejaculating?"
Resolution	"Do you have pain after sex?"
	"Do you smoke after sex?"

Reprinted from Sadovsky, *Am J Med* 2000;109:22S-28S, with permission from Excerpta Medica, Inc.

the skin on the front inner side of the thigh. To identify neurogenic ED, a history of multiple sclerosis; epilepsy; Parkinson's disease; multiple systems atrophy; spina bifida; or lower back injury, surgery, or trauma should also be assessed.[10] Saddle anesthesia, anal sphincter laxity, and absent bulbocavernous reflex may indicate a prolapsed intervertebral disc or intraspinal mass.[7] The bulbocavernous reflex can be elicited by squeezing the glans and noting contraction of the external anal sphincter.[11]

The medical history should focus on hypertension, smoking, and coronary artery disease because of the primarily vascular nature of ED and because, along with dia-

Information

ED preceded by loss of desire signals hormonal problems, relationship problems, medication side effects, depression

Distinguishes psychogenic from organic ED; indicates stress or anxiety as a trigger

Anxiety over quick or delayed (retrograde) ejaculation may lead to psychogenic ED

Reveals Peyronie's disease or pain disorder

Reveals risk factor for ED

---

betes, they are the most important risk factors for ED.[8] In addition to assessment of the penile vasculature, the peripheral arterial supply should be evaluated by assessing distal pulses, capillary refill, and peripheral arterial bruits. Vasculogenic ED is indicated by weak distal artery pulses, intermittent claudication, positive history of smoking, insidious onset, and lack of morning or nocturnal erections.

Hormonally based ED is usually indicated by small testes, loss of libido, gynecomastia, decreased spontaneous sex fantasy, decreased hair growth,[7] cognitive impairment, and osteoporosis.[4] Genital examination should include an evaluation of the consistency of the testes as well as an

Table 12-2: The Five-Item International Index of Erectile Function (IIEF-5) Questionnaire

Over the past 6 months:

1. How do you rate your confidence that you could get and keep an erection?	Very low (1)	Low (2)
2. When you had erections with sexual stimulation, how often were your erections hard enough for penetration?	Almost never/never (1)	A few times (much less than half the time) (2)
3. During sexual intercourse, how often were you able to maintain your erection after you had penetrated (entered) your partner?	Almost never/never (1)	A few times (much less than half the time) (2)
4. During sexual intercourse, how difficult was it to maintain your erection to completion of intercourse?	Extremely difficult (1)	Very difficult (2)
5. When you attempted sexual intercourse, how often was it satisfactory for you?	Almost never/never (1)	A few times (much less than half the time) (2)

The IIEF-5 score is the sum of the ordinal responses to the five items; thus, the score can range from 5 to 25. High scores (>22) indicate normal erectile function; low scores (<11) indicate moderate to severe erectile dysfunction.

Moderate	High	Very high
(3)	(4)	(5)

Sometimes (about half the time)	Most times (much more than half the time)	Almost always/always
(3)	(4)	(5)

Sometimes (about half the time)	Most times (much more than (half the time)	Almost always/always
(3)	(4)	(5)

Difficult	Slightly difficult	Not difficult
(3)	(4)	(5)

Sometimes (about half the time)	Most times (much more than half the time)	Almost always/always
(3)	(4)	(5)

Reprinted from Sadovsky, *Am J Med* 2000;109: 22S-28S, with permission from Excerpta Medica, Inc.

evaluation of their size.[11] Palpation of the length of the corpora for fibrotic plaques that typically appear as a hard scar on the dorsum is important to identify Peyronie's disease,[7,9] which may be a more common cause of ED in diabetic patients. Results of the Androgen Deficiency in the Aging Male (ADAM) questionnaire can help detect hypogonadism and can indicate that measuring hormone levels is required.[9] Patients should also be checked for obstructive sleep apnea, which has been linked with low testosterone levels. Treatment of this breathing disorder may normalize testosterone in some patients.[6] Use of anabolic steroids or antiandrogenic drugs such as spironolactone (Aldactone®) may induce hormonal ED, which can often be easily corrected by changing or discontinuing the offending agent.[11]

Because as many as 25% of ED cases are caused by drug side effects, the medication history should be thoroughly reviewed.[11] Erectile dysfunction as a drug side effect often has sudden onset,[9] and the use of common diabetic medications that can cause ED should be carefully noted. These include antihypertensives, particularly nonselective β-blockers, thiazide diuretics, and centrally acting α-adrenoceptor blockers such as clonidine (Catapres®).[7] The Treatment of Mild Hypertension Study, which included groups treated with acebutolol (Sectral®), amlodipine (Norvasc®), chlorthalidone (Hygroton®, Thalitone®), enalapril (Vasotec®), or doxazosin (Cardura®), found that the only antihypertensive that was not associated with ED was doxazosin.[1] Other medications implicated in ED include neuroleptics,[6] antipsychotics, anxiolytics, and antidepressants,[7] such as tricyclics, monoamine oxidase inhibitors (MAOIs),[11] and selective serotonin reuptake inhibitors (SSRIs).[9] Other common ED-inducers include cimetidine (Tagamet®), corticosteroids, finasteride (Proscar®), gemfibrozil (Lopid®),[11] digoxin (Digitek®, Lanoxicaps®, Lanoxin®), opiates,[7] recreational drugs, and alcohol.[8] Because obesity and inadequate exercise may also promote diabetic ED, they should be assessed as well.[7]

Laboratory Analysis

Complete blood count, urinalysis, and measurement of serum creatinine, blood glucose, and lipids can help identify systemic diseases contributing to ED.[8] Micro-albuminuria, elevated serum cholesterol level, or both may indicate penile atherosclerosis and endothelial dysfunction. Although a 2% incidence of hormonal ED has been reported,[11] one study of ED patients found that 19% had hypogonadism, 6% had thyroid abnormalities, and 4% had hyperprolactinemia. Therefore, total testosterone and thyroid-stimulating hormone levels should be measured in most male diabetic patients, particularly in those with decreased libido. Bioavailable testosterone should be measured in the elderly, the obese, or those with liver abnormalities because changes in sex hormone-binding globulin level may confound total testosterone measurement. Testosterone levels vary substantially depending on time of day, reaching their peak in the early morning. Because most normative data is based on peak morning levels, testosterone should be measured early in the morning.[7] If testosterone levels are low (ie, less than 300 ng/dL),[6] prolactin and pituitary gonadotropin levels should also be measured.[7] Excess prolactin impairs testosterone production and action, and almost all hyperprolactinemic patients have ED. High levels of follicle-stimulating hormone and interstitial cell-stimulating hormone (ICSH), the male counterpart of luteinizing hormone (LH) in women, may signal testicular failure, whereas low levels of these gonadotropins may indicate hypogonadotropic hypogonadism.[9]

Special Tests

If initial ED treatment fails or penile abnormality is suspected, specialized testing may clarify the cause of ED and enhance the therapeutic strategy.[7] Because nocturnal erections are not affected by psychologic factors, nocturnal penile tumescence studies can quantify organic erectile capacity and distinguish between psychogenic and organic ED. Positive results indicate that ED may be psychogenic, and negative results indicate that it may be organic. Such studies have found that 10% to 20% of diabetic men have normal nocturnal erections, and, therefore, their ED is psychogenic. A common means of detecting vasculogenic ED is diagnostic challenge with injected vasodilators, after which failure to achieve complete erection suggests vascular disease. However, its high false negative rate limits its value.[6]

Indications for Referral

Candidates for referral to urologists include young men who have never had an adequate erection, those with Peyronie's disease, or those in whom oral therapy has failed. However, ensuring that patients have received an adequate dose of an oral agent and have used it enough times appropriately is necessary before concluding that oral treatment has failed.[8] Especially when ED has a substantial psychogenic component, referral to a psychologist for marriage or couples counseling or to a psychiatrist for treatment of anxiety or depression may be effective.[6]

Communicating the Results

After the evaluation, its results, including a determination of the causes of ED and treatment options, should be discussed with the patient and, ideally, with his partner as well. This discussion enables the clinician to suggest lifestyle modifications that can improve both ED and general health.[8]

Treatment Options

Medication Adjustment

Adequate consideration should be given to changing medications that may contribute to ED.[11] If β-blocker or thiazide diuretic monotherapy is being used, switching to an angiotensin-converting enzyme inhibitor (ACEI) or an angiotensin receptor blocker should be considered. Diabetic patients with ED who are taking tricyclics, MAOIs, or SSRIs for depression may benefit from the antidepressant bupropion (Wellbutrin®, Zyban®) instead.[9]

Lifestyle Modification and
Intensive Medical Management of Diabetes

Diet and exercise, stress reduction, decreased consumption of alcohol and recreational drugs, and cessation of cigarette smoking can all improve erectile function.[8] Because smoking is such a strong ED risk factor in the presence of other cardiovascular risk factors and in itself is a major risk factor for cardiovascular disease, complete elimination of smoking should be the goal. Discussion of the harmful effects of smoking on sexual and cardiovascular health can be initiated while the physician is taking the sexual history.[5] The discussion should also explore methods of quitting smoking. The use of nicotine therapy as a bridge to cessation and referral to tobacco addiction programs may be appropriate for many patients.[11] Reducing the consumption of fat, cholesterol, and salt can reduce the progression of vascular insufficiency and help prevent vasculogenic ED from worsening. The patient should be encouraged to begin an exercise regimen to promote weight loss if overweight, increase cardiac output, improve peripheral circulation, and reduce ED risk.[5] Although losing weight, decreasing alcohol consumption, and decreasing or ceasing smoking did not affect ED incidence rates in the MMAS, the study found that patients with a sedentary lifestyle who began a regular moderate physical exercise program had the lowest ED risk.[2]

Data on the relation between glycemic control and ED in diabetic patients is sparse. However, clinical experience indicates that enhanced glycemic control can also enhance erectile function in diabetic patients with ED.[7] Finally, because of the association between cardiovascular disease and ED, UKPDS findings indicate that intensive treatment regimens designed to reduce cardiovascular risk in diabetic patients can reduce ED prevalence or severity.[1]

Psychosocial Counseling

Because psychosocial factors are an important contributor to all forms of ED, psychosocial counseling is often a key part of the treatment plan for diabetic patients with ED.[8] Although psychosexual counseling alone is frequently unable to resolve ED in diabetic patients, it may be helpful in particular cases.[7] Providing education about factors that contribute to a normal sexual response and about factors that contribute to ED can help patients cope more effectively.[8] Patients may need to be reminded of the importance of communication, romance, and foreplay in obtaining sexual satisfaction. They may also be reassured by education about the normal effects of aging on sexual function, such as diminished spontaneous erections.[5]

Androgen Replacement

Hypogonadism with testosterone deficiency is a common and potentially reversible cause of ED that can be ameliorated by hormone replacement therapy.[8] If gonadotropins are not appropriately elevated despite testosterone deficiency, cranial imagery should be performed to rule out a pituitary or hypothalamic lesion.[12] Even after androgen deficiency has been diagnosed and corrected, other ED treatment is usually needed.[4] Androgens are available in oral, parenteral, and transdermal forms[8] that include gels and body or scrotal patches. In addition, intramuscular injection of 200 mg of testosterone cypionate once every 2 to 3 weeks is one of the most common androgen regimens. Oral testosterone is absorbed poorly[12] and may cause liver damage, so it is not recommended. Patches are expensive and may cause skin irritation. Their results vary by patient because they may only increase testosterone levels by 400 to 500 mg/dL, which may be inadequate for some.[9] Although the results of gels also vary, applying them to the upper torso may be more effective and better tolerated than patch use.[4] Hormone replacement therapy may suppress endogenous androgen production and may also increase the risk of prostate hypertrophy and cancer.[8] However, one study found that the use of intramuscular testosterone for 3 years produced no clinically significant change in prostate-specific antigen (PSA) level or prostate cancer risk.[9] Other evidence indicates that testosterone therapy may protect against prostate cancer.[4] Nevertheless, normal prostate size and the absence of possibly malignant prostate nodules should be documented by digital rectal examination, and a baseline PSA level should be obtained before testosterone therapy for hypogonadism is started.[7] In addition, every 6 months, the patient should be monitored for response to androgen therapy, and signs of prostate malignancy, PSA, serum hematocrit, and lipid profile should be assessed.[8]

Vacuum-constrictor Devices

Vacuum-constrictor devices (VCDs) are noninvasive and reusable mechanical devices, which combine a negative pressure mechanism that increases corporeal blood flow with an occlusive constriction band applied to the base of the penis to prolong erection by decreasing venous drainage from the corpora.[7] They are approved by the US Food and Drug Administration (FDA) for nonprescription use and have been available since the 1960s. The typical VCD consists of a constriction band mounted on the end of a clear plastic cylinder attached to a battery- or hand-operated air pump. The flaccid penis is inserted into the cylinder, creating an airtight seal. Upon operation, the pump generates suction to remove the air from the cylinder and to create a partial vacuum that draws blood into the erectile tissue. After maximal engorgement is reached, the patient rolls the band over the cylinder and onto the base of the erect penis to keep the blood in the corpora and maintain the erection, then the patient removes the cylinder. However, because the band creates ischemia and ischemic complications begin to set in after approximately 15 minutes, patients can only use it continuously for 15 to 30 minutes at most.[10,12] Patients with diminished genital sensation who have left the band on for extended periods have sustained penile injury.[12] Penile skin necrosis has resulted after 6 hours of use, and urethral bleeding and possible worsening of fibrotic plaques or curvature in patients predisposed to Peyronie's disease may result from extended wear.

In diabetic patients, the VCD has a reported success rate of 70%,[10] which is similar to that reported for oral and injection therapy. However, VCD users report a lower discontinuation rate than injection therapy users do.[7] Common adverse effects of VCD therapy include bruising, pain, delayed ejaculation, and numbness.[8] In addition, VCD use reduces sexual spontaneity and can be perceived as cumbersome.[12] However, the VCD may be appropriate for men in stable relationships whose partners are willing to accept it.[5] Moreover, VCD manipulation requires sufficient manual dexterity. Thus, it may be ineffective in patients with limited hand function. It may also be difficult to use in obese patients whose suprapubic fat pad envelopes the penis and obstructs access to its base.[12] Although high cost has prevented more widespread use, new VCDs with design improvements are less expensive, making them more affordable than older models.[4]

ED-targeted Pharmacotherapy

Because tight glucose, blood pressure, and lipid control are crucial in diabetic patients, pharmacotherapy for ED should not worsen these parameters. The ideal ED treatment for diabetic patients should not interact with medications, such as glucose-control agents, antihypertensives, or lipid-lowering drugs.[9] In addition, because sexual activity increases cardiovascular event risk and diabetic patients are at high risk already, clinicians must manage this risk appropriately when making ED management decisions.[13] To pursue intercourse, patients should be able to generate about 4 to 6 metabolic equivalents of task as assessed by history data and results of a standard exercise stress test, when indicated.[9] Table 12-3 lists recommendations developed by the Princeton Consensus

Panel's international conference on cardiovascular assessment and ED treatment in patients with cardiovascular disease. Table 12-4 lists available ED therapies with details on their action, dosing, and effects.

Oral ED agents are noninvasive, easy to use, and convenient. As a result, most patients prefer them to other types of therapy.[13]

Sildenafil

Sildenafil (Viagra®) was the first oral ED treatment to receive FDA approval and has been in use for this indication in the United States since March of 1998. Between that time and the second half of 2002, more than 16 million men, worldwide, received more than 100 million sildenafil prescriptions.[14]

Mechanism of action. Sildenafil is a potent, selective inhibitor of phosphodiesterase 5 (PDE5), the enzyme produced by cyclic guanosine monophosphate (cGMP)-mediated signal transduction to convert cGMP into guanosine monophosphate in cavernosal tissue. By protracting cavernosal cGMP activity,[15] sildenafil enhances the relaxant effect of nitric oxide (NO) released by nonadrenergic, noncholinergic nerves and by the corporal endothelium in response to sexual stimulation. Thus, sildenafil can only augment an erection produced by sexual stimulation.[15] Sildenafil's action counteracts impaired cavernosal smooth muscle relaxation, a cause of ED.[1] By promoting this relaxation, sildenafil promotes the inflow of blood into the corpora, causing an erection (Figure 12-2).[5,8,10]

Effectiveness. In pooled data of 14 clinical trials using flexible dosing, 44% of sildenafil-treated patients in the diabetic subgroups reported improved erections vs 16% of placebo-treated patients, and 70% of those taking sildenafil had at least one successful attempt at intercourse during treatment vs 34% for placebo.[16] Analysis of sildenafil trial data based on diabetes type found that 63% of sildenafil-treated type 2 diabetic patients had improved

Table 12-3: Erectile Dysfunction Management Depending on Graded Cardiovascular Risk[9,15]

Risk Category	Patient Profile
Low Sexual activity not likely to be associated with specific cardiac risk ED treatment may be initiated without need for additional cardiovascular evaluation or treatment	• Asymptomatic, fewer than 3 CVD risk factors (gender excluded) • Controlled hypertension • Mild, stable angina • Coronary revascularization completed successfully • Uncomplicated myocardial infarction more than 6-8 wk ago • Mild valvular disease • Left ventricular dysfunction or NYHA Class I congestive heart failure
Intermediate or Indeterminate Cardiac risk from sexual activity is unknown ED treatment should not be initiated until risk can be restratified	• Asymptomatic, 3 or more CVD risk factors (gender excluded) • Moderate stable angina • Myocardial infarction more than 2 wk but less than 6 wk ago • Left ventricular dysfunction or NYHA Class II congestive heart failure • Arrhythmia, cause unknown • Cerebrovascular accident • Peripheral vascular disease

Recommended Management Strategy

- Primary care management
- Consider all first-line therapies
- Reassess every 6-12 months

- Defer ED treatment until high or low risk can be determined from cardiovascular assessment results
- Pursue specialized tests such as
  - Exercise treadmill test
  - Electrocardiogram

continued on next page

Table 12-3: Erectile Dysfunction Management Depending on Graded Cardiovascular Risk[9,15]
(continued)

Risk Category	Patient Profile
High Cardiovascular disease requires specialist consultation, evaluation, and priority management ED treatment should not be initiated until cardiac condition improves	• Unstable or refractory angina • Uncontrolled hypertension • Left ventricular dysfunction, NYHA Class III or IV congestive heart failure • Cardiomyopathy (hypertrophic obstructive, idiopathic hypertrophic subaortic stenosis) • Myocardial infarction less than 2 wk ago • High-risk arrhythmia • Moderate to severe valve disease • Cerebrovascular accident

CVD = cardiovascular disease; ED = erectile dysfunction; NYHA = New York Heart Association.

CVD risk factors include diabetes, obesity, hypertension, smoking, and sedentary lifestyle.

erections. Treatment discontinuation occurred primarily because of inadequate response, and discontinuation rates ranged from 5% to 17%.[7] In a dose-titration trial of patients with diabetic ED, in which 79% had type 2 diabetes,[13] 57% of sildenafil-treated patients reported improved erections vs 10% of placebo-treated patients.[17] Of those taking sildenafil, 61% had a least one successful attempt

Recommended Management Strategy

• Defer ED treatment until cardiac condition can be fully evaluated, treated, and stabilized

• Refer to specialist for consultation, evaluation, and management

The recommendations listed are those of the Princeton Consensus Panel on the Management of Sexual Dysfunction in Patients with Cardiovascular Diseases.

at intercourse vs 22% for placebo. Moreover, the frequency of having an erection sufficient for intercourse was statistically significantly increased in the sildenafil group vs the placebo group.[10] Diary data showed the rate of success of intercourse was 48% in the sildenafil group vs 12% in the placebo group.[13,17] All patients were taking 50 mg or 100 mg of sildenafil by study completion.[17] A small

Table 12-4: Erectile Dysfunction Agents: Action, Dosing, and Effects[1,6,7,8,11,13,15,16]

Drug Class, Agent, and Brand Name(s)	Mode of Action	Initial Dosage; Dosage Range	Administration and Follow-up Testing
PDE5 Inhibitors: Sildenafil (Viagra®)	Increases relaxation by inhibiting breakdown of cGMP	50 mg q.d.; 25-100 mg q.d.	100 mg often recommended as initial dose in diabetic patients; should decrease initial dose in patients older than 65 years and in renal/hepatic disease; do not use more than once daily or with other ED agents; take 1 to 4 h before intercourse; onset (typically 30 to 60 min) delayed if taken with fatty meal; sexual stimulation is still required for erection

PDE5 = phosphodiesterase 5; q.d. = once daily

Effectiveness % (vs Placebo %)	Main Side Effects	Contraindications
70 (34)	Headache, muscle/ backache, facial flushing, dyspepsia, nasal congestion, hypotension, dizziness, visual disturbance, upper respiratory or urinary tract infection, diarrhea, nausea	Poorly controlled diabetes; severe blood, kidney, or liver disease; heart failure; unstable angina; recent history (within less than 6 months) of stroke, myocardial infarction, life-threatening arrhythmia, or clinically significant cardiovascular disease; resting blood pressure less than 90/50 mm Hg or more than 170/110 mm Hg; untreated glaucoma or proliferative diabetic retinopathy; retinitis pigmentosa; active peptic ulcer; known hypersensitivity to any tablet components; consider risk:benefit in myelomatosis, leukemia, sickle cell anemia, or paraproteinemia

continued on next page

Table 12-4: Erectile Dysfunction Agents: Action, Dosing, and Effects[1,6,7,8,11,13,15,16] *(continued)*

Drug Class, Agent, and Brand Name(s)	Mode of Action	Initial Dosage; Dosage Range	Administration and Follow-up Testing
Prostaglandin E_1/ alprostadil: Intracavernosal (for injection) Caverject®, Edex®	Direct vasodilation	2.5 μg; 1-60 μg	Do initial dosing and dose adjustment in office; titrate dose up in 5-μg increments; typical dose range is 5 to 40 μg; maximum dose is 60 μg; use a maximum of 3 injections weekly; space injections at least 24 h apart
Intraurethral MUSE®	Direct vasodilation	125-250 μg; 125-1,000 μg	Few patients respond to less than 500 μg; adjust dose as indicated; available in 125-, 250-, 500-, and 1,000-μg pellets; use a maximum of twice in 24 h

MUSE® = Medicated Urethral System for Erection

Effectiveness % (vs Placebo %)	Main Side Effects	Contraindications
67-94	Penile pain, ecchymosis/ hematoma, fibrosis, prolonged erection, priapism	Penile deformity, those conditions that predispose to priapism (sickle cell anemia or trait, leukemia, multiple myeloma, poly- or thrombocythemia), known hyper-sensitivity to alprostadil
65	Penile pain, urethral discomfort, dizziness, symptomatic hypotension	Same as those for intracavernosal alprostadil; should not be used when partner is pregnant

Russian study of 100 mg sildenafil in diabetic patients found an even higher response rate, 68.5%, than the dose-titration trial did.

Postmarketing data indicate that 58% of diabetic patients were satisfied with sildenafil therapy, as indicated by a score of 4 or 5 on the 5-point IIEF.[8] Although men aged 65 years or younger had successful intercourse 60% of the time with sildenafil vs 46% for men older than 65 years, sildenafil resulted in significantly better outcomes in both younger and older patients.[16] This finding is particularly important because the prevalence of type 2 diabetes increases with age.[1] However, patients with the most severe ED are the poorest responders, which indicates that, in some patients, peripheral neuropathy and degeneration of NO-containing nerves may require alternate treatment.[10] Response to sildenafil may decrease over time because of drug tolerance or worsening vascular disease. However, studies of up to 3 years in duration showed consistent improvement in erectile function and response rates as high as 90% with sildenafil therapy.[8]

Adverse effects and safety. In one postmarketing study, although adverse effects occurred in approximately one third of patients, none was severe enough to require drug discontinuation.[8] These findings support premarketing study results that indicated that sildenafil's adverse effects are generally transient,[15] mostly mild to moderate, more frequent at higher doses, and generally comparable for diabetic patients and nondiabetic individuals.[16] Although one large study of diabetic patients found a greater incidence of mild adverse effects in the sildenafil group than in the placebo group, the incidence of cardiovascular events in both was similar.[11] Muscle pain, which was generally reported at dosages higher than those recommended, was more frequent in diabetic patients than in nondiabetic individuals.[15] However, a study of sildenafil in diabetic patients found no clinically significant changes in laboratory test results, which suggests that sildenafil does not

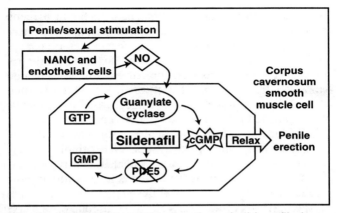

Figure 12-2: Mechanism of action of sildenafil showing the NO-cGMP mechanism of penile erection and the NO-enhancing effect of the PDE5 inhibitor sildenafil. NO = nitric oxide, cGMP = cyclic guanosine monophosphate, PDE5 = phosphodiesterase type 5, GTP = guanosine triphosphate, NANC = nonadrenergic, noncholinergic neurons. Reprinted from Levine, *Am J Med* 2000;109:3S-12S, with permission from Excerpta Medica, Inc.

impair metabolic control. An analysis of UK trials, in which 30% of sildenafil-treated patients had diabetes, found no treatment withdrawals because of abnormal laboratory test results. Thus, sildenafil does not appear to have any adverse effects on glucose control in diabetic patients. In a dose-titration trial of mostly type 2 diabetic patients with ED, no patients discontinued treatment because of adverse events, an encouraging finding given their multiple ED risk factors.[1]

For sildenafil therapy trials in the general population, the overall discontinuation rate related to any adverse event (2.5%) was nearly identical to that for placebo (2.3%). Meta-analysis of short-term trials found that patients taking sildenafil were less likely than patients taking placebo to drop out for any reason (7% vs 14%) and were no more likely to drop out from an adverse effect or abnormal laboratory test result (1.3% vs 1.2%).[16] Trials of long-term (2-year) treatment reported comparably low discontinuation rates from adverse effects for sildenafil and for placebo, and postmarketing data indicate a similar adverse event profile to that found in premarketing trials.[8]

Most adverse effects associated with sildenafil result from vasodilation and are apparently age-independent.[9] Adverse effects during sildenafil therapy, whose frequency was statistically significantly greater than that for placebo, include headache (11% vs 4%), facial flushing (12% vs 2%), and dyspepsia (5% vs 1%).[16] Less common vasodilatory adverse effects include nasal congestion (from mucosal hyperemia, 4% vs 2%), dizziness (2%),[8] and red eyes (from conjunctival suffusion, 1%).[15] Other reported adverse effects include upper respiratory infection (6%),[13] urinary tract infection (3%), diarrhea (2% to 3%), and nausea.[1,13]

The hypotensive effect of sildenafil has little impact on normotensive individuals or controlled hypertensive patients; however, data on the effects of sildenafil in uncontrolled hypertensive patients are sparse. PDE5 is not expressed in isolated cardiac myocytes,[13] and, thus, sildenafil has no direct effect on the contractility of myocardial tissue.[9] Its selectivity for PDE5 is about 4,000-fold greater than that for PDE3, the isoform involved in control of cardiac contractility. Studies have found that sildenafil has no inotropic effect and does not alter cardiac output.[13]

The incidence of any cardiovascular adverse event (except flushing) in the general population was found to be the same for sildenafil (3%) and placebo (3.5%). This finding also held true for diabetic patients, in whom a 3% incidence of cardiovascular adverse events was found for sildenafil vs 5% for placebo.[1] The incidence of death or serious cardiovascular events, such as angina and myocardial infarction, was infrequent in randomized trials of sildenafil and no more likely with sildenafil than with placebo. In pooled data from relevant trials of adequate quality for meta-analysis, the combined outcome of angina or possibly cardiogenic chest pain was 0.8% for sildenafil vs 0.5% for placebo ($P = 0.08$). In all 27 randomized sildenafil trials, myocardial infarction occurred in 0.1% for sildenafil vs 0.2% for placebo. Death occurred in the same percentage, 0.1%, in both groups, and all deaths occurred more than 7 days after the last dose. For men with ischemic heart disease or myocardial infarction who were not receiving nitrates, angina was reported in 2.4% for sildenafil vs 0.4% for placebo. However, no trial in this meta-analysis lasted more than 26 weeks.[16] Another meta-analysis that included trials lasting 6 weeks to 2 years found statistically similar rates of myocardial infarction and death for both sildenafil- and placebo-treated patients. Furthermore, its investigators determined that the relative risk of myocardial infarction during sildenafil-assisted intercourse was similar to that for the general population not taking sildenafil.[13] Postmarketing data do not provide conclusive evidence that sildenafil use is associated with excess cardiovascular risk. Although 635 deaths possibly associated with sildenafil use were reported from its introduction through January 14, 2000, via the FDA Adverse Event Reporting System, whether these deaths were related to sildenafil use, sexual activity, underlying disease, or all three is unclear. Preliminary UK data indicate that ischemic heart disease mortality in nearly 6,000 sildenafil users was no greater than that expected in a similar age group in the general population, although group differences may limit the value of this comparison.[16]

A 3% overall incidence of visual changes, which increased to 9% to 11% at 100 mg, was also reported.[13] Such changes include mild, transient blurring; increased brightness; more intense whiteness; and blue tinge, with difficulty in distinguishing blue from green.[15] These changes are related to sildenafil's inhibition of PDE6, which is active in retinal phototransduction, but long-term safety studies have not found any functional or structural alterations in the retina or optic pathway in patients taking sildenafil.[9]

Food and drug interactions. Because of its rapid effect, which can take as little as 12 minutes, sildenafil's onset may be delayed if it is taken with food, particularly if the food has a high fat content.[14] However, antacids do not affect absorption or bioavailability of sildenafil.[8,15] Coadministration of sildenafil and potent CYP3A4 inhibitors, such as erythromycin, cimetidine, saquinavir (Fortovase®, Invirase®), and ketoconazole (Nizoral®), interferes with its hepatic metabolism, decreases its clearance, and increases its plasma levels considerably.[8] Coadministration with phenytoin (Dilantin®, Phenytek®) has similar effects.[15] Because of these effects, the recommended dose of sildenafil, 50 mg, should be halved when any of these drugs is given with sildenafil or when sildenafil is used in patients with liver disease.[9] The CYP3A4 and CYP2C9 inhibitor ritonavir (Norvir®) had more marked effects than these agents, and no more than 25 mg of sildenafil should be given with this antiretroviral within 48 hours. The pharmacokinetics of sildenafil were unaltered by coadministration of CYP2C9 inhibitors, such as tolbutamide (Orinase®) and warfarin (Coumadin®), and sildenafil did not potentiate the increase in bleeding time caused by aspirin.[8]

CYP2D6 inhibitors, such as SSRIs, tricyclics, thiazides, calcium channel blockers and angiotensin-converting enzyme inhibitors, may also increase plasma sildenafil levels. However, a single dose of sildenafil rarely produces high enough plasma levels to interact substantially with other drugs,[15] and, despite sildenafil's mild vasodilatory effects, no clinically significant drug interactions have been found between sildenafil and any class of antihypertensive.[13] When the 100 mg, maximum dose of sildenafil was given with amlodipine 5 or 10 mg, only modest additional blood pressure reduction (8/7 mm Hg) occurred.[9] Blood pressure reduction from sildenafil of not more than 10 mm Hg is additive to that from antihypertensives and does not change the amount attributable to the antihypertensive.[15] Moreover, sildenafil does not potentiate the hypotensive effects of alcohol.[8] However, because patients who take nitrates have high plasma NO levels and sildenafil potentiates the vasodilatory effects of nitrates by inhibiting cGMP breakdown,[11] blood pressure reductions as great as 30 to 40 mm Hg have been reported from coadministration of sildenafil and nitrates.[9] If sildenafil therapy for nitrate-treated patients is desired, nearly 90% can be switched to β-blockers or calcium-channel blockers, which may improve long-term prognosis.[4]

Contraindications and precautions. Regular or intermittent use of nitrates in any form, whether by prescription as organic nitrates or other NO donors such as nitroprusside (Nitropress®, Nipride®) or for recreation as amyl nitrate or 'poppers,' is an absolute contraindication to sildenafil therapy.[13] A nitrate wash-out period of 24 hours is required before sildenafil can be used,[15] and this period is extended in patients taking other drugs metabolized by the CYP3A4 system or in those with renal or hepatic dysfunction.[11] Some of the most relevant sildenafil study exclusion criteria included diabetic patients with poorly controlled diabetes or severe kidney disease; heart failure or unstable angina; recent history (within less than 6 months) of stroke, myocardial infarction, life-threatening arrhythmia, or clinically significant cardiovascular disease; and resting blood pressure less than 90/50 mm Hg or more than 170/110 mm Hg.[13] Because sildenafil could precipitously decrease blood pressure in patients with cardiovascular disease, it must be used with caution in this setting and in persons with hypotensive symptoms related to antihypertensives.[15] The American College of Cardiology has recommended caution in combining sildenafil with complicated multi-drug antihypertensive regimens.[13] Sildenafil is still being studied in patients who have severe coronary artery disease, are taking multiple antihypertensives, or are undergoing hemodialysis.

Patients with untreated proliferative diabetic retinopathy were also excluded from sildenafil trials,[13] and sildenafil should be used with caution in patients with retinal ischemia, a poorly perfused optic nerve head, or untreated glaucoma.[15] However, clinical experience indicates that sildenafil is safe for patients with nonproliferative diabetic retinopathy, treated glaucoma, or macular degeneration. No safety data are available on sildenafil use in retinitis pigmentosa, but no clinically significant adverse effects of sildenafil occurred in patients with retinitis pigmentosa in anecdotal reports.[13]

Additional exclusion criteria were severe blood or liver disease; primary diagnosis of another sexual disorder, such as premature ejaculation, hyperprolactinemia, testosterone deficiency, or androgen therapy; major psychiatric disorder; trazodone (Desyrel®) use; or history of alcohol or substance abuse. Active peptic ulcer, also an exclusion criterion,[13] is a relative contraindication because sildenafil may decrease platelet aggregability and cause dyspepsia by inducing gastroesophageal sphincter relaxation and reflux.[15] Patients with substantial penile deformity, including Peyronie's disease, were excluded from sildenafil trials because Peyronie's disease could confound assessment of successful attempts at intercourse. No cases of penile fibrosis related to sildenafil use were reported during clinical trials. Neither were cases of priapism (defined as erection lasting 4 to 6 hours), although, after sildenafil approval, some prolonged erections were reported, mostly from combining sildenafil with other ED agents.[13] The ratio of risk to benefit should be considered in patients prone to priapism by myelomatosis, leukemia, sickle cell anemia, or paraproteinemia.[15] Sildenafil use is also contraindicated in patients with known hypersensitivity to any of its components, although reports of allergic reactions are sparse.[13]

Tadalafil

Another potent selective PDE5 inhibitor, tadalafil (Cialis®) received regulatory approval for the treatment of ED in November 2002 in Europe and became available there in February 2003. In April, 2002, the FDA stated that, although tadalafil was approvable, it needed additional confirmatory clinical studies before the FDA would proceed to approve it in the United States. As a result, US regulatory approval of tadalafil for treating ED is anticipated for the second half of 2003. Because tadalafil's mean onset of action (45 min) is longer than that of sildenafil (less than 30 min), its absorption is not delayed or decreased when it is taken with food, unlike sildenafil. In phase III clinical trials, 81% of patients taking tadalafil, 20 mg, reported improved erections vs 35% for placebo (P <0.001), and 60% of tadalafil patients had successful intercourse 30 to 48 hours after dosing vs 30% for placebo.[18] In contrast, sildenafil remains effective for about 4 hours after dosing.[4]

The most common adverse events reported with tadalafil use in clinical trials were headache, dyspepsia, flushing, and muscle pain or backache, and most were mild to moderate and transient. No visual disturbances were reported, which reflects tadalafil's 1,000-fold greater selectivity for PDE5 than for PDE6,[13] for which it has virtually no affinity.[4] However, tadalafil does have fairly high selectivity for PDE11. The function of this isoform is currently unknown, although it is widely distributed throughout skeletal muscle as well as organs, such as the testes, heart, prostate, kidney, liver, and pituitary. Unlike sildenafil, tadalafil has a methyldione structure and may, therefore, result in different clinical effects when taken by large numbers of patients. Some investigators have suggested that the presence of a methylene-dioxyphenyl group on the tadalafil molecule could increase drug-drug interactions substantially and have neurotoxic and hepatotoxic effects in rare cases. Information on potential drug interactions with tadalafil is limited. However, because tadalafil is hepatically eliminated and has a longer half-life (17.5 hours) than sildenafil does (3.7 hours), caution in coadministering potent CYP3A4 inhibitors may be even more important, and greater dosing intervals may be required for tadalafil than for sildenafil.[14]

Vardenafil

Vardenafil (Levitra®) is another, more potent inhibitor of PDE5 in vitro than either sildenafil or tadalafil. However, whether its greater in vitro potency will translate into greater clinical efficacy is unclear at this stage of development of vardenafil, whose FDA approval is estimated to follow tadalafil's by several months. Vardenafil and sildenafil have similar chemical structures and appear to share a similar clinical profile. However, vardenafil's mean onset of action (26 min) appears quicker than that of sildenafil, and its duration of action seems to be longer.[14]

Apomorphine

A D1/D2 dopamine receptor agonist in the aporphine (nonopiate) class,[13] apomorphine hydrochloride acts on the central nervous system (CNS)[10] by activating *c-fos* gene expression in the hypothalamic paraventricular and supraoptic nuclei, thereby inducing erection and yawning in animals. Given subcutaneously in humans, it produces non-sexual erections that can be enhanced by erotic stimulation, without changing libido, but it also produces clinically significant side effects, especially nausea. A sublingual form (Uprima®) with a rapid onset of action (15 to 25 minutes) has been developed to treat ED. This form has received regulatory approval in Europe; however, in the United States, its New Drug Application was withdrawn after submission to the FDA so that data could be accumulated from optimal-dose-titration studies instead of fixed-dose studies. Such dose-optimization data are associated with a lower incidence of adverse events, particularly nausea, than the fixed-dose data are. Fixed-dose studies found that, at the 4-mg dose, slightly more patients (54.4%) obtained an erection firm enough for intercourse than at 2 mg (45.6% vs 31% for placebo, $P <0.001$ for both comparisons). However, incidence of nausea was substantially greater at 4 mg (20.7%) than at 2 mg (2.1% vs 0% for placebo), although nausea diminished with repeated dosing. Incidence of sweating, dizziness, and somnolence was similarly increased in the 4-mg group relative to the 2-mg and placebo groups. The most serious adverse event was syncope (0.8%), but all episodes resolved spontaneously without sequelae. No apomorphine-related priapism was reported.[13]

In Europe, sublingual apomorphine is available in 2- and 3-mg doses, which are effective in about one half of all cases of mild to moderate ED. Transient treatment-related nausea was seen in about 4% of European patients and syncope in 0.2%, a much lower rate than that reported for α-adrenoceptor blockers.[4] Phase II trials of an intranasal formulation for ED have been completed in the United States. In these trials, intranasal apomorphine was 80% effective (vs 67% for sildenafil and 39% for placebo) and well tolerated. No serious side effects such as dizziness, sweating, vomiting, hypotension, or syncope were reported.[19] Because of its central action, apomorphine may enhance orgasm, which may benefit older men with delayed ejaculation. Although apomorphine therapy is not contraindicated by nitrate therapy, it should be initiated with caution if nitrates are being taken.[4]

Other Therapies

A combination of the NO donor L-arginine and yohimbine may be emerging from phase III trials shortly.[13] L-arginine is an important factor in the production of NO by NOS,[3] and yohimbine is a presynaptic α_2-adrenoceptor blocker that decreases outflow of blood from the corpora and may increase libido via a CNS effect. A yohimbine dose of 5.4 mg three times daily has improved erectile function in some cases. However, yohimbine is only effective in less than one half of ED cases and may be even less effective in patients with diabetes.[1] Moreover, yohimbine may cause palpitations[7] and increase blood pressure, which poses particular problems for hypertensive patients and those with cardiovascular disease,[1] and its use is contraindicated by renal insufficiency. Because outcome data indicate that yohimbine has marginal efficacy, the American Urological Association (AUA) has recommended against its use for ED. Like yohimbine, the nonselective α-adrenoceptor antagonist phentolamine has also been used as an oral agent for ED but is more commonly used in ED injection therapy.[7] Phentolamine may ameliorate ED mainly by inhibiting ejaculation.

Another established agent, the antidepressant serotonin antagonist and reuptake inhibitor trazodone,[7] has been known to cause priapism, which led to its use for ED. It may exert its effects via α-adrenoceptor antagonism and antiserotonergic action. Recommended dosages range from 50 mg at night to 50 mg three times daily.[12] Although trazodone can treat premature ejaculation and improve erectile function in men with psychogenic ED, it is only marginally effective for organic ED[7] and generally ineffective in the elderly and those with long-standing ED. Side effects, which include dizziness, lightheadedness, and somnolence, are minimal at this dosage. Oral agents for diabetic neuropathy, such as bethanechol (Duvoid®, Myotonachol®, Urecholine®) and nerve growth factor, which has under late-stage drug development, may also assist in managing neurogenic ED in diabetic patients.[12] In addition to oral ED therapies, several topical ED therapies are being developed. However, the relative impermeability of the tunica albuginea hampers their absorption and may restrict their eventual use to cases of mild ED.[4]

Injection and Intraurethral Therapy
Injection therapy

More invasive therapies in which vasoactive agents are administered within the penis to decrease vascular resistance and, thereby, allow blood to enter erectile tissue have been in worldwide use since the middle of the 1980s.[12] Because they target the penile vasculature, they have a predictable clinical effect and decrease the chance of adverse effects from systemic absorption.[7] Unlike sildenafil, they produce erections independent of sexual stimulation.[6] They are effective to some degree in most patients but work best for neurogenic or psychogenic impotence. Training in their use is required, and some patients find their use difficult or stressful.[1] Use of these therapies is not recommended in patients with severe psychiatric disorders, poor manual dexterity or eyesight, or morbid obesity, and use is contraindicated by an implanted penile prosthesis.[12]

The vasoactive agents most commonly used in this approach include prostaglandin E_1 (PGE_1), or alprostadil (Caverject®); the PDE inhibitor papaverine;[12] VIP; and phentolamine,[1] whether in various combinations or as monotherapy.[12] Combination therapy using smaller amounts of synergistic agents may be preferred over monotherapy because of increased efficacy and a more favorable adverse-effect profile.[7] However, because alprostadil has a lower incidence of related priapism and fibrosis, AUA guidelines have recommended Caverject® as a first-line ED injection monotherapy.[12] Injectable alprostadil complexed with α-cyclodextrin is also available (Edex®).[10] Only these two injectable alprostadil compounds (Caverject®, Edex®), as well as the intraurethral alprostadil suppository and its applicator, Medicated Urethral System for Erection (MUSE®), have received FDA approval.[6] These forms of alprostadil have been used in patients with various types of neurogenic impotence, including diabetic patients. Through the interaction of PDE with specific receptors on cavernosal smooth muscle,[10] alprostadil stimulates adenylcyclase[6] and increases cAMP levels, reducing intracellular calcium and, thereby, inducing the muscle to relax. As a result, alprostadil can dilate corporal smooth muscle directly in many patients, regardless of the functional status of penile neurons, and alprostadil's direct ac-

401

tion on smooth muscle ensures that tumescence will occur unless veno-occlusive dysfunction is sufficient to hamper rigid erection.[10]

Penile injection therapy uses a small-gauge needle and syringe such as those used for insulin to inject the agent at the base of the penis on the lateral aspect to avoid nerves and blood vessels. Alternate sides are used for the injection site. The dose is titrated to achieve an erection rigid enough for intercourse. Onset of action is usually about 5 to 10 minutes, and erection lasts about 30 to 60 minutes. Patients with neurogenic impotence typically require a lower dose than other patients.[12] Although such patients may have reflexive erections or tumescence, they may lack sufficient rigidity for penetration, and their erection may not last long enough to complete intercourse. Therefore, although patients with vasculogenic ED may require an alprostadil dose of 20 μg, patients with neurogenic ED may require a dose of only 5 μg. Moreover, initial dosing of these patients in the office is crucial to allow treatment of priapism that may result from overdose.[10]

Dosing should be limited to twice weekly to avoid fibrosis, which results from the trauma of injection as well as the agent itself.[12] The incidence of fibrosis (5% to 10%)[7] is directly related to treatment duration, and fibrotic plaque formation requires treatment discontinuation. Injection of excessive doses may cause prolonged erection or priapism in about 1% to 4% of injectors.[12] Erection lasting more than 60 minutes should be treated with 30 mg of pseudoephedrine to induce detumescence. Lack of response to such oral therapy should be promptly addressed by aspiration of the corpora and then by monitored injection of α-adrenoceptor agonists such as phenylephrine (Neo-Synephrine®) in the emergency department.[7,11] Occasionally, surgical treatment may also be necessary.[11]

Initial rates of acceptance of injection therapy are only about 50% because of penile pain[12] (in 10% to 20% of patients),[7] inconvenience, decreased efficacy, and lack of interest in sex.[12] Moreover, in one study, the discontinuation rate after 1 year of injection therapy was reported to be 56%, and, after 2 years, the discontinuation rate was 68%.[11] The success rate for injection therapy in all patients is estimated at 73%.[10] Some clinical trials have reported even higher success rates. In a 6-month study of injection therapy in patients with ED of varying causes, 94% reported sexual activity after injection that was satisfactory for both partners about 87% of the time. The mean dose at study end was 20.7 μg. Although penile pain occurred after only 11% of injections, one half of the patients reported it after at least one injection. Other complications included hematomas or ecchymoses in 8%.[6] Such complications are more common in anticoagulated patients. A case of penile necrosis from fulminant corporal infection resulting from intrapenile injection was reported in a diabetic patient.[12] These results suggest that, although more patients respond to injection therapy than to sildenafil, injection conveys a risk of discomfort and traumatic side effects.[6]

Intraurethral Therapy

In intraurethral therapy, a polypropylene applicator delivers a semisolid pellet of alprostadil into the penile urethra.[8] With this method, alprostadil acts in the same manner as it does when injected, although the agent is delivered by absorption through the urethra into the corpora. Erection results within 10 to 20 minutes,[12] and treatment is effective in 40% to 65% of patients.[6,12] However, much higher doses of alprostadil (125 to 1,000 μg) are required in intraurethral therapy than in injection therapy, and most patients require 500 or 1,000 μg. Intraurethral alprostadil therapy may cause urethral discomfort, dizziness (2%),[6] and symptomatic hypotension (3%)[11] and has an incidence of penile pain (11% to 32%)[11] similar to that of injection therapy.[6] However, unlike injection therapy, it does not cause fibrosis and priapism.[12] Both forms of alprostadil therapy are contraindicated in patients with penile deformity; those with conditions that predispose them to priapism, such as sickle cell anemia or trait, leukemia, multiple myeloma, polycythemia, or thrombocythemia; and those with known hypersensitivity to alprostadil. In addition, intraurethral alprostadil should not be used with a pregnant partner.[11] When intraurethral therapy, injection therapy, and oral pharmacotherapy are contraindicated or ineffective, patients are left with the choice of either VCD therapy or penile implantation surgery.[10]

Surgery

Surgical implantation of a penile prosthesis is the most invasive form of ED therapy and therefore is considered a last resort. Rates of satisfaction with penile prostheses are similar for patients with diabetes and those without. Although the rate of prosthesis infection is high (18%),[12] and although such infection can be an especially serious problem in patients with diabetes,[10] carefully selected diabetic patients do not appear to have a higher reoperation rate than patients without diabetes.[12]

References

1. Cummings MH, Alexander WD: Erectile dysfunction in patients with diabetes. *Hosp Med* 1999;60:638-644.

2. Lewis RW: Epidemiology of erectile dysfunction. *Urol Clin North Am* 2001;28:209-216.

3. Sullivan ME, Thompson CS, Dashwood MR, et al: Nitric oxide and penile erection: is erectile dysfunction another manifestation of vascular disease? *Cardiovasc Res* 1999;43:658-665.

4. Hackett GI: Managing erectile dysfunction. *Practitioner* 2001;245:820, 823-824, 827-828.

5. Sadovsky R: Integrating erectile dysfunction treatment into primary care practice. *Am J Med* 2000;109:22S-28S.

6. Hirshkowitz M, Cunningham GR: Erectile dysfunction in diabetes. In: Taylor SI, ed. *Current Review of Diabetes*. Philadelphia, PA: Current Medicine; 1999:95-103.

7. Dey J, Shepherd MD: Evaluation and treatment of erectile dysfunction in men with diabetes mellitus. *Mayo Clin Proc* 2002; 77:276-282.

8. Levine LA: Diagnosis and treatment of erectile dysfunction. *Am J Med* 2000;109:3S-12S.

9. Carbone DJ Jr, Seftel AD: Erectile dysfunction. Diagnosis and treatment in older men. *Geriatrics* 2002;57:18-24.

10. Nehra A, Moreland RB: Neurologic erectile dysfunction. *Urol Clin North Am* 2001;28:289-308.

11. Viera AJ, Clenney TL, Shenenberger DW, et al: Newer pharmacologic alternatives for erectile dysfunction. *Am Fam Physician* 1999;60:1159-1172.

12. Yang CC, Bradley WE: Treatment of diabetic sexual dysfunction and cystopathy. In: Dyck PJ and Thomas PK, eds. *Diabetic Neuropathy*. 2nd ed. Philadelphia, PA: W.B. Saunders Co.; 1999:530-540.

13. Padma-Nathan H, Giuliano F: Oral drug therapy for erectile dysfunction. *Urol Clin North Am* 2001;28:321-334.

14. Corbin JD, Francis SH: Pharmacology of phosphodiesterase-5 inhibitors. *Int J Clin Pract* 2002;56:453-459.

15. Lim PH, Moorthy P, Benton KG: The clinical safety of viagra. *Ann N Y Acad Sci* 2002;962:378-388.

16. Fink HA, Mac Donald R, Rutks IR, et al: Sildenafil for male erectile dysfunction: a systematic review and meta-analysis. *Arch Intern Med* 2002;162:1349-1360.

17. Nissen D: Mosby's Drug Consult 2002. St. Louis, MO: Mosby, Inc: 2002.

18. Eli Lilly and Company Investment Community Update. Eli Lilly and Company, November 8, 2002. pp 83-89.

19. Nastech technology. Nastech Pharmaceutical Company Web site. Available at: http://www.nastech.com/nastech.htm. Accessed January 8, 2003.

Index

NOTES

NOTES

NOTES